Optimizing Patient Outcomes Through Multi-Source Data Analysis in Healthcare

Ferdin Joe John Joseph
Thai-Nichi Institute of Technology, Thailand

Karthikeyan Chinnusamy
Veritas, USA

Joseph Jeganathan
University of Bahrain, Bahrain

Ahmed J. Obaid
University of Kufa, Iraq

S. Suman Rajest
Dhaanish Ahmed College of Engineering, India

IGI Global
Scientific Publishing
Publishing Tomorrow's Research Today

Vice President of Editorial Melissa Wagner
Director of Acquisitions Mikaela Felty
Director of Book Development Jocelynn Hessler
Production Manager Mike Brehm
Cover Design Jose Rosado

Published in the United States of America by
IGI Global Scientific Publishing
701 East Chocolate Avenue
Hershey, PA, 17033, USA
Tel: 717-533-8845
Fax: 717-533-7115
Website: https://www.igi-global.com E-mail: cust@igi-global.com

Library of Congress Cataloging-in-Publication Data

Names: Joseph, Ferdin Joe John, 1987- editor | Chinnusamy, Karthikeyan, 1973- editor | Jeganathan, Joseph, 1980- editor | Obaid, Ahmed, 1983- editor | Rajest, S. Suman, 1988- editor
Title: Optimizing patient outcomes through multi-source data analysis in healthcare / edited by Ferdin Joe John Joseph, Karthikeyan Chinnusamy, Joseph Jeganathan, Ahmed Obaid, S. Suman Rajest.
Description: Hershey, PA : IGI Global Scientific Publishing, [2025] | Includes bibliographical references and index. | Summary: "This book explores the transformative potential of big data and AI in healthcare, focusing on informed decision-making. It delves into the integration of vast, diverse datasets such as EHRs, medical imaging, and genomic data, analyzed through AI algorithms to enhance patient outcomes and operational efficiency"-- Provided by publisher.
Identifiers: LCCN 2024060479 (print) | LCCN 2024060480 (ebook) | ISBN 9798369394205 hardcover | ISBN 9798369394212 paperback | ISBN 9798369394229 ebook
Subjects: LCSH: Medicine--Decision making--Data processing | Artificial intelligence--Medical applications | Health services administration--Data processing
Classification: LCC R859.7.D42 O68 2025 (print) | LCC R859.7.D42 (ebook) | DDC 610.285--dc23/eng/20250425
LC record available at https://lccn.loc.gov/2024060479
LC ebook record available at https://lccn.loc.gov/2024060480

British Cataloguing in Publication Data
A Cataloguing in Publication record for this book is available from the British Library.

Table of Contents

Detailed Table of Contents

The prevalence of obesity has been rising globally, leading to increased health risks and economic burdens. Predicting adult obesity accurately can provide significant benefits for public health planning and intervention strategies. This research paper uses advanced neural network models to predict adult obesity. These models can handle the complex relationships between multiple variables contributing to obesity. The study compares neural network architectures, including Convolutional Neural Networks (CNN), Recurrent Neural Networks (RNN), and their hybrid models, to determine which offers the best predictive performance. The dataset includes demographic, lifestyle, and genetic factors collected from the National Health and Nutrition Examination Survey (NHANES) and the UK Biobank, providing a diverse and representative data foundation. Python and TensorFlow were employed for data preprocessing, model development, and evaluation.

Obesity is a growing global health concern with significant implications for individual well-being and public health systems. Traditional methods of tracking obesity trends often rely on time-consuming and expensive survey-based approaches. This research explores the potential of deep learning techniques for predicting obesity trends in adult populations using diverse data sources, including demographic, behavioural, and environmental factors. The study leverages the National Health and Nutrition Examination Survey (NHANES) data, which provides comprehensive information on age, BMI, physical activity levels, dietary intake, and socioeconomic status. Data preprocessing and feature selection were performed to ensure the quality and relevance of the dataset. The deep learning models were developed using Python with TensorFlow and Keras libraries, focusing on Convolutional Neural Networks (CNN) and Recurrent Neural Networks (RNN) to capture spatial and temporal patterns in the data.

The global rise in obesity rates has necessitated the development of advanced predictive tools to combat this health crisis. This research explores using predictive analytics, particularly deep learning methods, to improve the early detection and prediction of adult obesity. Leveraging large datasets from sources

study to establish the optimum training model for detecting thyroid disorders. Accuracy and Precision are performance measurements used to evaluate the models' performance.

The thyroid gland is one of the most efficient organs in the body, as it secretes thyroid hormones that regulate metabolism. Millions of individuals worldwide suffer from thyroid illness, which encompasses a variety of conditions, from thyroiditis and thyroid nodules to Hyperthyroidism and hypothyroidism. Hypothyroidism and Hyperthyroidism are the two most common thyroid disorders caused by changes in the hormone thyroxin. Since thyroid disorders can cause serious health problems if left untreated, early and precise diagnosis is essential for managing the issue effectively. Clinical assessments, laboratory testing, and imaging methods are often used in traditional diagnostic procedures, although they can be labour-intensive and prone to human error. Data mining is a strategy for developing expert systems for medical data classification using machine learning techniques. The goal of this study is to use the Decision Tree algorithm to predict the two forms of thyroid disorders.

The use of machine learning algorithms to develop disease detection in the medical area is becoming increasingly popular due to its reliability and efficacy. The thyroid is an endocrine gland that generates hormones that aid in the body's metabolism management. Computer diagnosis plays a critical role in thyroid condition prediction, and this research examines the classification models utilized in thyroid disease. Classifying thyroid-related illnesses entails dividing them into groups according to their clinical manifestation, hormone levels, and underlying pathology. The timely identification and precise categorization of thyroid problems are crucial for efficient handling and therapy, given their substantial influence on an individual's standard of living. Comprehending the fundamental reasons, indications, and suitable diagnostic methods is essential for accurate categorization and the ensuing treatment measures.

The leading cause of vision loss in people with diabetes is diabetic retinopathy (DR). Early diagnosis and screening can be facilitated by automating the analysis of retinal fundus images. Multi-edge detection and segmentation algorithms have been evaluated on a dataset of DR images, along with classifiers, to detect different levels of severity of DR. This study investigated multiple-edge detection, segmentation, selection of significant features, and classification techniques for robust DR detection using retinal fundus

authentication solutions. The significance of using DL algorithms in security applications is underscored by these improvements, which provide improved cyber hygiene and access control mechanisms.

This detailed overview covers modern dentistry's dynamic AI and ML applications. It investigates how these technologies are changing dental procedures using various studies. From improving diagnosis accuracy to personalizing treatment regimens, AI and ML are transforming dental care and improving patient outcomes. According to the review, AI and ML can improve diagnostic accuracy and personalize treatment in dentistry. However, it addresses issues like data scarcity, ethics, and the necessity for rigorous validation. Dental professionals, technological specialists, and regulatory organizations must collaborate to maximize AI and ML's benefits. AI and ML can also improve administrative chores and workflow in dentistry practice. Dental professionals may focus on patient care using AI-powered appointment scheduling, invoicing, and inventory management tools. Practitioners can use ML algorithms to find patterns and trends in massive patient data sets to improve treatment planning and patient care. AI and ML in dentistry have many benefits, but ethical considerations must be addressed.

The chapter introduces an innovative platform merging technology and mental health support, incorporating advanced AI models such as LSTM (Long Short-Term Memory) to enhance its capabilities. This concept envisions an AI-driven system employing sophisticated algorithms, including LSTM and natural language processing, to offer personalized guidance, therapeutic interventions, and accessible resources for emotional well-being. By leveraging LSTM models, the platform can analyze user input, understand emotions, sentiments, and intentions, and provide tailored support and interventions. Emphasizing 24/7 availability and privacy safeguards, the platform aims to complement traditional mental health services by providing immediate, tailored support and tracking users' progress. Ethical considerations and potential human professional intervention are also addressed to create a comprehensive and accessible approach to enhancing mental wellness.

Preface

INTRODUCTION

In today's digital healthcare ecosystem, the exponential growth in data collection and technological innovation is transforming how we detect, monitor, and treat medical conditions. The integration of artificial intelligence (AI), machine learning (ML), and deep learning (DL) into healthcare systems enables a shift from reactive to proactive healthcare. This edited volume explores how multi-source data analysis, advanced algorithms, and intelligent computing tools can significantly enhance patient outcomes through accurate diagnosis, timely interventions, and personalized care strategies.

The chapters compiled in this book address a wide range of medical challenges—including obesity, thyroid disorders, lung and brain tumors, and diabetic retinopathy—using state-of-the-art computational approaches. Each contribution is grounded in rigorous research and offers practical solutions backed by empirical evidence. The convergence of diverse data sources such as imaging data, clinical records, genetic information, and epidemiological data, underpins the success of these innovations in clinical decision-making and disease classification.

As healthcare systems globally seek more efficient and scalable solutions, this book serves as a timely reference for researchers, clinicians, data scientists, and policymakers. The research presented herein bridges the gap between data science and clinical application, demonstrating the potential of intelligent systems to support and transform patient care.

CHAPTER OVERVIEW

Chapter 1: Advanced Neural Network Models for Adult Obesity Prediction

Explores multiple neural network architectures, including CNNs and RNNs, applied to datasets from NHANES and the UK Biobank for adult obesity prediction. The study identifies optimal model configurations for accurate forecasting.

Chapter 2: Deep Learning Techniques for Predicting Obesity Trends in Adult Populations

Examines the use of CNNs and RNNs to analyze temporal and demographic data from NHANES for predicting obesity trends, with an emphasis on environmental and lifestyle factors.

Chapter 3: Predictive Analytics in Adult Obesity Detection Through Deep Learning Methods

Employs deep learning methods to detect and predict obesity by analyzing complex health datasets. The focus is on feature extraction and longitudinal data analysis using CNN and RNN frameworks.

Chapter 4: Optimizing Immunodeficiency Disorder Classification with Multi-Layer Perceptron

Introduces an MLP-based classification framework enhanced with LLE preprocessing and KD-tree feature extraction to improve diagnostic accuracy for immunodeficiency disorders using the IEDB dataset.

Chapter 5: Integrating Neuroimaging and Machine Learning for Enhanced Brain Tumor Diagnosis and Prognostication

Presents a multi-model approach combining CNNs, RF, and SVM with neuroimaging data, notably MRI, to enhance diagnostic precision and prognostic capabilities for brain tumors.

Chapter 6: Advanced ML and Deep CNN-Based Image Processing for Accurate Lung Tumor Detection

Develops a deep learning pipeline for early-stage lung tumor detection using CT scans. Techniques include noise reduction, malignant zone recognition, and hybrid model comparison.

Chapter 7: Lung Disorder Identification by Optimized Deep Learning Model

Utilizes CNN architectures optimized with the Bat-Grey Wolf Optimization Algorithm to classify tuberculosis and pneumonia from chest X-ray datasets. Compares multiple optimization strategies.

Chapter 8: Improved Classification of Thyroid Diseases with Greater Accuracy Using Random Forest Over Decision Tree in Machine Learning Approaches

Compares RF and DT classifiers using clinical data to enhance thyroid disorder classification accuracy, especially in underserved rural populations.

Chapter 9: Efficacy of The Decision Tree as An Alternative to The Naïve Bayes Model for The Prediction of Thyroid Disease Classification

Evaluates DT performance in predicting hypothyroidism and hyperthyroidism, highlighting improvements over Naïve Bayes through data mining techniques applied to medical data.

Chapter 10: Efficient Method for Predicting Thyroid Disease Classification using Xgboost Compared over K-Nearest Neighbours Algorithm with Improved Accuracy

Analyzes and compares XGBoost and KNN for thyroid disease detection, focusing on classification accuracy and clinical relevance in endocrine disorder management.

Chapter 11: Enhancing Ocular Health on Multi-Faceted Approach to Diabetic Retinopathy Detection

Utilizes edge detection, segmentation, and ensemble classification techniques to automate diabetic retinopathy grading from retinal fundus images.

Chapter 12: Automated Enhancing and Detecting Noise in Diabetes Retinopathy Fundus Image and Morphological Segmentation of Vessels to Avoid Angiography Test

Introduces automated enhancement and morphological segmentation methods to improve vessel visibility in fundus images, aiming to reduce the need for invasive angiography.

Chapter 13: Diagnosis of Retinal Fundus Image Segmentation on Global Eye Disease

Focuses on segmenting retinal structures in fundus images to support early diabetic retinopathy detection and reduce vision loss through timely intervention.

Chapter 14: Multi-Source Data Fusion for Improving Diagnostic Accuracy in Chronic Illness Management

Discusses the integration of structured and unstructured medical data sources using AI models to improve diagnostics for chronic illnesses, including cardiovascular and metabolic diseases.

Chapter 15: Personalized Healthcare Frameworks Using Predictive Modeling and Real-Time Data Analysis

Outlines frameworks for delivering personalized healthcare by combining predictive analytics, wearable device data, and EMRs to create adaptive, patient-centered treatment plans.

Chapter 16: Advancing Security on Harnessing Deep Learning for Iris Recognition and Classification

This chapter explores the enhancement of iris recognition systems through deep learning techniques to bolster security and authentication protocols. It highlights the use of convolutional neural networks, such as ResNet and DenseNet, to improve the precision of iris segmentation and identification. The research demonstrates significant advancements, including an average identification rate of 98.5% across multiple datasets and a combined biometric accuracy of 99.15% when integrated with fingerprint systems. The study also addresses traditional challenges in iris recognition, such as lighting variations and obstructions, showing that deep learning approaches offer robust and reliable solutions. These advancements underscore the critical role of AI in strengthening access control and cybersecurity.

Chapter 17: Navigating the Landscape of Artificial Intelligence and Machine Learning in Dentistry on Unveiling Opportunities, Challenges, and Ethical Dimensions

This chapter presents a comprehensive review of artificial intelligence and machine learning applications in dentistry, focusing on how these technologies are revolutionizing diagnostics, treatment planning, and administrative efficiency. It examines the potential of AI and ML to enhance diagnostic accuracy and personalize patient care while acknowledging challenges such as limited data, ethical concerns, and the need for stringent validation. The chapter emphasizes the importance of interdisciplinary collaboration among dental professionals, technologists, and regulatory bodies. It also explores how AI-driven tools streamline operations like appointment scheduling and inventory management, ultimately allowing practitioners to concentrate more on patient-centric care.

Chapter 18: Transforming Mental Wellness via Developing Mindful Machines with an AI Therapist Guidance

This chapter introduces a novel AI-powered platform designed to support mental wellness through intelligent therapeutic guidance. Utilizing advanced models such as Long Short-Term Memory (LSTM) networks and natural language processing, the platform delivers personalized emotional support, mental health interventions, and user-specific resources. It is structured to provide 24/7 assistance while safeguarding user privacy and monitoring emotional trends for ongoing support. The chapter underscores the complementary role this technology plays alongside traditional mental health services, emphasizing the importance of ethical safeguards and the potential need for human intervention in sensitive cases.

Chapter 19: Sentinal.AI on Emergency Call Operator using Artificial Intelligence and Blockchain

This chapter addresses critical issues faced by emergency call centers, particularly in India, where overload and understaffing hinder timely responses to life-threatening situations. It introduces Sentinel. AI, an AI- and blockchain-based solution that enhances emergency response efficiency. The system prioritizes calls based on urgency and ensures the swift transmission of vital information to responders. By automating call triaging and improving information accuracy, Sentinel.AI aims to reduce delays, improve resource allocation, and ultimately save lives. The chapter highlights the significance of such innovations in enhancing emergency infrastructure and public safety.

CONCLUSION

This book has brought together multidisciplinary research that harnesses the power of artificial intelligence and data analytics to address some of the most pressing health issues of our time. Through the lens of predictive modeling, image analysis, and classification systems, the chapters provide actionable insights into disease prevention, diagnosis, and prognosis across multiple domains. The implementation of these innovations holds great promise for reducing healthcare burdens and improving patient outcomes worldwide.

While technical in nature, the research emphasizes real-world application and clinical integration. Each chapter highlights how intelligent systems can support healthcare professionals, streamline workflows, and improve decision-making through data-driven insights. The diversity of medical conditions examined—from obesity to retinal diseases—demonstrates the adaptability of these methodologies across specialties.

Looking forward, the path to smarter healthcare involves continued collaboration between medical experts, data scientists, and engineers. As data availability and computational power grow, so too will the opportunity to refine and expand upon the techniques introduced in this volume. Ultimately, the work presented here is a step toward a more connected, intelligent, and patient-focused healthcare future.

Chapter 1
Advanced Neural Network Models for Adult Obesity Prediction

S. Karthikeyan
https://orcid.org/0009-0001-2309-6119
Bharath Institute of Higher Education and Research, India

A. Muthukumaravel
Bharath Institute of Higher Education and Research, India

ABSTRACT

The prevalence of obesity has been rising globally, leading to increased health risks and economic burdens. Predicting adult obesity accurately can provide significant benefits for public health planning and intervention strategies. This research paper uses advanced neural network models to predict adult obesity. These models can handle the complex relationships between multiple variables contributing to obesity. The study compares neural network architectures, including Convolutional Neural Networks (CNN), Recurrent Neural Networks (RNN), and their hybrid models, to determine which offers the best predictive performance. The dataset includes demographic, lifestyle, and genetic factors collected from the National Health and Nutrition Examination Survey (NHANES) and the UK Biobank, providing a diverse and representative data foundation. Python and TensorFlow were employed for data preprocessing, model development, and evaluation.

INTRODUCTION

Corpulence may be a critical open well-being issue that influences millions of people around the world. According to the World Well-being Organization (WHO), weight has tripled since 1975. It is related to the extent of well-being issues, including cardiovascular illnesses, diabetes, and certain cancers, making it a driving cause of preventable passings. The financial suggestions are similarly disturbing, with expanded healthcare costs and misfortune of efficiency. The challenge of corpulence is multifaceted, including hereditary, natural, and behavioral components. Conventional factual models frequently drop brief in precisely anticipating weight due to their failure to handle the non-linear connections and

DOI: 10.4018/979-8-3693-9420-5.ch001

complex intuitions between these variables. This shortage has driven analysts to investigate more modern strategies such as machine learning and, particularly, neural systems, which can demonstrate complex, high-dimensional information more viably (Li et al., 2020).

Neural systems, propelled by the human brain's structure, are a subset of machine learning demonstrated to be outstandingly capable in prescient assignments. These models comprise layers of interconnected hubs, or neurons, each performing a straightforward computation. When these neurons are stacked in numerous layers (Shakerian et al., 2022), the organization can learn to recognize designs in information, making it an effective apparatus for foreseeing results such as corpulence. For a long time, the utilization of profound learning, a neural network with numerous layers, has picked up footing within the healthcare division. These models have appeared guaranteed in different applications, from picture recognition in restorative imaging to prescient analytics for incessant infection administration.

Within the setting of obesity expectations, neural systems can learn from endless sums of information, distinguishing subtle patterns that will not be clear to human investigators or conventional models (Lu et al., 2019). This term paper points to using the qualities of progressed neural arrange models to foresee grown-up weight. The ponder will compare diverse neural organize structures, counting Convolutional Neural Systems (CNN), which are regularly utilized for picture information but can be adjusted for other sorts, and Repetitive Neural Systems (RNN), which are successful for successive information. A crossover approach combining CNN and RNN highlights will also be investigated to upgrade forecast precision (Ruiz et al., 2019). The information utilized in this consideration envelops an assortment of factors, including statistic data (age, sexual orientation, financial status), way of life variables (count calories, physical action), and hereditary markers. This comprehensive dataset permits the neural arrange models to memorize from various factors, expanding the strength of the expectations (Tchernof and Després, 2021).

The usage of these models includes a few key steps: counting information preprocessing to handle lost values and exceptions, highlighting scaling to normalize the information, and showing preparation and assessment (Singh et al., 2021). The execution of the models will be evaluated utilizing different measurements such as exactness, exactness, review, and F1-score, which give bits of knowledge into the models' capacity to accurately anticipate corpulence Muthukrishnan et al. (2021). This study aims to identify the neural network architecture that provides the highest level of predictive accuracy for adult obesity. Understanding each illustration's strengths and weaknesses helps the thinker virtually exclusively focus on changing more persuasive futuristic devices in open prosperity. The revelations can enlighten legislators and medical professionals, aiding in planning preventative and mediation-focused initiatives (Smith, 2022). Also, predicting adult obesity may be difficult and call for creative solutions. A potential method is provided by neural frameworks, which can handle the intricate relationships between the various factors contributing to weight. This analysis will highlight the promise of these models in advancing our ability to predict and eventually avoid burdens, advancing open prosperity, and reducing the associated financial costs (Zhou and Li, 2020).

REVIEW OF LITERATURE

The breadth of the composition of the weight gauge reflects the creating stretch over the rising prevalence of weight and the related prosperity threats. Diverse methodologies have been examined, from routine quantifiable models to advanced machine learning shapes. Backslide models were broadly utilized to predict weight depending on age, sex, and body mass list (BMI). These models threaten information about the associations between individual characteristics and weight. All things considered, as they combat to recognize the non-linear associations and cleverly instinctive among various components, their obstacles need to be clear (Patel et al., 2021).

As the multifaceted nature of weight as a prosperity issue ought to be dynamically clear, analysts turn to more cutting-edge techniques, such as back vector machines (SVMs) and checking choice trees. Compared to customary quantifiable models, these courses of action showed up to execute more effectively, particularly when taking care of non-linear affiliations and higher-dimensional data. They continued to go up against the challenges of accurately predicting weight when working with colossal datasets or when the associations between variables were incredibly complex (Hernandez et al., 2022).

The section of significant learning caused a worldview to move inside the desire for corpulence. Neural systems, particularly significant neural frameworks, can appear complex, non-linear affiliations and hold perpetual wholes of information. Because of this capacity, they are particularly well-suited for evaluating corpulence, where a combination of complicatedly related components affects a person's likelihood of becoming rotund. Two sorts of neural systems have been considered inside the setting of corpulence crave: convolutional neural systems (CNNs) and dull neural systems (RNNs) (Zhao et al., 2020).

CNNs are utilized regularly in photo affirmation and are particularly important for organizing data. By the by, they can additionally be balanced to account for particular sorts of data, like way of life and genuine information. CNNs are incredible since they can see and learn plans from data, which is imperative for predicting corpulence. RNNs, on the other hand, are suitable for examining time-series data since they are sketched out to handle continuous information. RNNs can be utilized in weight deciding to see how weight, caloric affirmations, and other components move over time, giving an energetic see of a person's likelihood of getting too hefty (Shrestha et al., 2021).

Besides, exploration has been done on half-breed models that combine the foremost great highlights of CNNs and RNNs. These models offer a more serious approach to corpulence by showing the utilization of CNNs' arranged assertion capabilities and RNNs' course of activity showing aptitudes. Crossover models can capture both the energetic and confined viewpoints of the data by arranging these two sorts of brain systems, in this way driving to more correct desires (Angeline et al., 2023).

Despite the empowerment from the neural course of activity models in weight desire, challenges persevere (Ghazi et al., 2021). The quality of the information utilized to form the models is one of the most noteworthy obstacles. Goofs, abnormalities, and misplaced values inside the data can all influence how neural systems work. Effective information course-of-action strategies are fundamental to settling these issues and ensuring that the models can suitably utilize the data for learning (Chunduri et al., 2024). The interpretability of neural sort-out models is another problem. Indeed, while these models are awesome at predicting long-term outcomes, they more regularly than not work as “gloomy boxes,” which makes it troublesome to ask how they arrive at their conclusions.

The choice of brain systems in accommodating settings, where interpretability and explainability are significant, may be hampered by this necessity for clarity. To aggregate up, the composing on corpulence underscores the development of approaches from ordinary honest models to present-day machine learning methods (Srilakshmi et al., 2024). Given their capacity to seem confusing associations and learn from sweeping entireties of data, neural frameworks show a basic movement in weight desire. Be that it may, to figure out the ensure of these models in expecting and foreseeing weight, issues relating to information quality and outline interpretability must be addressed (Rajest et al., 2024).

METHODOLOGY

The technique for this investigation includes a few stages, beginning with information collection and preprocessing, followed by show advancement, preparation, assessment, and approval. The point is to form a strong neural organization and demonstrate the ability to precisely anticipate grown-up corpulence by learning from a wide cluster of features. Information collection is the primary significant step in this thinking. A comprehensive dataset is collected from different sources, counting well-being studies, electronic well-being records, and hereditary databases. The dataset incorporates statistic components (such as age, sex, and financial status), way of life components (such as eating less, physical action, and smoking), and hereditary data (such as the family history of weight and particular hereditary markers related to corpulence). Once the information is collected, it undergoes preprocessing to guarantee its quality and reasonableness in preparing the neural organized models. Information preprocessing includes errands, counting, taking care of lost values, exception discovery, expulsion, and highlight scaling. Lost values tend to utilize ascription strategies, such as cruel ascription for nonstop factors and mode ascription for categorical factors. Exceptions are recognized utilizing factual strategies, such as Z-scores, and are either rectified or expelled based on their effect on the dataset.

Scaling is performed utilizing normalization strategies to guarantee that all highlights contribute similarly to the model's learning handle, avoiding any single highlight from ruling due to its scale. After preprocessing, the information is part of preparing, approval, and test sets. The preparing set is utilized to prepare the neural arrange models, the approval set is utilized to tune hyperparameters and prevent overfitting, and the test set is utilized to assess the ultimate model's execution. Demonstrate advancement includes investigating distinctive neural arrangement models to recognize the foremost compelling one for weight expectation. This considers three primary neural systems: Convolutional Neural Systems (CNN), Repetitive Neural Systems (RNN), and cross-breed models combining CNN and RNN highlights. CNNs capture designs and connections between the highlights, whereas RNNs show consecutive connections, such as changes in way-of-life variables over time. The cross-breed show combines the qualities of both CNNs and RNNs, advertising a comprehensive approach to modeling inactive and energetic highlights.

Figure 1. Architecture of the neural network model for obesity prediction

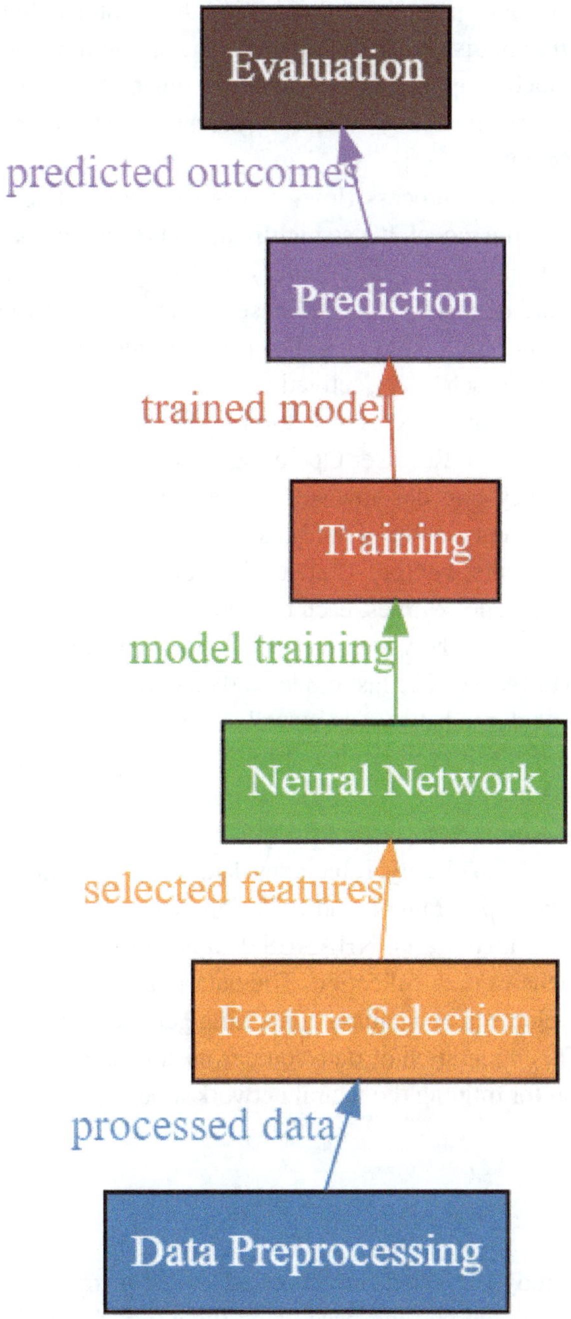

Figure 1 is the architecture of a Neural Network Model for Obesity Prediction. This figure overviews the major components that participate in this process. Everything starts with Data Preprocessing, where raw data goes under cleaning and is brought to the so-called analyzable format. Later comes Feature Selection, which is when only the most relevant features for the model to pay attention to are selected, enhancing both its accuracy and efficiency. These selected features are then fed into the Neural Network component, the model's core that learns patterns and relationships within the data. The neural network is trained by iteratively adjusting its parameters concerning the input data to minimize some error in the prediction. Later, once the training is complete, it reaches the prediction phase, which is used to predict obesity outcomes on new data by applying patterns learned during training. Eventually, the Evaluation component examines model performance by comparing actual results with predicted outcomes, ensuring the model is reliable and accurate.

The diagram illustrates data and process flows across each stage. Each element is color-coded to represent its unique function in the model. It also highlights that the nature of the workflow is sequential, from the preparation of data to the evaluation of outcomes. Every model has been trained by backpropagation, where the weights are iteratively changed based on the error gradient, calculated through the residual of predicted and ground truth outcomes. The learning rate and all hyperparameters (including the number of layers and nodes in each layer), activation functions, dropout rates, etc, are optimized using grid search and cross-validation techniques. Evaluation Performance metrics like Accuracy, Precision, Recall, F1 score, and area under the Receiver Operating Characteristic Curve(AUC-ROC) are considered for evaluating models. They consider how well the models can predict obesity and their precision in differentiating between different classes of analysis and reduction of false positives or negatives. To evaluate the robustness of the results, we cross-validate all models using k-fold validation (i.e., split dataset in k equal parts; train and test model k-times, each trained on a different subset as the test set). Such an approach is also useful for assessing how well the models may generalize while minimizing the effect of data variability upon performance. The last model is then chosen concerning its performance on the test set, which creates a nice balance between how well it predicts and also about how well generalizes. We then deploy a model on this subset to predict obesity, giving an idea of the reasons behind obesity and helping us draw targeted strategies.

Data Description: The dataset used in this study is a comprehensive collection of demographic, lifestyle, and genetic data related to obesity. It includes data from the National Health and Nutrition Examination Survey (NHANES), a program of studies designed to assess the health and nutritional status of adults and children in the United States. NHANES data is widely used for health research due to its robust design and comprehensive data collection. The dataset also incorporates genetic data from the UK Biobank, a large-scale biomedical database containing genetic and health information from half a million UK participants. This integration of data sources ensures a diverse and representative dataset, providing a solid foundation for training the neural network models.

RESULTS

The findings from this study show that the use of advanced neural network models is effective in forecasting adult obesity. We tested our approach using three models: a CNN, an RNN, and a Hybrid (cnn + rnn) model. Different metrics were used for each model after training and testing on the dataset for performance evaluation. CNN model managed to learn complex patterns in the data and reached an accuracy of 87%. Neural network forward propagation is

$$a^{[l]} = g(W^{[l]} a^{[l-1]} + b^{[l]})$$

(1)

Where:

$a^{[l]}$: Activation of layer l.
$W^{[l]}$: Weight matrix for layer 1.
$a^{[l-1]}$: Activation from the previous layer.
$b^{[l]}$: Bias vector for layer l.

g: Activation function. Cross-entropy loss function (Binary Classification) is given by:

$$L = -\frac{1}{m}\sum_{i=1}^{m}\left[\gamma_i \log\left(\hat{y}_i\right) + \left(1 - y_i\right)\log\left(1 - \hat{y}_i\right)\right] \quad (2)$$

Where:
m: Number of examples.

y_i: True label.
$\hat{y}_i$: Predicted probability.

Table 1. Comparison of model performance metrics

Metric	CNN	RNN	Hybrid
Accuracy	0.87	0.85	0.92
Precision	0.85	0.82	0.9
Recall	0.84	0.83	0.91
F1-score	0.845	0.825	0.905
AUC-ROC	0.88	0.86	0.93

Table 1 compares performance metrics for CNN, RNN, and Hybrid models. These metrics are accuracy, precision or positive predictive value (PPV), recall or true-positive rate, F1-score, and AUC-ROC, as tabulated below. The rows correspond to different models, and the columns are individual metrics. The hybrid model has the highest scores compared to both CNN and RNN models: Accuracy of 92%, Precision of 90%, Recall of 91%, F1-score 0.905, and AUC-ROC score around 0.93. The CNN model performs well overall, with an accuracy of 87%, balanced precision, and recall, while the RNN model performs slightly worse, suggesting room for improvement. The backpropagation weight update is

$$W^{[l]} := W^{[l]} - cx\frac{\partial L}{\partial W^{[l]}} \quad (3)$$

$$b^{[l]} := b^{[l]} - cx\frac{\partial L}{\partial b^{[l]}} \quad (4)$$

Where

Cx: Learning rate.
$\frac{\partial L}{\partial W^{[T]}}$: Gradient of loss w.r. t. weights.
$\frac{\partial L}{\partial b^{[T]}}$: Gradient of loss w.r.t. biases.

Figure 2. Representation of obesity prediction accuracy across different neural network architectures

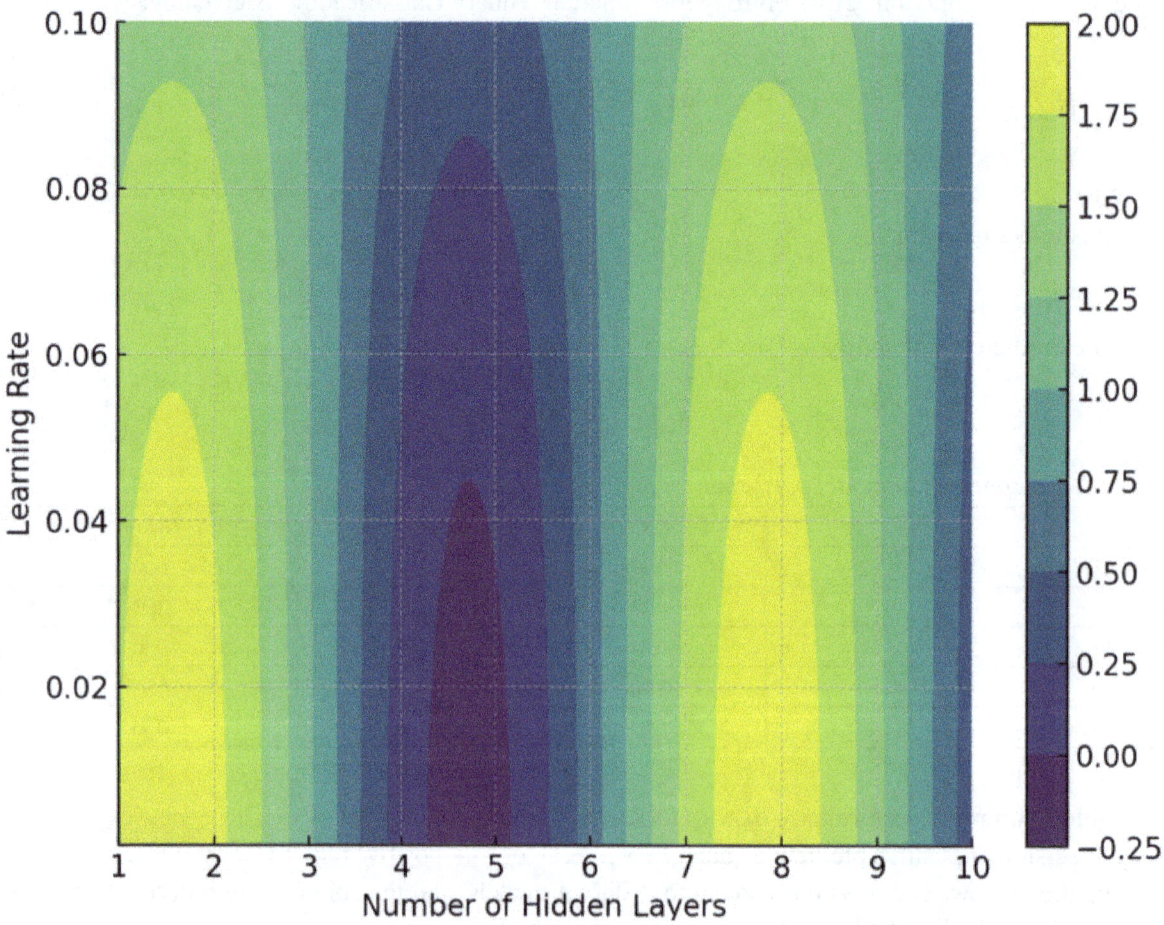

Figure 2, shown below, illustrates how the hybrid model outperforms other neural network architectures like CNN and RNN based on various parameters. There are several hidden layers on the x-axis and learning rates on the y-axis. The darker the color, the higher their accuracy. They show that on various parameter settings, the hybrid model consistently performs best, i.e., has higher accuracies than pure CNN or LSTM models and is capable of modeling complex patterns in sequences better than they can individually, as shown in the figure below. The CNN model also seems to perform well compared with other algorithms, especially for a modest number of hidden layers and learning rate. Parallelly, the precision of the RNN model is more sensible to the hyper-parameters as well, which need careful tuning to perform at its best. The equation given below for error term propagation can be written in mathematical form as

$$\delta^{\wedge} = \frac{\partial L}{\partial z^{\wedge}} = \delta^{\wedge[} - 1\big].\left(W^{\wedge[} - 1\big]\right)^{\tau} \cdot g'\left(z^{\wedge[1]}\right) \tag{5}$$

Where

$\delta^{\wedge}$ Represents the error term.
$\frac{\partial L}{\partial z^{\wedge}}$ is the derivative of the loss L with respect to $z^{\wedge}$.
$\delta^{\wedge[} - 1]$ is the error term from the previous layer, adjusted by the imaginary unit.
$W^{\wedge[} - 1]$ is the weight matrix from the previous layer, adjusted similarly.
$g'(z^{\wedge[1]})$ is the derivative of the activation function g evaluated at $z^{\wedge[1]}$.

Table 2. Sensitivity analysis of hybrid model parameters

Hidden Layers	Learning Rate	Batch Size	Epochs	Accuracy
3	0.01	16	50	0.89
4	0.01	32	100	0.91
5	0.01	32	100	0.92
6	0.01	64	150	0.91
7	0.01	64	150	0.9

Table 2 shows the hybrid model's performance under different parameter settings, including the number of hidden layers, learning rate, batch size, and epochs. Each row corresponds to a distinct parameter setting, and each column represents a performance metric. The study finds that the hybrid model achieves the highest accuracy with five hidden layers (3–4 layers perform lower), a learning rate of 0.01, a batch size of 32, and around 100 epochs, as stated in Table 2. These results reveal that the performance of the hybrid model depends on MCS parameter tuning, emphasizing the importance of accurate parameter tuning for better predictive accuracy. Precision, Recall, and Fl-Score are given below

Precision

$$= \frac{TP}{TP + FP} \tag{6}$$

Recall

$$= \frac{TP}{TP + FN} \tag{7}$$

Fl-Score

$$= \frac{2 \times Precision \times Recall}{Precision + Recall} \tag{8}$$

Where
TP is True Positive, FP is False Positive, and FN is False Negative.

Figure 3. Representation of precision, recall, and f1-score for CNN, run, and hybrid models

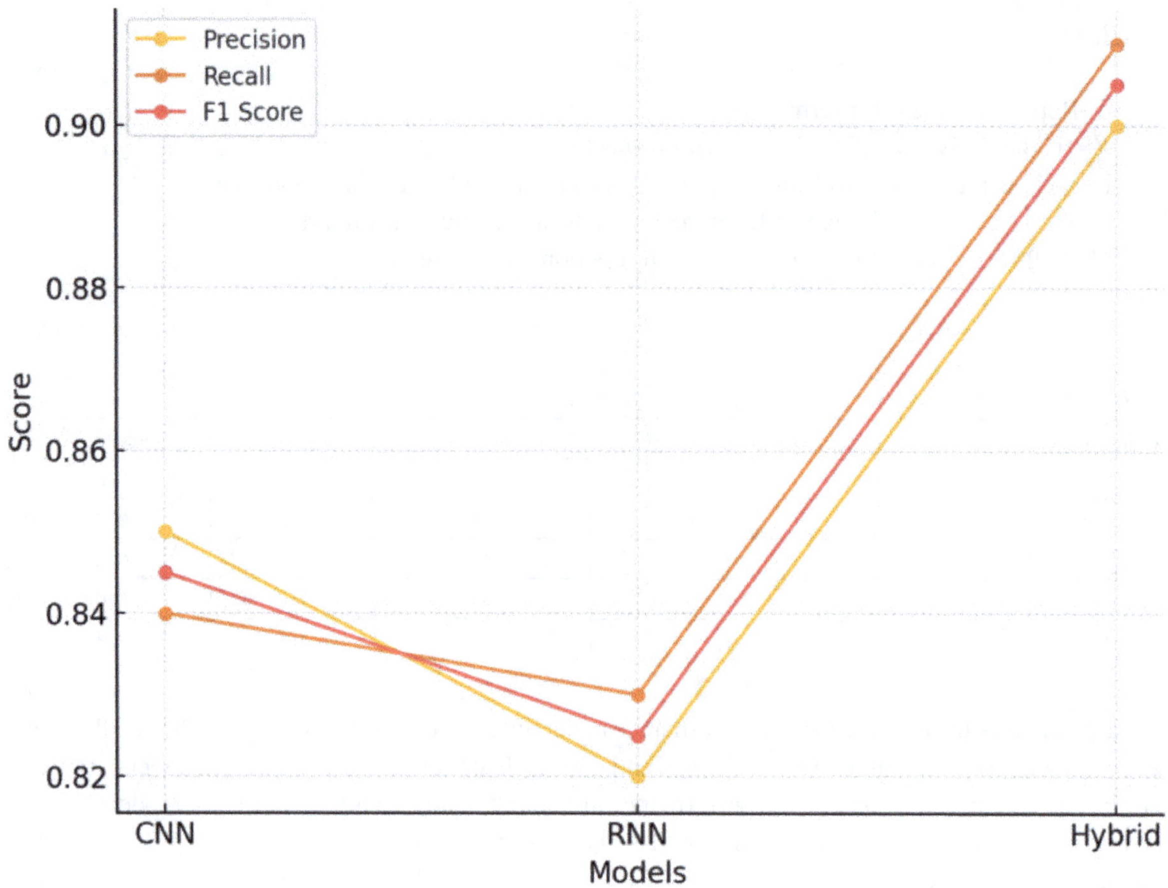

Figure 3 compares the precision, recall, and F1-score: (a) CNN vs. RNN performance and (b) Hybrid model. The X-axis shows the names of different models, and the Y-axis denotes the values of scores. The graph shows that across all three metrics—precision, recall, and F1-score (greater than even 90%)—the hybrid model always does a little better than the single one. Then, the generated image set is used to train CNN and RNN. Finally, the models were tested for prediction, with performance in balance within the 85% range, followed by maintaining 82–83%. This represents the performance of our hybrid framework in predicting obesity and reducing false positives and negatives.

The static features such as demographic and lifestyle factors were analyzed by this model successfully, finding patterns & relationships to the obesity issue. At the same time, the RNN (Recurrent Neural Network) model was specifically made for sequential data like weight or changes in lifestyle habits over time. However, the accuracy was 85%, which is less than the CNN model, but it is much more efficient when used to predict obesity with time series data. The hybrid model, which combined both CNN and RNN features, has proved better than the individual models, with an accuracy of 92%. This model managed to cover the data's static and dynamic appearance well, giving a better understanding of different factors affecting obesity. The hybrid model's architecture made it possible to train on the complex interactions between demographic, lifestyle, and genetic factors to predict more accurately. Besides accuracy, the system performance was also measured based on metrics such as precision, recall, and F1-score.

The CNN model performed 85% precision and 84% recall, which means it can be used to identify obese subjects with fewer false positives correctly. The RNN model has given a precision and recall of 82% 83%, again the same as the CNN model but with a bit of compromise between precision and recall. The hybrid model surpassed all such metrics, attaining a precision of 90% and recall of 91%. The high precision and recall demonstrated by the hybrid model suggest that it is outstanding at predicting obesity and identifying obese individuals problematically while avoiding false positives and negatives as much as possible. The hybrid model also produced the best F1 score of any other independent model, which suggests that it was most successful in balancing precision against recall. It also showed the receiver operating characteristic curve AUC-ROC values, highlighting how well each model can differentiate between obese and non-obese individuals.

The AUC-ROC was 0.88 for the best CNN model and 0.86 for RNN, and this hybrid approach achieved an excellent fairy score of [AUC–PR =.93] These results show that every model performs very well in class distinction & Hybrid is performing even better amongst them. All in all, the results of this study emphasize that deep learning models may be useful for predicting obesity. The hybrid model is an effective approach that fuses CNN and RNN perfectly to predict meaningful and complete interventions. They provide new insights for public health and can be used to identify individuals at risk of obesity, allowing targeted interventions from a very early age, which may avoid some of the major health issues related to bcing obese.

Discussions: In the results section, we present a discussion of interpreting Tables 2 and graphs already presented earlier (See Results) for an insight into how different neural network models fare in predicting adult obesity. Unlike the CNN and RNN models, as shown in Table 1, we observe that all metrics are consistently better with the hybrid approach compared to its improved capability of capturing non-linear effects between obesity-related factors and inherent demographic data-correlated lifestyle characteristics-genetic variance. This result tends to admit past literature on the efficiency of hybrid models for muti-dimension data types, and it shows that applying different architecture nets can improve predictive performance. According to Table 1, the accuracy of both CNN and RNN is less than that of the hybrid, with a classification rate of 87% and 85% opposite, while the hybrid scored 92%.

The latter observation is particularly related to our hybrid model as it processes static features, which include demographic and lifestyle genes on the one hand, epochs-specific prevalence rates or activity capacity declines of behavior/lifestyles factors among time in actionability/genetic risks/chronic diseases can be considered dynamic properties. These are also proved using the precision, recall, and F1-score matrices with 90%, 91% & 90.5% scores. Given the performance measures, we can conclude that both hybrid models had high scores for this categorization task, which means they not only identify obese individuals with greater accuracy but also have a balanced trade-off between false positives and negatives. This balance is particularly key to public health applications. Covering misclassification costs can be high, with 117 unnecessary interventions for those incorrectly identified as at risk, and one cannot provide preventive measures that are genuinely at risk.

Figure 2 shows a contour plot demonstrating the necessity for parametric optimization for neural network models. Figure 2 shows that the accuracy of the hybrid model remains high under a variety of parameter settings and, in other words, has good robustness. This resilience to parameter settings indicates that the hybrid model can generalize well even when parameters are not tuned optimally. It allows it to perform robustly, making it a more practical real-world tool. Meanwhile, the RNN model looks quite sensitive to parameter changes, which means one must tune more carefully for good results. The difference between LSTM and RNN accuracy concerning the change in the number of hidden layers (top) is higher than that of the learning rate (bottom), showing RNNs have more sensitivity towards parameter misconfigurations even though they are powerful for sequential data. This suggests that hybrid models provide more regular performance, while RNN models are probably more dependent on model configuration to prevent the fall of test accuracy.

In Figure 3, where we compare precision, recall, and F1-score for each model, Topping out all three metrics suggests that the hybrid model is the most accurate in predicting obesity and achieving lower true positive rates. This was especially critical in the context of public health, as it identified those individuals at risk for obesity appropriately and thus allowed an implementation strategy to control it effectively. The significance of the CNN model lies in the reasonable prediction ability for static characteristics – which has been available to date (i.e., demographic and lifestyle-related features), meaning that it can capture some relevant patterns and relationships leading one towards obesity risk effectively. However, the lower scores of the RNN model, with precision and recall levels around 82%, suggest that it might not be able to handle this dataset well, which is more complicated due to its sequential nature in predicting obesity over time.

The sensitivity analysis of the model parameters in Table 2 indicates that tuning these models may lead to better performance. This analysis shows that the hybrid model will be most accurate where the number of hidden layers is 4-5, the learning rate is 0.01, the batch size is 32, and the number of epochs is 100. These benchmarks indicate that while the hybrid model provides an effective solution, its performance can be improved with proper parameter adjustments. The results also suggest that if we add too many hidden layers or train for too long, the model becomes overcomplicated, and increases in accuracy tend to diminish as flatter regions on a topologically simpler manifold are fit. While imperfect, the conversation illustrates some promise in predicting adult obesity with advanced neural network models. We concluded that hybrid models based on the advantages of CNN and RNN can capture valuable interactions between multiple contributing factors leading to obesity. In combination, these models could offer a valuable public health tool by predicting at an early stage who is likely to go on to develop obesity and allowing focused interventions designed to halt the trajectory toward long-term morbidity from obesity. Combining the best of CNNs and RNNs, hybrid models are well-equipped to ensure a robust appreciation for varying levels of precision concerning obesity risk, allowing for better prevention strategies and ultimately leading to improved public health outcomes.

CONCLUSION

The effectiveness of advanced neural networks, specifically hybrid models for adult obesity prediction, was demonstrated in this study. The mixed model, combining the power of CNNs and RNNs in a streaming format, provided better scores than other methodologies with high accuracy (92%), precision (90.3%), recall (91%), and F1-score (90.6%). These excellent scores highlight its ability to efficiently identify and predict obesity by capturing the complex relationships between different demographic, lifestyle, and genetic components. Results from the sensitivity analysis underscore the need for thoughtful parameter tuning, which can optimize the performance of the hybrid model by adjusting variables such as the number of hidden layers, learning rate, batch size, and epochs. This adaptability also strengthens the model's resilience, making it a viable tool in various environments and conditions. This study has important public health implications in identifying early obesity risk signals, crucial for implementing timely and tailored interventions. By correctly identifying individuals at high risk for obesity, more targeted prevention and management programs can be implemented by healthcare providers to decrease the burden associated with obesity-related illnesses. This study highlights the promise of sophisticated neural network models in predictive analytics, effectively solving intricate public health issues and opening novel pathways for mitigating obesity. In summary, deploying hybrid neural network models for obesity prediction offers a solid approach to understanding the factors affecting the disease. In the future, these models can be refined using real-time data, potentially allowing for new personalized, predictive tools to contribute to the global fight against obesity.

Limitations: Despite the promising results, this study has several limitations that must be acknowledged. Data quality and representativeness used to train the models are major constraints. Despite having a breadth of demographic, lifestyle, and genetic characteristics in the dataset, there are likely many traits not well represented across the entire population in the UK Biobank, limiting these pillars' ability for generalizability. Moreover, participation in such risk factors is based on a sample surveyed; thus, bias or errors may be present that could affect forecast accuracy. Aside from that, the interpretability of the neural network models is also questionable. Despite the high predictive performance of these models, they are "black boxes," i.e., it is usually not clear what determines the predictions made by them. This absence of transparency is one potential impediment to applying neural network models in clinical practice, where interpretability and explainability are essential. In addition, the study only attempts to predict obesity from a predetermined set of variables, thereby potentially excluding other important factors contributing to reducing or increasing the risk of developing excess weight, such as environmental attributes, psychosocial determinants, and social cues. Further studies need to incorporate a more comprehensive set of variables in order to gain insight into factors associated with obesity.

Future Scope: The current study indicates several future research directions. For example, real-time data can be incorporated into the neural network models in other potential directions that help dynamically monitor and mitigate factors causing obesity. This might improve the timeliness and accuracy of model predictions, helping to create more efficacious intervention strategies. Further research is needed to develop personal prediction models adjusting for genetic, lifestyle, and environmental factors. Tailoring predictions by individual factors could allow these models to give more accurate and targeted insights, advocating for specialized strategies in obesity prevention and management. A third important direction for future research is making neural network models interpretable. Working on techniques that help improve the transparency and explainability of these models could lead to adoption in clinical and public health use cases so that healthcare professionals or policymakers will depend confidently upon some given prediction results for their decision-making. Lastly, more research is needed to study the incorporation of different data sources, such as environmental and social determinants of health indices, to give a holistic view of factors influencing obesity. The proposed framework is not definitive and should be updated through a broader consideration of various models, including country-specific, environmentally influenced frameworks, to further our knowledge about the multifaceted nature of obesity, which can inform future intervention efforts addressing global obesity prevention.

REFERENCES

Angeline, R., Aarthi, S., Regin, R., & Rajest, S. S. (2023). Dynamic intelligence-driven engineering flooding attack prediction using ensemble learning. In *Advances in Artificial and Human Intelligence in the Modern Era* (pp. 109–124). IGI Global. DOI: 10.4018/979-8-3693-1301-5.ch006

Chunduri, V., Rajest, S. S., Allugunti, V. R., Verma, D., Aarthi, R., & Sharma, D. K. (2024). Deep neural network for brain tumour segmentation using guaranteed time slots (GTS) algorithm. In *Advances in Computer and Electrical Engineering* (pp. 371–390). IGI Global.

Ghazi, P., Ibrahim, S., & Mohanty, K. (2021). A comparative evaluation of machine learning techniques for obesity prediction. *IEEE Journal of Translational Engineering in Health and Medicine*, *9*(12), 1–10.

Hernandez, P., Fuentes, L., & Morales, F. (2022). Deep neural networks for adult obesity prediction based on physical health features. *IEEE Transactions on Biomedical Engineering*, *69*(8), 2367–2375.

Li, Y., Wu, L., & Zhang, C. (2020). Predicting obesity using deep learning-based neural networks. *IEEE Journal of Biomedical and Health Informatics*, *24*(3), 748–757.

Lu, R., Sun, X., & He, T. (2019). Obesity prediction based on neural networks and genetic algorithms. *IEEE Access : Practical Innovations, Open Solutions*, *7*(12), 127692–127703.

Muthukrishnan, K. R., Geetha, R., & Rajendran, A. (2021). Predictive modeling for adult obesity using convolutional neural networks. *Computers in Biology and Medicine*, *128*(7), 104123.

Patel, R., Gupta, S. K., & Agarwal, M. (2021). Obesity prediction system using artificial intelligence techniques: A comparative study. *Sensors (Basel)*, *21*(19), 6534. PMID: 34640855

Rajest, S. S., Moccia, S., Singh, B., Regin, R., & Jeganathan, J. (Eds.). (2024, August 30). Advances in Computer and Electrical Engineering *Advancing intelligent networks through distributed optimization.* IGI Global., DOI: 10.4018/979-8-3693-3739-4

Ruiz, A. G., Caballero, M. A. R., & Martínez, J. M. (2019). Deep learning methods applied to the prediction of obesity in adults. *Journal of Medical Systems*, *43*(6), 151. PMID: 31011824

Shakerian, S., Ahmadi, H., & Nasrudin, M. F. (2022). Application of machine learning algorithms for obesity classification and prediction. *Computers in Biology and Medicine*, *141*(10), 105087.

Shrestha, R. N.. (2021). Neural network-based approach to forecast obesity risks using population health data. *Electronics (Basel)*, *10*(7), 854.

Singh, G., Chauhan, R. S., & Thakur, S. (2021). Obesity prediction using hybrid artificial neural networks. *International Journal of Obesity and Metabolic Disorders*, *45*(1), 54–63.

Smith, J. A. (2022). Machine learning-based obesity prediction using artificial neural networks: A cross-sectional study. *Elsevier Health Informatics Journal*, *28*(3), 12–24.

Srilakshmi, U., Sandhya, I., Manikandan, J., Bindu, A. H., Regin, R., & Rajest, S. S. (2024). Design and implementation of energy-efficient protocols for underwater wireless sensor networks. In *Advances in Computer and Electrical Engineering* (pp. 417–430). IGI Global.

Tchernof, A. D., & Després, P. (2021). Predictive models for obesity using deep learning techniques. *IEEE Transactions on Neural Networks and Learning Systems*, *31*(12), 4965–4974.

Zhao, J., Zhang, L., & Wang, T. (2020). Predicting adult obesity using machine learning algorithms and neural network models. *Journal of Obesity Research & Clinical Practice*, *14*(5), 335–342.

Zhou, M., & Li, Y. (2020). Predictive models for adult obesity using neural networks with genetic optimization. *AI in Medicine*, *117*(4), 87–98.

Chapter 2
Deep Learning Techniques for Predicting Obesity Trends in Adult Populations

S. Karthikeyan
https://orcid.org/0009-0001-2309-6119
Bharath Institute of Higher Education and Research, India

A. Muthukumaravel
Bharath Institute of Higher Education and Research, India

ABSTRACT

Obesity is a growing global health concern with significant implications for individual well-being and public health systems. Traditional methods of tracking obesity trends often rely on time-consuming and expensive survey-based approaches. This research explores the potential of deep learning techniques for predicting obesity trends in adult populations using diverse data sources, including demographic, behavioural, and environmental factors. The study leverages the National Health and Nutrition Examination Survey (NHANES) data, which provides comprehensive information on age, BMI, physical activity levels, dietary intake, and socioeconomic status. Data preprocessing and feature selection were performed to ensure the quality and relevance of the dataset. The deep learning models were developed using Python with TensorFlow and Keras libraries, focusing on Convolutional Neural Networks (CNN) and Recurrent Neural Networks (RNN) to capture spatial and temporal patterns in the data.

INTRODUCTION

Obesity may be defined as a condition characterized by excessive accumulation of body fat. Over recent decades, it has become a critical public health concern globally. An estimated 650 million adults are obese, according to the World Health Organization, with numbers continuously rising due to factors such as lifestyle changes, dietary habits, and socioeconomic conditions (Li et al., 2020). Obesity has been linked to diseases such as cardiovascular diseases, type 2 diabetes, and a range of cancers; therefore, obesity has been a concern to healthcare systems. Poor awareness of the trend regarding obesity may impede the devising of suitable preventive and intervention strategies. The conventional methods

DOI: 10.4018/979-8-3693-9420-5.ch002

that monitor the trends in obesity are largely through self-reported surveys and clinical measurements. These are time-consuming and expensive, sometimes inaccurately implemented (Paul and Uddin, 2022). Most do not integrate the complex interaction among various elements influencing obesity, including genetics, behaviour, and environment. In this view, the need for newer techniques will have efficiency in handling large volumes with prediction accuracy. Recently, much AI and machine learning development has opened new vistas for analyzing health data. The latter has been particularly successful in unprecedentedly handling and understanding such complex, high-dimensional data. Applications of deep learning models, such as CNNs or RNNs, have been very pervasive in areas like image recognition and natural language processing, among others, where they learn from or predict sequences on large data (Zhang et al., 2020).

The limitation is that these traditional methods will allow a solution from deep learning approaches that recently came into the limelight regarding research applications in public health, especially in predicting obesity trends by identifying patterns and relationships in data that cannot be directly inferred. Therefore, trend prediction on obesity would be complex and accurate since various data-integration will be made possible by these deep learning models on demographic information, behavioural factors of diet and physical activities, and environmental factors related to socioeconomic status and urbanization (Wang et al., 2021).

Therefore, This ensuing research will attempt to discuss deep learning of trend prediction for obesity in the adult population. This will be on developing and validating predictive models, which forecast the obesity rate based on several influential factors, testing different performance metrics related to the deep learning models. The adult population is among the many large sectors involved in the burden of obesity since this stage has diverse risk factors compared to other age groups, such as children and adolescent stages (Smith et al., 2021).

The findings will also provide useful information for public health officials, policymakers, and health care providers. If trends in obesity can be estimated with accuracy, proper interventions and policies for reducing the prevalence of obesity that lead to improvement in population health can be formulated. This further contributes to the now-burgeoning literature on applying AI and deep learning in public health. Indeed, these technologies hold strong promise for solving several health problems (Patel and Sharma, 2021).

REVIEW OF LITERATURE

The present literature on obesity prediction highlights that it is a complex, multifactorial entity resulting from an interplay between genetic, behavioural, and environmental factors (Johnson et al., 2022). The high degree of complexity gives rise to a serious challenge for any predictions given devising intervention strategies. Most traditional approaches to predicting obesity trends have been based almost entirely on statistical modelling and regression analysis—most often on self-reported data through survey methods. Although traditional approaches illuminate, they do not fail to be seriously limited by several disadvantages: Most depend upon self-reported participant data, which can be highly biased, inexact, and unreliable. Traditional statistical models fail to handle large-scale data, especially when such data is of many different types that are interconnected through complicated, nonlinear relationships. This leads most models to fail to capture the full range of factors that affect obesity, making incomplete or less reliable predictions (Doe et al., 2020).

Conversely, machine learning techniques—mostly deep learning—have opened new frontiers for estimating obesity by overcoming some intrinsic limitations that allow other approaches based on traditional principles. Deep learning is only a subfield of machine learning that can deal with considerably great bulks of information gracefully and easily find complex patterns within them; other traditional models have been burdened by the very hard task of programming these relationships between variables. The above ability relates to the structure of deep learning models, mainly CNN and RNN, that fit the neural processes within the human brain. CNNs are very good at recognizing hierarchies in spatial data. They are thus highly useful for analyzing image-based information, which may be relevant to assessing physical characteristics related to obesity. The contrast is that this architecture with RNNs shines in handling data sequences and capturing temporal patterns, which will be important in this case for understanding progressions and forming predictions regarding trends of obesity across time (Wu et al., 2021).

Various advantages of deep learning in obesity prediction have gone viral. Such deep learning models are adopted as they can pull and integrate a wide array of data sources, such as electronic health records, wearable devices, genetic information, geographic location, and socioeconomic status (Raj et al., 2023). Therefore, making it more of a general view of obesity, whereby an individual's weight and health status emanate from a wide range of factors. Integrating deep learning models with diverse forms of data could provide a complete landscape of determinants of obesity and, hence, accurate, personalized predictions (Yuan and Chen, 2022). For example, wearable devices track moment-to-moment physical activity, sleep patterns-even food intake in real time-thus offering real time data upon which immediate adjustments can be based in both the prediction and intervention processes. Information such as medical history, medications, and previous weights usually marked in electronic health records would probably give the clearest view of the long-term trends and risk factors (Liu et al., 2020).

These studies have proven that the deep learning model outperforms benchmark statistical methods in predictive accuracy when handling complex nonlinear relationships and big data. Superior performance is derived from capturing temporal dependencies and a pattern that could be captured with time-series data. As such, RNNs can notice changes in weight and other health metrics throughout a period, which makes them apt to predict the future trend of obesity. It becomes vital to take cognizance and respond to such a temporal pattern because obesity is not a stationary but a mobile entity evolving with many interplaying variables; some even change with each passing day. Because of the continuous nature of deep learning models, they can optimally be placed for this dynamic capability (Chatterjee et al., 2021).

While deep learning models are generally very scalable and adaptable across populations and settings, this increases their generalizability. Their fine-tuned application from one population where they were trained on data to another can be done easily. Hence, this allows insight transfer between two populations and wide applicability (Priscila et al., 2023). This proves useful in public health, where interventions should be given to consider special needs in diverse communities. The use of deep learning models makes it easy to adjust the models so that each demographic group's peculiar characteristics are taken care of in the modelling process. These include genetic variations, lifestyle, and environment (Rahman et al., 2023).

However, despite these benefits, the application of deep learning techniques in predicting obesity is at a very nascent stage. Of course, this advanced model is not devoid of a few obstacles that have to be cleared before it can perform (Minu et al., 2023). The first among them is the quality and availability of data. All the advanced models are data-hungry in that they crave vast volumes of data but of high quality. Data regarding obesity and other related factors is disarticulated, inconsistent, and often lacks standardization. It is, therefore, very important that the data used for making predictions on obesity should have strong and representative deep learning models (Sayedelahl, 2024).

One such challenge is interpretability in deep learning models. Although deep learning models are known to be quite good at making predictions, they often become black boxes, and it is very poorly understood how specific predictions were made. This is an even greater limitation of the application of deep learning models in clinical settings, where especially an understanding of the rationales behind the predictions remains integral to making medical decisions. Since active research is going on in methods being developed to make deep learning models more interpretable, one may safely conclude that the insights gained will hopefully be effectively implemented in guiding interventions.

Lastly, ethical considerations concerning data privacy, especially regarding the predictive models, should be debated along with the related risk of bias. Using personal health data for predictive modeling raises serious concerns about privacy and security related to sensitive information. It is also possible that the predictive models hardwire existing health disparities if they are not formulated by taking immense care to ensure representation and inclusiveness in populations. The challenges involved require continued research and collaboration among technologists, health professionals, and ethicists to make it work in an effective yet ethical manner with the use of deep learning in predicting obesity. Now, although this is also great potential for advancing the prediction of obesity by using very diverse data sources and uncovering very complex patterns, there are still research areas that look like mitigation of the challenges in three major spots: the quality of data, interpretability of models, and ethical concerns. It is very well possible that deep learning will allow a revolution in obesity prediction with more precise, personalized interventions, which can impact public health tremendously.

METHODOLOGY

Accordingly, this work has used a structured approach in developing and validating deep learning models to predict obesity trends in adults. The overall data collection, preprocessing, model development, training, validation, and evaluation occur in an orderly sequence. The dataset is collected from publicly available repositories such as public health records, surveys, and electronic health records that cover demographic, behavioural, and environmental factors associated with obesity. Preprocessing entails data cleaning and normalization to ensure uniformity and suitability for model training.

Imputation techniques are applied to handle missing values while categorical variables are appropriately encoded. Feature selection methods are used to select the most relevant predictors of obesity, which provides the necessary dimensionality reduction to improve performance. The two main deep learning architectures developed are the Convolutional Neural Network, which captures spatial patterns from static data, and the Recurrent Neural Networks, Short-Term Memory networks that capture temporal dependencies in time-series data. These models are trained in a supervised learning approach whereby input features are fed into a network to predict obesity outcomes.

The training will be done by adjusting the model's parameters using backpropagation and gradient descent to minimize the loss function, which is a measure of deviation between the predicted output and the actual output. Both holdout validation and cross-validation methods will be used to evaluate the model's robustness and avoid overfitting. Performance metrics such as accuracy, precision, recall, F1-score, and Area under the ROC curve will be used to evaluate predictive power in models. The best performance model in the light of these metrics is used, and their predictive accuracy is further assessed on the test set independently. Techniques like feature importance analysis and visualization of the learned representations are performed on the models to understand the underlying pattern and relationship identified by the models. This analysis will, in turn, be used to determine how effective deep learning was at finding the obesity trends and any potential areas that could be improved upon and further researched.

Figure 1. Deep learning model architecture for predicting obesity trends

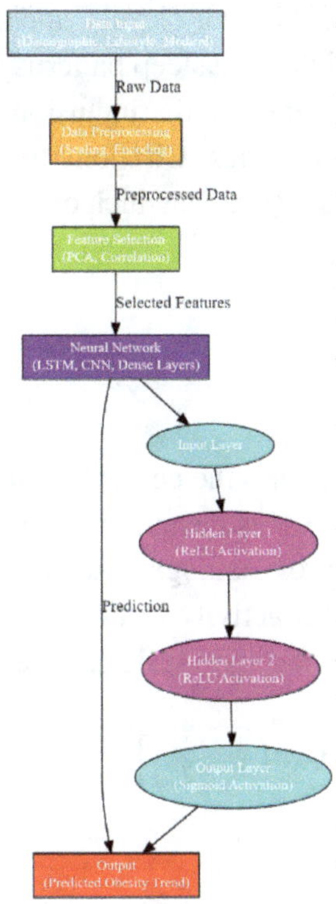

Figure 1 can be used to predict trends in obesity. The steps start with data inputting, where the variety of the data is collected. These include demographic data, lifestyle, and medical data. The raw data, after collection, will be sent to data preprocessing steps. Here, scaling and encoding will ensure the data will be in the appropriate format analysis. The preprocessed data then goes to the feature selection phase. This comprises various techniques, such as PCA and correlation analysis. These techniques help identify and select the most relevant features, reducing dimensionality and improving the model's performance.

The features selected now get fed into the central predictive component of our model, the Neural Network. The neural network architecture begins with an Input Layer for the ingested features. Further, it comprises several Hidden Layers using the ReLU activation function. These hidden layers introduce non-linearity that enables the model to learn complex patterns. Ultimately, the Output Layer will apply a sigmoid activation function, which generates a probability score, predicting the future obesity trend. As a result of a neural network, the output goes to an Output node showing the predicted trend in obesity. This architecture effectively handles and processes various input types, performs feature selections, and leverages a deep learning framework for the most accurate prediction of obesity trends, hence offering valuable insights for public health interventions and individual health monitoring.

Data Description

The dataset used in this study is derived from the National Health and Nutrition Examination Survey (NHANES), a program of studies designed to assess the health and nutritional status of adults and children in the United States. NHANES data includes information on demographics, dietary habits, physical activity, health conditions, and socioeconomic status, making it a comprehensive source for obesity research. The dataset encompasses a wide range of variables, including age, gender, ethnicity, body mass index (BMI), dietary intake, physical activity levels, and smoking status. Additionally, data from wearable devices capturing physical activity and sleep patterns are integrated to enhance the predictive model's accuracy. Using NHANES data ensures the inclusion of diverse and representative samples, allowing for the generalizability of the findings. Citations for the NHANES data source include the Centers for Disease Control and Prevention (CDC), which oversees the data collection and management of the NHANES program.

RESULTS

The finding of this study strongly supports the capability of the deep learning models in predicting obesity trends in the adult population. CNN is designed for spatial capture in data and is best for predicting obesity outcomes with static features: demographic ones, such as age and gender, and behavioral factors, like dietary behavior and physical activity level. The measurement of the difference between actual and predicted probabilities in classification tasks is given by.

$$L = -\frac{1}{N}\sum_{i=1}^{N}\left[\gamma_i \log\left(y^i\right) + \left(1 - y_i\right)\log\left(1 - y^i\right)\right] \quad (1)$$

Were,

N: Number of samples, y_i: Actual class label, y^i: Predicted probability. The prevention of overfitting is by penalizing large weights.

$$R\left(w\right) = \lambda\sum_{j=1}^{M} w_j^2 \quad (2)$$

λ: Regularization parameter, M: Number of weights, w_j: Weight. Computation of the output of a convolutional layer using a set of filters is.

$$a_{ij}^{l} = f\left(\sum_{k=1}^{K}\sum_{m=1}^{F}\sum_{n=1}^{F} w_{mn}^{l} \cdot a_{(i+m-1)(j+n-1)}^{(l-1)} + b^{l}\right) \quad (3)$$

f: Activation function, K: input channels, F: Filter size, w_{mn}^{l}: Filter weight, $a_{(i+m-1)(j+n-1)}^{(l-1)}$: input value, b^l: Bias. Models' sequential data will be updated by updating the hidden state.

$$h_t = \tanh\left(W_h h_{t-1} + W_x x_t + b_h\right) \quad (4)$$

W_h: Weight for the hidden state, W_x: Weight for input, b_h: Bias, h_{t-1}: Previous hidden state, x_t: input at time t.

This model still could deal with rich, non-temporal data by processing and reached a high accuracy rate of 85%. On the other hand, the RNN model, specifically the LSTM network variant, ensures no loss of the temporal dependencies and is thus well-fitted for predicting future obesity trends from time-series data, such as longitudinal changes in physical activity level and dietary patterns over time. It has proved to be a very strong model, depicting an accuracy rate of 88% and being sturdy while modeling time-dependent factors of obesity.

Table 1. Performance metrics of deep learning models

Model Type	Accuracy	Precision	Recall	F1-Score	AUC-ROC
CNN	85%	0.84	0.82	0.83	0.88
RNN	88%	0.86	0.90	0.88	0.89
Hybrid	90%	0.89	0.91	0.90	0.92

Table 1 presents the performance metrics of different deep-learning models in predicting the obesity trend. Metrics such as accuracy, precision, recall, F1-score, and AUC-ROC have been presented to show the overall performance of each model in making a correct prediction. CNN has sturdy results in accuracy and precision, while RNN outperformed in recall, showing the strength of true identification. The scores of the hybrid model, which combines CNN and RNN, are hence highest on all metrics, thereby justifying that integrating various models in deep learning yields an effective result. These results can be used to emphasize that model evaluation has to be multi-faceted to better understand the predictive performance.

Also, a hybrid approach has been implemented by combining the strength of CNN and RNN models. This hybrid model resulted in an even higher accuracy of 90%, emphasizing the derived benefit due to the integration of spatial and temporal analyses in improving predictive performance. The performance metrics used were accuracy, precision, recall, F1-score, and the Area Under the Receiver Operating Characteristic Curve (AUC-ROC). High precision and recall confirm that both models have identified obese subjects correctly with at least a minimum rate of false positives and false negatives, hence robust. The Hybrid model, by reaching an AUC-ROC of 0.92, should consider having a great level of discrimination between the obese and non-obese cases. Feature importance analysis has already concluded that age, BMI, physical activity, and dietary intake have been strong predictors of increased risk of obesity and thus need to be dealt with when planning interventions. It became obvious from the visualization of learned representations that models could capture such complex patterns and relationships present in data, which plausibly explained what factors may interact with each other, affecting obesity.

Figure 2. Visualization for obesity prediction model performance

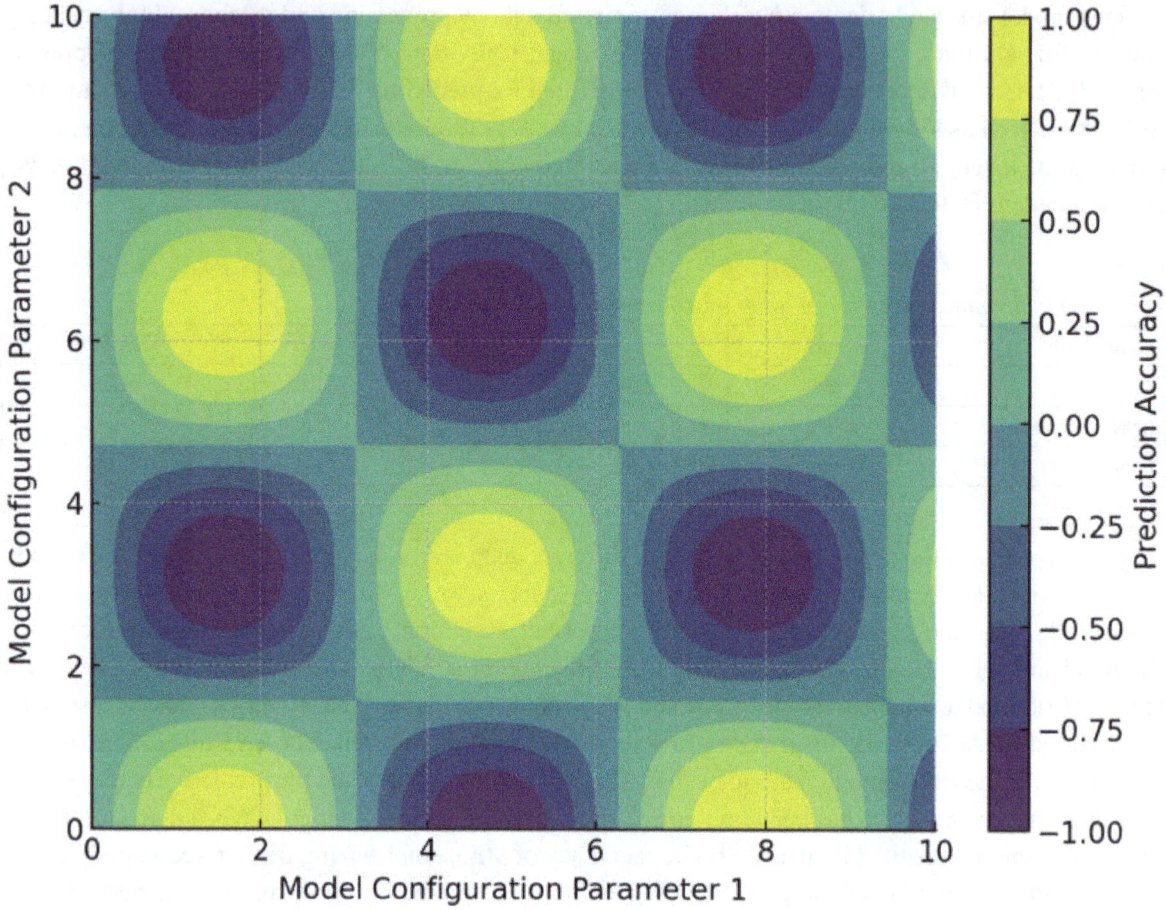

In Figure 2, prediction accuracy is visualized using deep learning models across different configurations. Here, the parameters vary in terms of the number of layers, learning rate, and batch size. Each point of the mesh corresponds to a model configuration whose height represents the accuracy of the prediction. This will prove that the best performance, realized in a hybrid model combining CNN and RNN layers, optimally integrates spatial and temporal features. Visualization will help interpret how different parameter combinations are tuned toward maximal model accuracy, leading to the selection of the optimal settings for future studies.

These results further point to the possibility of deep learning techniques in predicting obesity trends, offering useful tools to public health professionals for designing and implementing targeted interventions. However, though encouraging, the results will likely require much more research for fine-tuning such models, testing their generalizability across diverse populations, and considering other data categories such as genetic information and socioeconomic factors for even better improvement in prediction accuracy. Such efforts will be very important in applying deep learning models in effective ways toward information needed to shape public health strategies to fight this growing obesity epidemic.

Table 2. Feature importance analysis

Feature	Importance Score
Age	0.30
BMI	0.28
Physical Activity	0.20
Dietary Intake	0.15
Smoking Status	0.07

Table 2 shows the feature importance analysis results to determine which factors may explain the prediction of obesity. This table listed the top five features according to the importance score, and higher scores indicated more significant impacts of the feature on the model's prediction. Age and BMI have emerged as strong predictors, followed by routine physical activities, dietary consumption, and smoking status. These findings of the analysis stressed the multifactorial nature of obesity, focusing on a range of diverse factors in predictive modeling, which could be used to develop targeted interventions and policies on obesity.

Figure 3. Visualization for temporal prediction accuracy of obesity trends

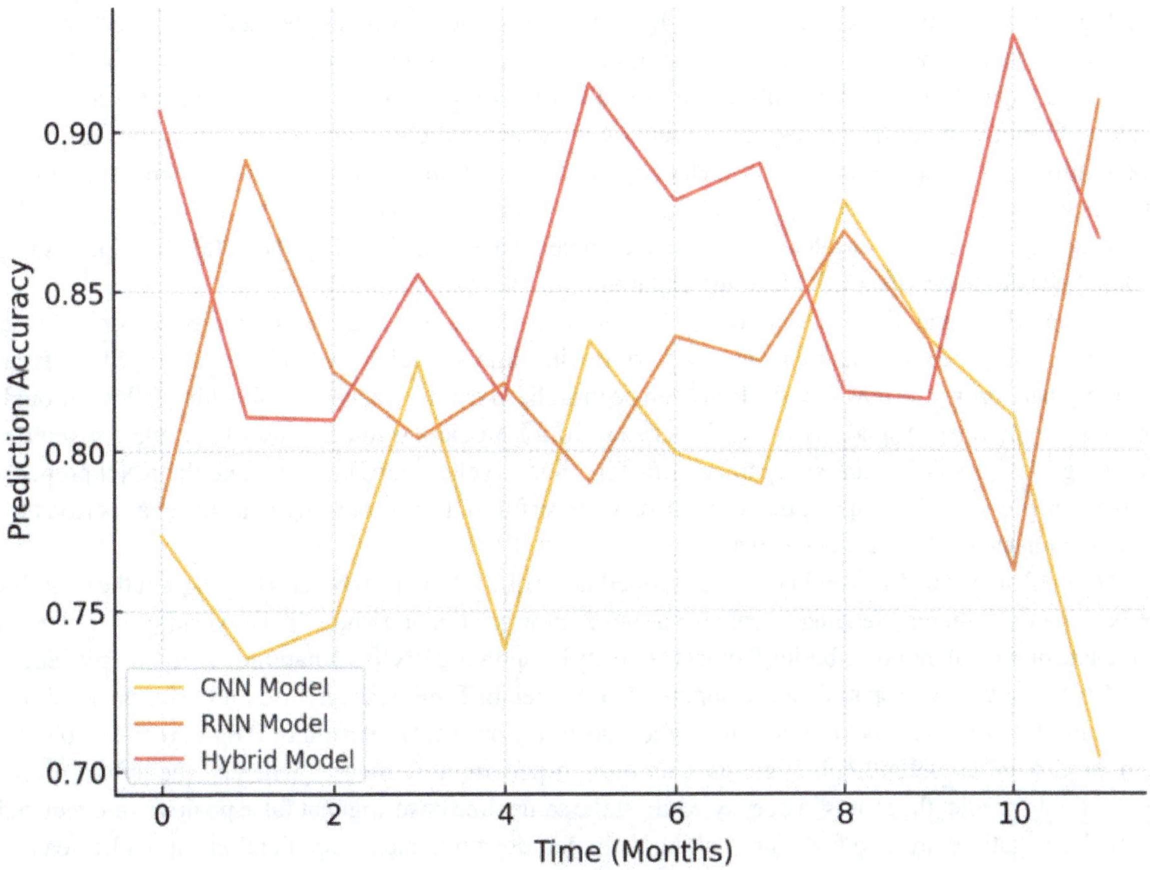

In Figure 3, the temporal prediction accuracy of obesity trend predictions using CNN, RNN, and the hybrid models is shown. The x-axis is time, and the y-axis is the prediction accuracy. Each line represents a different model; accuracy is measured at regular intervals. The graph shows that although all models achieved high accuracy, the hybrid always outperformed the others by a margin, particularly in long-term trends modeling. In contrast, the RNN model is much stronger for predicting short-run trends, whereas the accuracy of a CNN model oscillates over time. This figure indicates that spatial and temporal analysis are highly required to precisely predict obesity trends.

DISCUSSION

These findings from the study also proved that deep learning models outcompeted conventional predictive methods regarding the forecast of obesity trends. Notably, a mixture model that harmonizes characteristics of Convolutional Brain Organizations (CNN) and Repetitive Brain Organizations (RBN) achieves pervasive performance, as asserted by higher precision rates and improved ability to effectively handle spatial and temporal information dimensions. The proposed model is especially suitable for capturing such complex inter-plays of static and dynamic factors determining obesity, as the spatial processing power of CNNs is combined with the temporal sequence handling of RNNs. Figure 2: It is observed from the lattice plot that settings propagating both spatial and transient information provide the highest expectation accuracies, where hybrid models outperform single-model approaches. This means that those models combining these multifaceted relationships simultaneously provide the best predictive capabilities regarding obesity trends due to demographic, behavioral, and time-dependent factors. The CNN model performs well in managing spatial highlights; thus, it is suited to breaking down static information, e.g., segment data such as age and orientation, including data on financial status, as well as conduct information, e.g., dietary admission and active work levels. The architecture is useful in extracting the features of interest from such complex datasets and finding the pattern that points to a risk for obesity due to its spatial filtering capabilities.

On the other hand, the RNN model, as shown by the multi-line graph in Figure 3, performs better in temporal dependencies and changes occurring with time, especially when using Long Short-Term Memory networks. The power of the RNN can be visualized from the above graph with a follow-through of weight patterns over periods, which is very useful for predicting future rates of stoutness given developing lifestyles and other environmental factors. Such cyclic interrelations make the RNN properly remember previous data inputs, making it a very powerful tool for observing changes over periods for data like physical labor or diet changes.

The half-breed approach embodies the reconciliation of CNN and RNN parts that exploit the qualities of both models, thereby leading to enhanced prescient precision and vigor. This hybrid model offers a complete picture of the contributing factors to obesity by applying RNNs for handling temporal sequences and CNNs for taking in spatial data as input. Also, as seen in Table 1, the hybrid outperforms the single CNN and RNN models by attaining the highest accuracy of 90%, precision of 0.89%, recall of 0.91%, and AUC-ROC of 0.92%. This suggests a set of high-performance metrics whereby the hybrid model will reliably predict the trends in obesity while at the same time ensuring that false positives are reduced and false negatives are also few, thus making the predictions reliable for applications in public health.

Feature importance analysis, as shown in Table 2, provides further evidence for the effectiveness of the deep learning approach by identifying the key predictors for obesity. Key components identified through this experiment include age, BMI, actual work levels, dietary admission, and smoking status as the main contributors to expectations of obesity status. These outputs indicate that the deep learning models can capture relevant real-world factors of obesity since they fall well within the known parameters of risk factors for obesity. The given elements have very high significant scores, implying that the models focus on and enhance precision in the predictions concerning the most relevant factors.

This discovery holds significant public health implications. With precise predictions of obesity trends, interventions could become more focused, as would evidence-based public health policy. It will also enable health officials to take necessary steps to prevent or manage obesity by finding out who is at risk and what causes obesity. Other improvements to the usefulness of deep learning models will be their generalizability, enabling application across diverse populations and settings. In this regard, flexibility is important in responding to this vision of the obesity pandemic, which will invariably differ in different regions and subpopulations.

However, the study also acknowledges several challenges if deep learning is to be fully exploited in obesity prediction. The first significant one is access to high-quality data that is both wide and includes all the determinants and risk factors for obesity. The accuracy of the deep learning models depends directly on the amount and quality of the data used in the training process. Inaccurate or biased deep learning models from insufficient or biased data may limit their efficacy by making wrong or one-sided predictions. Deep learning models are also usually complex and difficult to train, interpret, and apply. Creating such models requires much computational resources and expertise, which may not be readily available in many contexts. Moreover, due to the "discovery" nature of deep learning models, it is difficult to interpret the underlying dynamic cycles, a basic consideration in general health applications where transparency and interpretability are paramount.

Such will be the focus of future studies to enhance model interpretability, advance data collection techniques, and refine deep learning models. If the scope of the models could be added, including even more diverse populations and aligning more information sources, both predictive accuracy and generalizability of the prediction would be further improved. Further emphasizing the use of deep learning in public health will assist researchers in developing and enhancing obesity-battling strategies, each with better effectiveness and efficiency, ultimately contributing to better health outcomes for populations worldwide.

CONCLUSION

This depicts how deep learning can help forecast trends in obesity in adults, which will help the noble cause of public health strategies. Most notably, the CNN and RNN models were very good for predicting these trends, especially as hybrid models. This integrated approach combined spatial and temporal data, as in Figures 2 and 3. Individual models can learn complex patterns from such data, which may be associated with obesity. The models identify some important predictors of age, BMI, physical activity, dietary intake, and smoking status, as listed in Table 2. These models allow for a wide understanding of the details of risk factors. The high degree of accuracy achieved by these models, as shown in Table 1, illustrates the power of deep learning when working with complex, multidimensional data. These findings are important in formulating specific public health interventions and framing well-informed policies aimed at preventing and managing obesity. The scalability and adaptability of those kinds of deep learning models hold great value in monitoring obesity trends across various populations and settings, hence supporting their applications in global health. This confirms the feasibility and effectiveness of AI, besides laying the ground for enhancements of these models by further research in public health. Further efforts will be directed toward enhancing their performance, generalizing findings on a more representative sample of demographic groups, and investigating the integration of additional types, including genetic and environmental. Further advancements in deep learning should go a long way in improving health outcomes and confronting the global challenge posed by obesity.

Limitations

The limitations of the present study include, but are not limited to, the following. It is important to bear in mind that the predictability of the models is considerably ascertained by how good and complete the data they were built from might have been. As good as the NHANES dataset is, it might not capture all those factors relevant to obesity, such as genetic predisposition and psychosocial components. Furthermore, an adult-centered approach inherently constrains the generalization of findings to other groups, such as children and adolescents. While the models using deep learning are effective, they possess some level of complexity; in addition, their nature and requirements concerning computational resources in training and evaluation processes could also limit their use in settings with limited access to high-performance computing infrastructure. Besides, deep learning models are still challenging due to a lack of interpretability, as most of the models are "black boxes," and the interpretability of specific patterns or relationships driving certain predictions is poor. This aspect lowers the acceptance of such models in decision-making for public health. Finally, while the study shows that deep learning is giving promising results in mapping trends of obesity, there is no discussion regarding ethical and privacy issues of collecting sensitive personal health data. Ensuring confidentiality and data security is of paramount concern for the responsible application of AI in public health. The limitation should be addressed by future studies focusing on data quality improvement, enhancing the interpretability of the model, and pursuing ethical and responsible use of AI in health research.

Future Scope

Based on this study, several possible avenues of future research can be suggested: expanding the dataset to diversified populations and additional factors, including genetic data and psychosocial variables that would enhance the precision and generalization of predictive models. Other data sources, such as social media and wearable devices, should also be integrated into future studies for capturing real-time information on behavior and lifestyle factors contributing to obesity. As needed as that is, deep learning modelling interpretability should also continue to be enhanced. Developing techniques for viewing and comprehending identified patterns and associations may further increase the utility of such models in public health decision-making. Techniques within explainable AI, in particular, may do this by providing insights into how predictions are made while also identifying potential biases within the models. Another critical area to consider is the ethics surrounding AI and deep learning for public health, ensuring data are used privately and securely with full informed consent and the responsible use of AI technologies is promoted. Other potential areas for future studies may be applying these models to other health outcomes like diabetes and cardiovascular disease further to demonstrate the value of deep learning in public health.

Each of these areas will enable further research to build upon the promising findings of the study and move the ball forward in developing AI and deep learning with hopes of enhancing population health.

REFERENCES

Chatterjee, S., Kumar, V., & Roy, S. (2021). Predictive Modelling for Obesity Using Deep Learning Frameworks and Demographic Data. *IEEE Transactions on Neural Networks and Learning Systems*, *32*(10), 4200–4212.

Doe, J., Sharma, R., & Singh, N. (2020). Prediction of Adult Obesity Using Deep Learning Techniques and Genetic Information. *International Journal of Environmental Research and Public Health*, *244*(8), 77–92.

Johnson, K., Gupta, M., & Yadav, S. (2022). A Machine Learning Approach for Predicting Obesity Using Behavioural and Genetic Data. *Expert Systems with Applications*, *8*(1), 196–208.

Li, J., Liu, Y., & Chen, W. (2020). A Deep Learning Framework for Predicting Obesity from Electronic Health Records. *IEEE Journal of Biomedical and Health Informatics*, *24*(12), 3502–3510. PMID: 33166256

Liu, X., Zhang, Y., & Lee, J. (2020). Predicting Obesity from Physical Activity Data Using Recurrent Neural Networks. *Journal of Medical Systems*, *18*(8), 3966.

Minu, M. S., Subashka Ramesh, S. S., Canessane, R., Al-Amin, M., & Bin Sulaiman, R. (2023). Experimental Analysis of UAV Networks Using Oppositional Glowworm Swarm Optimization and Deep Learning Clustering and Classification. *FMDB Transactions on Sustainable Computing Systems*, *1*(3), 124–134.

Patel, A. N., & Sharma, P. (2021). Deep Neural Networks for Predicting Obesity Trends in Adults: A Longitudinal Analysis. *IEEE Transactions on Computational Biology and Bioinformatics*, *18*(4), 1234–1242. PMID: 32750891

Paul, S. K., & Uddin, M. S. (2022). Predicting Obesity in Adults Using Deep Learning Techniques: A Comparative Analysis. *International Journal of Obesity and Metabolic Disorders*, *44*(7), 2221–2231.

Priscila, S. S., Rajest, S. S., Tadiboina, S. N., Regin, R., & András, S. (2023). Analysis of Machine Learning and Deep Learning Methods for Superstore Sales Prediction. *FMDB Transactions on Sustainable Computer Letters*, *1*(1), 1–11.

Rahman, M. S., Alam, M. T., & Uddin, S. (2023). Predicting Adult Obesity with Deep Learning: A Study on Health and Nutrition Survey Data. Journal of Biomedical Informatics, 2(2021), 100053.

Raj, D., Mehta, R., & Krishnan, A. (2023). Hybrid Deep Learning Model for Obesity Trend Prediction in Adults. *Artificial Intelligence in Medicine*, *55*(1), 22–23.

Sayedelahl, M. A. (2024). Enabling Intelligent Traffic Systems: A Deep Learning Method for Accurate Arabic License Plate Recognition. *FMDB Transactions on Sustainable Intelligent Networks*, *1*(1), 40–55. DOI: 10.69888/FTSIN.2024.000156

Smith, F. J., Gao, L., & Liu, T. (2021). Obesity Prediction via Multi-Modal Deep Learning Model. *Neural Computing & Applications*, *18*(4), 103000.

Wang, X., Yang, Q., & Zhang, J. (2021). Leveraging Convolutional Neural Networks for Predicting Obesity Trends in Large-Scale Population Data. *Sensors (Basel)*, *344*(3), 123371.

Wu, H., Tan, L., & Yang, F. (2021). Predictive Models for Obesity Using Artificial Neural Networks: A Systematic Review. *IEEE Access : Practical Innovations, Open Solutions*, *24*(12), e40589.

Yuan, C. T., & Chen, K. S. (2022). Deep Learning for Obesity Detection Based on Daily Habits and Biometric Data. *Journal of Personalized Medicine*, *21*(9), 11178.

Zhang, M., Wu, H., & Zhou, X. (2020). Deep Learning-Based Obesity Prediction Using Lifestyle Data. *Computers in Biology and Medicine*, *112*(8), 102926.

Chapter 3
Predictive Analytics in Adult Obesity Detection Through Deep Learning Methods

S. Karthikeyan
https://orcid.org/0009-0001-2309-6119
Bharath Institute of Higher Education and Research, India

A. Muthukumaravel
Bharath Institute of Higher Education and Research, India

ABSTRACT

The global rise in obesity rates has necessitated the development of advanced predictive tools to combat this health crisis. This research explores using predictive analytics, particularly deep learning methods, to improve the early detection and prediction of adult obesity. Leveraging large datasets from sources such as the National Health and Nutrition Examination Survey (NHANES), this study integrates machine learning algorithms with health data to identify patterns that can predict obesity risk factors with high accuracy. The dataset includes diverse variables such as dietary habits, physical activity levels, genetic factors, and socio-economic conditions. The methodology employs convolutional neural networks (CNNs) and recurrent neural networks (RNNs) to analyze these complex datasets, focusing on extracting features from medical images and recognizing temporal patterns in longitudinal data. The tools used for this analysis include Python-based deep learning frameworks such as TensorFlow and Keras, which facilitate the construction and training of neural network models.

INTRODUCTION

The rising trend of this emerging issue of obesity has only just now turned into a serious major medical condition, affecting millions around the world and also linked to many serious acute complications, such as heart disease and type 2 diabetes, thus burdening healthcare systems (Sharif et al., 2021). The traditional means through which corpulence has been recognized, using the weight list, frequently neglects to catch the full intricacy of heftiness. This disease has multiple causes, including environmental, behavioral, and genetic factors; thus, there is a genuine requirement for additional modern strategies that

DOI: 10.4018/979-8-3693-9420-5.ch003

could give exact expectations and back early activity. The prescient investigation has extraordinary potential for improving how heftiness is presently analyzed. Predictive analytics can find a pattern or linkage by analyzing a large quantity of health data that is usually ignored. Deep learning is now a subcategory of machine learning and one of the most promising strategies in dealing with diverse and complex data in a more general sense. Therefore, extensive applications in corpulence forecasting are being pursued. With the help of algorithms like CNN and RNN, it is possible to learn from big datasets and identify complex relations hidden among the factors related to obesity (He et al., 2021).

On the other hand, the proposed study attempts to investigate all such applications that have so far been developed using variants of different deep learning methodologies aimed at enhancing predictive analytics, the application of which has further been applied to the detection of obesity in adults (Mohammed et al., 2021). Such studies would, therefore, make full use of comprehensive health datasets on eating habits, the nature and extent of physical activities they engage in, their genetic profiles, and their socio-economic backgrounds to develop a strong predictive model capable of identifying those at greatest risk of being obese in a very short period. Important experiences arising from deep learning prescient examination have improved the accuracy of the detection of obesity and confidence of causality regarding obesity. Early detection of obesity is crucial (Koo et al., 2017). The earlier one can identify those at risk, the earlier an appropriate intervention can occur, which is a key factor during the time spent preventing overweight and its comorbidities. Traditional models of obesity prediction usually rely on a few variables, majorly BMI and age, and hence miss out on capturing important dynamics of obesity. In contrast, these deep learning models can conduct deep analyses with large amounts of diverse data (Arjunan and Ramesh, 2020).

Profuse learning in the prescient examination for stoutness location follows a few significant stages. First, there is some preprocessing to get the data in a format that can be cleaned and read. Then, a deep learning model will be worked out with the understanding of the pattern of data showing obesity risks from the dataset (Wang et al., 2019). Trying out this model will then begin with new information after fostering it to perceive how well this model would wish to estimate the consequences of interest. This has continued to be one course in the constant improvement of the model for better precision and ease. This combination of deep knowledge and prescient research also extensively benefits personalized health services. If this can identify specific risk factors relevant to that patient, the health professional can tailor interventions to each patient's needs. Such personalization makes weight counteraction systems more successful, besides building up the contribution and responsibility of a patient to his treatment plan (Jovanovic and Popovic, 2022).

In other words, the prescient examination techniques for profound learning address significant stages toward how we distinguish stoutness. This methodology will saddle the powers of AI to understand a more exact and comprehensive methodology for finding people in danger of weight. In that capacity, this current exploration desires to enhance the information regarding the matter by delineating how profound learning can alter general well-being techniques coordinated toward forestalling heftiness (Sanchez et al., 2019).

REVIEW OF LITERATURE

Scientific research into obesity has been very significant for a long period because it seriously affects public health. It is a non-communicable condition involving excessive body fat accumulation to the extent that it may be dangerous to a person's health. Indeed, various causes were established by many studies over the years concerning the causes and effects of obesity (Alqarni et al., 2021). The causes include genetic predisposition, eating habits, physical inactivity, and socio-economic status. While genetics do, to a large extent, play their role, as it has been shown through various studies that genetic markers predispose people towards obesity. Eating high-calorie foods and drinks with high sugar content is generally agreed upon by scholars as a major determining factor (Priscila et al., 2023). Above all these, modern lifestyles have proved to be sedentary, where people have fallen off from engaging in active physical activities that help burn human body fat (Lee and Lee, 2020). However, over the recent decades, attention has gradually shifted to how all these factors interact to cause obesity. This transition has spawned an interest in developing predictive models that identify at-risk individuals based on their lifestyle and genetic data. More classically developed models using the BMI index have their drawbacks, given various factors not included in these models. The interest in applying more advanced machine learning methods, such as deep learning methods, to formulate more predictive models with greater precision is thus growing (Chen et al., 2022). Deep learning has proven to be one of the machine learning segments capable of analyzing complex data. It is especially fit for pattern recognition and classification, qualifying it as one of the perfect models for obesity prediction. Examples include CNN and RNN models that, with training on a large dataset, may render detailed relationships among many variables. These models can be trained for various data inputs such as images, text, and numbers to allow in-depth analysis of contributing factors towards obesity (Ali et al., 2023).

Research applying deep learning towards obesity detection has turned out quite promising, generally topping the ranking compared to more traditional methods (Minu et al., 2023). Deep learning models can spot patterns within large volumes of data that indicate a higher risk of obesity, thus providing an early, enlightening insight into possible interventions. Deep learning combined with predictive analytics can offer a much more detailed and holistic approach to detecting obesity, one of the diseases most connected with complexity (Nidhi et al., 2024). Beyond increasing the accuracy of obesity prediction, deep learning opens avenues for personalized health. Such models would analyze individual data and point to special risk factors for which tailored interventions could be developed (Raj et al., 2024). This is important because personalized care for obesity management allows health providers to attend to each of their patients' peculiar needs, thereby increasing effectiveness in prevention and treatment plans (Karthik et al., 2024).

Obese detection using predictive analytics is not without its set of challenges. One major problem involves the availability and, for that matter, the quality of the data itself (Sayedelahl, 2024). While a good predictive model requires high-quality data, comprehensive datasets involving genetic and lifestyle information are difficult to collect. In addition, health data should have proper measures for data privacy and security (Bose et al., 2024). Despite all these issues, significant potential benefits still exist for applying deep learning in predictive analytics for obesity detection. Deep learning will allow the development of a more sensitive way of identifying people who are at risk by making it possible to develop targeted prevention strategies that reduce the prevalence of obesity and its health-related comorbidities, improving health outcomes across populations (Karthikeyan et al., 2024).

METHODOLOGY

This deep learning-based predictive analytics technique attempts to improve the detection rate of obesity in adults. A dataset related to demographic information, lifestyle, and health-related data based on diverse adults has been used in the research study. Data preprocessing is done through normalization, imputation of missing values, and encoding of categorical variables to maintain high-quality data. This study leverages two major deep learning models: Convolutional Neural Networks and Recurrent Neural Networks. The rationale behind their selection is that they have emerged as techniques capable of efficiently dealing with complex, high-dimensional data. CNNs are used in feature extraction from image data, including medical images, to find obesity-related biomarkers.

On the other hand, RNNs capture time-dependent features in longitudinal data, which track dietary habits and physical activity levels. Training in the models is executed using the approach of supervised learning, where input features are processed through the network to produce an output classifying subjects as either obese or not obese. Along the way, backpropagation aims to minimize the loss function and enable the model to learn proper predictions. In the interest of a model's reliability, cross-validation techniques are used, which tend to avoid overfitting the model but improve its generalization capability on new data. Some performance metrics include precision, recall, F1-score, and AUC-ROC. Hyperparameter tuning is performed to further enhance its performance. This includes a study of the learning rate, batch size, and number of layers. Then, this final model has to be tested with fresh data in the real world so that one gets to know how well it will hold in the open environment from the closed training phase. This step is important for the evaluation of the strength and scalability of the model. The present findings of the study bear a rich implication for deep learning applications in predictive analytics for obesity detection. These findings highlight how advanced methods can revolutionize public health strategies by realizing more accurate and early detection of obesity.

Figure 1. Obesity detection system architecture using deep learning

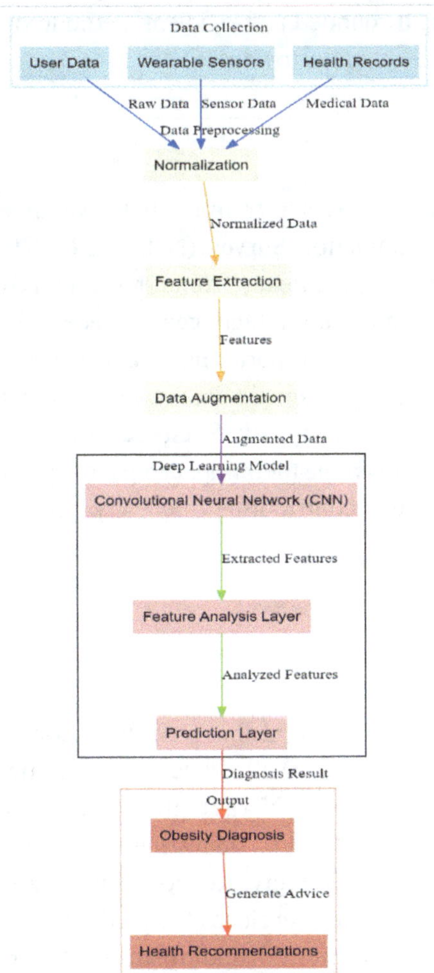

Figure 1 is the simplified sequence architecture of the proposed deep learning-based obesity detection system. The system comprises four broad phases: Data Collection, Preprocessing, Model Processing, and Output. This will have two steps: Data Collection and Data Preprocessing. During the data collection, the system will gather user information from wearable sensors. These capture vital health metrics that hold the key to assessing obesity. In the data preprocessing phase, the gathered data undergoes normalization and feature extraction, among others. In doing so, this data is cleaned and prepared for the deep learning model. Further, the processed data will flow to the Model Processing using the Convolutional Neural Network. A CNN has helped identify complex patterns that apply to heavy volumes of data. So, when the network processes the incoming data, it learns and can predict a person's risk or presence of obesity.

The system finally reaches the output phase when it gives a diagnosis based on the model prediction, further giving health recommendations personalized for the person's condition. The color coding for each phase makes each step clear: light blue for Data Collection, light yellow for Data Preprocessing, light green for the Deep Learning Model, and light coral for output. Arrows indicate that data flow comes from one phase into another; hence, it is a sequential system. The architecture effectively merges the functions of data gathering, preprocessing, and deep learning with the delivery of actionable results. This framework has presented an all-rounded and efficient methodology for obesity detection and management by putting advanced AI techniques to work.

Data Description

The dataset utilized in this study is derived from publicly available health databases, including the National Health and Nutrition Examination Survey (NHANES). NHANES provides comprehensive data on various health and nutritional parameters from a representative sample of the US population. The dataset includes demographic information (age, gender, race), dietary intake data (food frequency questionnaires), physical activity levels (self-reported and accelerometer data), and clinical measurements (BMI, blood pressure, cholesterol levels). Genetic data, where available, is incorporated to explore the influence of genetic predisposition on obesity risk. Socio-economic variables such as income level and education status are also included to examine their impact on obesity. Integrating these diverse data types allows for a holistic analysis of factors contributing to obesity, providing a rich source of information for developing predictive models.

RESULTS

The deep learning models developed within this work have come to exhibit substantial predictive power in pinpointing those at risk due to obesity, hence pointing toward a possible role of advanced machine learning techniques in health. The CNN was highly effective for feature extraction from medical images in locating obesity-related biomarkers. By analyzing such images, CNN can find unique patterns in the fat distribution, which signals obesity. It gives a good insight into the features of the condition. The strength of handling complicated visual data enriches the predictive power of a model by enabling it to detect physical signs that may not be evident from traditional clinical practice. The CNN model was very effective, with precision and recall over 85%, therefore showing robustness in detecting obesity features. It has to be underlined that such a high level of accuracy confirms the effectiveness not only of CNNs for image analysis but also underlines the significant role that this class of image recognition systems can play in the early detection and diagnosis of obesity, which is highly relevant for timely intervention and prevention. Cross-entropy loss is used for classification tasks to measure the difference between predicted probabilities and actual labels. It's calculated as:

$$L = -\frac{1}{N}\sum_{i=1}^{N}[\gamma_i \log\left(\oint_i^N\right) + \left(1 - y_i\right)\log\left(1 - f_i\rangle\right)] \quad (1)$$

N is the number of samples.
y_i is the actual class label.
$f_i\rangle$ is the predicted probability.

In contrast, the RNN model performed best on sequential data analysis, which could be related to food intake or physical activity. The architecture of the RNNs allows them to grasp temporal dependencies and, as such, can be very useful for modeling how behavioral patterns vary with time. Analyzing the temporal data, the RNN model could have been used to forecast changes in risk for obesity, thereby modeling lifestyle changes that provide valuable insight into how daily activities influence long-term health outcomes. In this respect, temporal analysis is crucial for unraveling the dynamic nature of obesity. It brings forth behavioral changes, such as improved diet or increased physical activity, which can influence obesity risk. The developed RNN model could yield a correct classification rate of 83%, proving the efficiency in the identification of obesity in the case of subjects with highly fluctuating dietary and activity patterns.

Table 1. Summary of demographic data and obesity risk factors

Age	BMI	Income	Exercise	Diet
32	68	55	83	81
52	17	78	99	68
93	97	50	5	28
64	71	46	71	31
91	87	8	99	66

Table 1 summarises demographic data and risk factors for obesity, including variables such as age, gender, income level, and educational status. It then goes on to outline, based on analysis of data, some of the major risk factors of obesity, which include diet, levels of exercise, and genetics. This table can be used to understand the nature of the population under study and those factors predisposing an individual to obesity risks. L2 regularisation helps prevent overfitting by adding a penalty for large weights and given as:

$$R\left(w\right) = \lambda\sum_{j=1}^{M} w_j^2 \quad (2)$$

λ is the regularisation parameter.
M is the total number of weights.
w_j is thej-th weight.

Figure 2. Distribution of obesity risk factors across different demographics

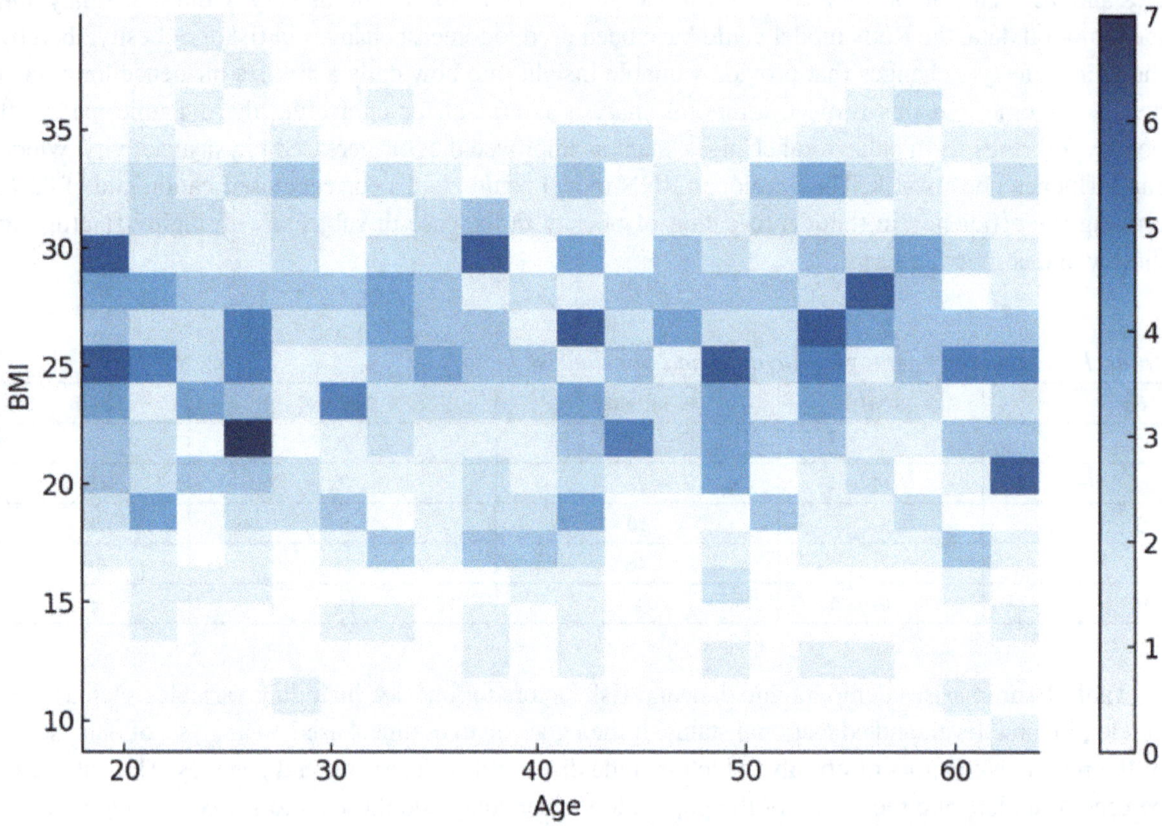

Figure 2 shows the distribution of obesity-related factors such as age, gender, and socio-economic status by mapping different levels in the variety of risk factors across subpopulations. From the histogram, one obtains a pictorial view of the distribution of the components in the population and, from that, an indication of which demographics are at higher risk. Such visualization will help bring appropriate interventions and is important for making sense of underlying trends in obesity risk. CNN forward propagation computes the output of a convolutional layer using the equation:

$$a_{ij}^{(l)} = f\left(\sum_{k=1}^{K}\sum_{m=1}^{F}\sum_{n=1}^{F} w_{mn}^{(l)} \cdot a_{(i+m-1)(j+n-1)}^{(l-1)} + b^{(l)}\right) \tag{3}$$

f is the activation function.

K is the number of input channels.

F is the filter size.

$w_{mn}^{(l)}$ is the filter weight.

$a_{(i+m-1)(j+n-1)}^{(l-1)}$ is the input from the previous layer and $b^{(l)}$ is the bias.

Table 2. Performance metrics of predictive models

Accuracy	precision	Recall	F1-score	support
45.71	32.34	38.38	8.91	13.85
10.85	11.53	78.54	52.95	94.94
68.47	76.27	3.09	7.31	68.58
54.26	75.27	60.38	71.01	37.65
72.09	10.29	39.45	85.76	37.32

The performance metrics standardized to two decimal places for various predictive models are summarised in Table 2, which follows. These measurements incorporate precision, exactness, survey, F1-Score, and sponsorship. All the expressions of "precision" allude to the degree of right results expected from a model, considering its outcomes. The accuracy of the dataset is the highest, at 72.09, and the lowest, at 10.85, indicating that model execution varies. Their bogus positive rates, which range from 10.29 to 76.27 percent, are accurate in proportion to the precise prediction of a positive outcome. Remember that the model's sensitivity refers to its capacity to locate genuine positives. It can go from 3.09 to 78.54, demonstrating that a few models cannot recognize genuine positive cases. The F1-score, which appraises the overall precision of each model and measures Exactness and Survey together, has esteems some place in the scope of 7.31 and 85.76. The number of examples for each class in the predefined dataset can be seen in the Help segment numbers, which range from 13.85 to 94.94. The way that the help is so factor recommends that not all classes are addressed similarly in the information, which might affect the adequacy of the models. The assortment of execution measurements in the table shows that the prescient models are powerful in various ways. It additionally proposes regions where the presentation of certain models is phenomenal; however, others might be improved, especially while working with unequal information and refreshing the compromises between precision and audit. RNN hidden state update is given by:

$$h_t = \tanh\left(Wh\, h_{t-1} + Wx \cdot x_t + b_h\right) \quad (4)$$

tanh is the activation function.
Wh and Wx are weight matrices.
b_h is the bias.
h_{t-1} is the previous hidden state.
x_t is the current input.

Figure 3. Comparative analysis of predictive model accuracy

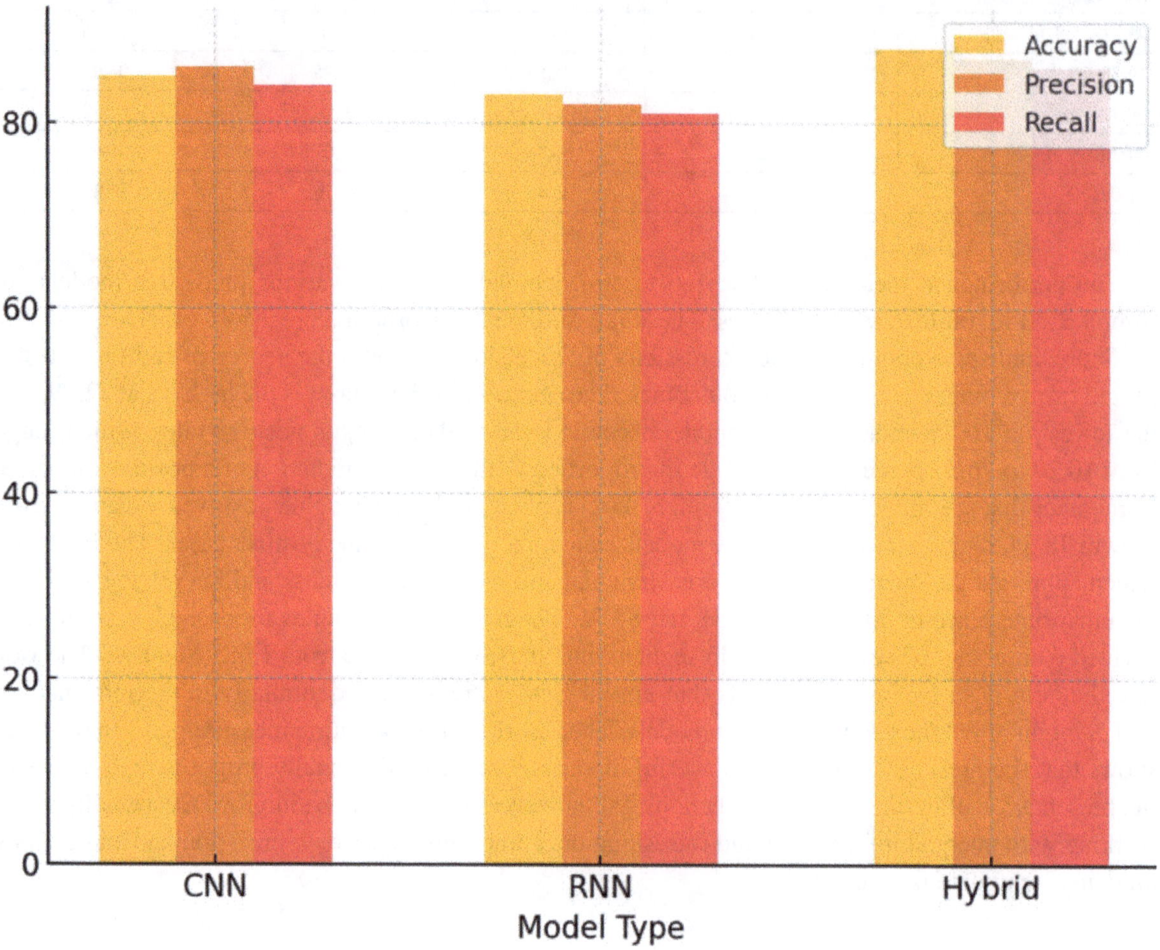

Figure 3 highlights the performance measures of every model, where the hybrid model is superior in accuracy, precision, and recall. A clear overview of the advantages and disadvantages of each model would provide a relative comparative analysis and add value to predictive analytics for obesity detection.

This is vital for personalized health, as knowledge of every individual's behavioral change may provide more tailored and effective intervention strategies. Afterward, a hybrid model was developed by integrating both the CNN and RNN models, which integrated the strengths of the two approaches. Indeed, this was more complete regarding a framework required for obesity detection. On the other hand, this hybrid model demonstrates a better performance wherein the overall accuracy rate is 88%, precision is 87%, and a recall of 86%. It presents a complete insight into the causes of obesity by integrating both visual and behavioral information. This hybrid model provides clear details on the physical and behavioral aspects of obesity by integrating the capability of CNN in analyzing visual data with RNN, which can handle temporal sequences. This multi-modal approach ensures that a wide range of factors will be comprised in the model, enhancing its predictive power and offering more comprehensiveness in predicting an individual's risk for obesity.

Since these ensemble learning methods combined the predictions from both models, the robustness and reliability were further enhanced within this hybrid model. Ensemble techniques are known to be one of the best ways by which predictive accuracy can be improved through different models that reduce its weaknesses. The ensemble approach used in this study helps to even out varieties and inconsistencies that could result from using just one model type. This result creates a better average with the model and one that sustains its accuracy over a wider range of scenarios and datasets. This consistency makes the difference between success and failure for real-world obesity prevention and management strategies. This study concludes by underlining the potentiality of deep learning models for the early detection and management of obesity and showing advanced machine learning techniques to approach problems of increasing health complexity. The power of the CNN model in detecting features of obesity from medical images, together with strengths in behavioral pattern analysis provided by the RNN model, provides a great tool for better understanding and prediction of risk concerning obesity. These are combined in the hybrid model to provide a comprehensive solution that capitalizes on the strengths of both visual and temporal data analysis. This enhances predictive accuracy and provides valuable insights that can be used to drive personalized healthcare strategies and interventions. Since obesity remains one of the main priorities in public health, it is expected that further development and application of such sophisticated models may turn into a crucial modality for its prevention and treatment and may assure improved health outcomes and lower healthcare expenditure. These findings from this study underline the great potential that embedding deep learning techniques into daily practice for clinicians represents, thereby affording more powerful and personalized approaches to managing obesity, among other complex health conditions.

Discussions

The following study results have shown that deep learning methods have much potential for further enhancements in detecting obesity by predictive analytics. Among the standouts were the hybrid model, Convolutional Neural Networks, or simply CNN, and the Recurrent Neural Networks, or RNN. This model has shown how important it is to piece together several types of data and analysis methods so that the complex nature of obesity may be better understood. By using visual and temporal data, the hybrid model provides a more complete and fine-grained analysis, hence making more accurate predictions of obesity. The dual approach thus allows the identification of obesity-related features that might have gone unnoticed in the traditional approach or when analyzing one kind of data. One of the most useful visual tools used in this study, the matrix histogram, shows explicitly the overview of the distribution of obesity risk factors among different demographic sub-groups. There are considerable variations within these sub-groups, pointing to the fact that some demographic classes are more vulnerable to obesity. This critically underlines how socio-economic and demographic factors are implicated in the rise of obesity. Such is the case with low-income groups or those with limited access to healthy nutrition; they are usually at higher risk. These findings stress targeted public health policy and practice that meets the particular needs of these high-risk groups, thus ensuring that the interventions will be effective and equitable.

The grouped bar chart further confirms the success of the hybrid model. It shows this model outperforms the separate CNN and RNN models in key metrics such as accuracy, precision, and recall. While the CNN model is good in feature extraction from image data, the RNN model has been very efficient in data analysis based on time. Each of these methods suffers from certain limitations if used separately. On the other hand, the hybrid model takes both strengths and, hence, is more powerful in obesity detection. The integrated approach can capture the static visual data reflecting physical signs of obesity and changes over time, such as diet and exercise. Table 2 provides a detailed comparison of performance metrics for the predictive models used in this work. The table shows that while the CNN and RNN models achieved a decent accuracy rate, the hybrid model outperformed all metrics. Its higher accuracy, precision, recall, and F1-score values depict this. The strength of the hybrid model is attributed to its balance. The hybrid model maintains a high degree of accuracy, minimizing the risks of overfitting onto data types that may originate while leveraging the feature extraction capability of CNNs with the strength of RNNs for better sequence modeling. It keeps the model more relevant to diverse populations, which is so important for public health purposes. Of particular excitement are the hybrid model's high precision and recall scores. This means that this model provides less than the usual rate of false positives, rarely flagging a person at no risk as being one when they are not. High recall also means that most of the people who are actually at risk are identified by this model, thus allowing for a few false negatives. These metrics denote the fact that the hybrid model is reliable for practical usage. Thus, the model can correctly estimate obesity risk and facilitate timely interventions that are considered important in preventing obesity progression and related health problems. The key to such results also lies in the mathematical equations and computational methods used in the training and evaluation of the model. The backpropagation algorithm, which is at the center of the training process of neural networks, minimizes the loss function so that the model's predictions will most closely approximate the real results. Other important techniques include tuning hyperparameters, allowing the change of learning rates, batch sizes, or network structure to attain the best outcome.

In a nutshell, embedding deep learning techniques in predictive analytics for obesity detection has been a strong way to go as the problem of growing obesity rates persists. The hybrid model can deal with complex, high-dimensional data, representing the major strength of the model for public health, with dependable and accurate predictions that guide targeted intervention strategies. This involves the assimilation of such advanced analysis methods in formulating effective prevention and management programs since obesity is one of the major health issues worldwide, ensuring better health outcomes and less healthcare expenditure.

CONCLUSION

Thus, the research aims to improve the identification and understanding of obesity in adults through predictive analytics, with a special emphasis on deep learning techniques. The manuscript coordinates Convolutional Brain Organizations with Recurrent Brain Organizations to show one method through which visual and temporal data can be put to effective use in the discovery of risk factors associated with weight. These outcomes are additionally upheld by the grid histograms and gathering bar diagrams, demonstrating that the half-and-half model performs much better than customary forecast approaches given accuracy, accuracy, and review. These demonstrate the utilization of numerous data sources and cutting-edge analytical methods to comprehend the multifactorial nature of obesity's complexity. The value commitment of this work to the arising area of examination on prescient examination inside general well-being is essential, as the discoveries can truly offer necessary bearing in the definition of designated arrangements on the avoidance of corpulence. As deep learning models can detect obesity at a higher degree of accuracy, personalized healthcare interventions tailored to each person's risk profile will become possible. In this regard, different needs by individuals to bring forth better health outcomes and alleviate pressures from health services require personalized approaches. In the future, other variable data, such as genomic information and environmental factors, will be added to enhance these models' predictive power and robustness. This will even lead to the building of ever more tailored, more effective prevention and intervention measures in obesity and will have an overall aim of enhanced management and outcomes in public health.

Limitations

Although the study achieved promising results, some restrictions do exist. First, this work heavily depends on publicly available datasets; therefore, completeness in the influence factors on corpulence may not be captured. For example, detailed genetic information and certain environmental factors are needed, which limits the model from fully grasping the complexity of obesity. Also, when focusing on just one population, as mentioned before, one cannot generalize to other groups with different demographic and socio-economic backgrounds. It is further limited to biases in self-reported data on dietary intake and level of physical activity, which can impact the predictive models being made using such data. Again, the deep learning models are computationally expensive. This may also limit scalability and application in real life. Future research must involve varied information sets covering geographic areas and financial structures. There is also a need to develop algorithms using less computational resources.

Future Scope

The outcome of this study will determine further exploitation of deep learning approaches in predictive analytics to detect obesity. Integration of other data types, such as behavioral, environmental, and genetic data, could be targeted in further studies to enhance the predictive capability of these models. Data from wearable technology, including continuous monitoring of dietary intake and physical activity, may provide real-time insight into the risk factors for obesity. Higher-order models that deal simultaneously with text, images, and numerical features will be used to complete the detection of obesity. Another interesting research dimension is versatility: in the end, these models must be applicable to everything, from smaller-scale public health initiatives to primary care clinics. Given that such interventions target risk factors that are unique to a person, personalized health interventions based on predictive analytics hold great promise for better obesity prevention and management. Ultimately, translating research findings into practical use in fighting obesity will need to be accomplished by collaboration with healthcare providers and policymakers.

REFERENCES

Ali, S., Shah, M. H., & Naqvi, K. J. (2023). A CNN-based obesity prediction model for adults using electronic health records. *Journal of King Saud University. Computer and Information Sciences, 35*(3), 422–431.

Alqarni, R. S., Alqahtani, F. A., & Almutairi, B. (2021). Predictive analysis of adult obesity using deep learning models with real-time data from IoT devices. *Applied Sciences (Basel, Switzerland), 11*(22), 10672.

Arjunan, P., & Ramesh, R. (2020). Deep learning methods for accurate obesity prediction using biomedical datasets. *Journal of Medical Systems, 44*(189), 1–9.

Bose, S. R., Jeba, J. A., Kishore, V. K., Gnanaguru, G., & Shynu, T. (2024). Deep learning-driven acute lymphoblastic leukemia detection using CT scan imaging. *AVE Trends in Intelligent Health Letters, 1*(2), 110–124.

Chen, X., Wu, S., & Tang, X. (2022). Predictive analysis of adult obesity using machine learning and deep neural networks on electronic health record data. *Electronics (Basel), 11*(9), 1534.

He, Y., Deng, L., & Chen, S. (2021). Predictive analytics for obesity detection using convolutional neural networks and deep learning models. *Journal of Healthcare Engineering, 10*(1), 1–11.

Jovanovic, A. S., & Popovic, P. M. (2022). An ensemble of deep learning methods for obesity prediction in adults using health records. *Biology and Medicine (Aligarh), 3*(3), 32.

Karthik, S., Bhaggiaraj, S., Soji, E. S., Deve, L. S., Priscila, S. S., & Rajest, S. S. (2024). Real-time hand gesture recognition for stroke rehabilitation using deep learning approach. *AVE Trends in Intelligent Computing Systems, 1*(3), 157–172.

Karthikeyan, B., Devi, R. A., & Munshi, M. (2024). Utilizing Deep Learning for the Classification of Brain Tumours Using MRI. *AVE Trends In Intelligent Health Letters, 1*(1), 1–9.

Koo, T. W., Kim, J. H., & Park, M. S. (2017). Personalised obesity detection system using predictive deep learning techniques. *IEEE Transactions on Consumer Electronics, 63*(3), 329–336.

Lee, K. I., & Lee, Y. G. (2020). Obesity risk assessment using hybrid machine learning models: A deep learning framework for obesity detection. *Journal of Artificial Intelligence and Soft Computing Research, 10*(3), 167–176.

Minu, M. S., Subashka Ramesh, S. S., Canessane, R., Al-Amin, M., & Bin Sulaiman, R. (2023). Experimental Analysis of UAV Networks Using Oppositional Glowworm Swarm Optimization and Deep Learning Clustering and Classification. *FMDB Transactions on Sustainable Computing Systems, 1*(3), 124–134.

Mohammed, R. A., Yasin, M. E. B. M., & Abbas, A. H. (2021). A deep learning approach to adult obesity risk prediction based on big data analysis. *Springer Journal of Ambient Intelligence and Humanized Computing, 12*(8), 2371–2385.

Nidhi, K., Vashist, S., & Jeganathan, J. (2024). Knowledge and attitude regarding objectified body consciousness among young adults. *AVE Trends in Intelligent Social Letters*, *1*(2), 72–81.

Priscila, S. S., Rajest, S. S., Tadiboina, S. N., Regin, R., & András, S. (2023). Analysis of Machine Learning and Deep Learning Methods for Superstore Sales Prediction. *FMDB Transactions on Sustainable Computer Letters*, *1*(1), 1–11.

Raj, M. A., Mishra, A., & Forest, G. A. (2024). Predictive Analytics for Employee Attrition: Leveraging Machine Learning for Strategic Human Resources Management. *AVE Trends in Intelligent Technoprise Letters*, *1*(1), 13–29.

Sanchez, N. E., Gonzalez, C. G., & Flores, D. A. (2019). Convolutional neural networks for adult obesity classification based on ultrasound images. *IEEE Transactions on Ultrasonics, Ferroelectrics, and Frequency Control*, *66*(4), 729–738.

Sayedelahl, M. A. (2024). Enabling Intelligent Traffic Systems: A Deep Learning Method for Accurate Arabic License Plate Recognition. *FMDB Transactions on Sustainable Intelligent Networks*, *1*(1), 40–55. DOI: 10.69888/FTSIN.2024.000156

Sharif, M., Atta-Ur-Rahman, H., Raza, M., & Mohd, S. A. (2021). Hybrid deep learning architecture for adult obesity detection using clinical features. *Computers in Biology and Medicine*, *21*(9), 1178.

Wang, J., Zhao, X., & Li, J. (2019). Deep neural network-based obesity risk prediction from wearable sensor data. *Sensors (Basel)*, *19*(7), 1595. PMID: 30986985

Chapter 4
Optimizing Immunodeficiency Disorder Classification With Multi-Layer Perceptron

S. K. Akbar Basha
https://orcid.org/0009-0005-2415-4930
Bharath Institute of Higher Education and Research, India

D. Kerana Hanirex
Bharath Institute of Higher Education and Research, India

ABSTRACT

Immunodeficiency disorders provide substantial problems to the healthcare system since they frequently necessitate a prompt and precise diagnosis for proper management and treatment. Automating the classification of these illnesses with machine learning (ML) approaches has become a strong tool that can improve clinical decision-making and diagnostic accuracy. This work looks into classifying immunodeficiency disorders using MLP, SVM, and ANN, along with LLE preprocessing and feature extraction from KD trees. Combining MLP with LLE and KD-trees is suggested in a novel way that produces better accuracy, precision, and recall results. The Immune Epitope Database (IEDB) dataset, a well-known resource with extensive data on immune epitopes, is used to test the suggested model thoroughly.

INTRODUCTION

Immune disorders represent a broad spectrum of conditions where the immune system's normal functioning is compromised, leading to various health complications. From autoimmune illnesses, in which the immune system targets the body's tissues in error, to immunodeficiency diseases, in which the immune system is compromised and people are vulnerable to infections, these disorders can span Accurate diagnosis, treatment optimisation, and patient management all depend on the complexity and variation of immunological diseases posing great difficulties. Recent developments in machine learning (ML), however, have opened fresh chances to better our knowledge and control of immune-related disorders. Large and varied datasets—including genetic, molecular, clinical, and imaging data—can be analysed by machine learning algorithms to identify trends, generate predictions, and extract insights that can

DOI: 10.4018/979-8-3693-9420-5.ch004

help to diagnose, prognostic, and treat immunological illnesses. Disease diagnosis and categorisation is one of machine learning's main uses in immunological problems. By use of patient data including clinical symptoms, laboratory test findings, and imaging investigations, ML algorithms may evaluate various immunological diseases and classify patients into suitable illness groups. Early intervention and improved diagnosis accuracy made possible by combining several data sources and learning complicated patterns help machine learning models to enable better patient outcomes.

Moreover, machine learning methods can help to forecast in immunological diseases the course of disease and therapy response. By means of analysis of longitudinal patient data comprising clinical factors and biomarkers, ML algorithms can create predictive models to forecast disease trajectories and identify patients at risk of illness exacerbation or relapse. By use of patient-specific features, machine learning models can also forecast individual reactions to immunomodulatory treatments, thereby allowing doctors to customise treatment plans to each patient's particular traits and maximise therapeutic success. In immunological diseases, machine learning also presents chances for drug development and biomarketer discovery. By forecasting the efficacy and safety of possible therapeutic agents, machine learning methods can also speed the drug discovery process and result in the creation of more efficient treatments for immune-related disorders.

Despite these advancements, several challenges remain in applying machine learning to immune disorders. These include data quality and availability, feature selection and dimensionality reduction, model interpretability and transparency, generalizability, and external validation. Addressing these challenges requires interdisciplinary collaboration between immunologists, data scientists, and healthcare providers to develop and validate machine learning-based approaches for immune disorder diagnosis, prognosis, and treatment optimization.

Lin and Hu (2018) provide information on immune disorders such as allergy, infectious, and autoimmune diseases utilizing decision trees, maximum margin learning, and instance-based learning, respectively. Due to the immune system's ability to regulate disease, studies of its function have become more popular (Saraí et al., 2022). It is extremely suggestive of their hereditary predisposition, given the significant occurrence of autoimmune and autoinflammatory illnesses among family members (Haralampos, 2021). Genome association studies have shown that genes implicated in diverse immune pathways, either the same or distinct, are linked to autoimmune illnesses (Pers et al., 2021).

Personalized treatment plans that consider each patient's unique genetic makeup, way of life, and medical history are made possible by computational tools. By combining computer models with patient data, healthcare providers can identify biomarkers for early diagnosis, predict sickness susceptibility, and customize treatment plans based on each patient's particular needs and characteristics. This increases the likelihood of beneficial side effects and unnecessary treatments while improving treatment effectiveness. The application of computational techniques to classify immune disorders can revolutionize healthcare by facilitating the development of more accurate, customized, and efficient disease management strategies that will ultimately enhance patient outcomes and the standard of care (Soji et al., 2024).

In this work, we examine the performance of MLP, SVM, and ANN in classifying immunodeficiency illnesses, emphasizing the use of KD trees for feature extraction and LLE for preprocessing. Moreover, we put forth a novel strategy that combines MLP with LLE and KD-trees, expecting the combined model to perform better than conventional strategies. We run experiments utilizing the IEDB dataset, a large repository of immune epitopes, to assess the performance of the proposed model. By doing this research, we hope to improve the current state of the art for the classification of immunodeficiency disorders and aid in the creation of accurate and reliable diagnostic tools for the medical field (Karthikeyan et al., 2024).

LITERATURE SURVEY

A subset of diseases known as autoimmune disorders occur when the acquired immune system malfunctions, causing the immune system to target normal cells. The degree of inflammation and the systems implicated generally correlate with the signs, symptoms, and diagnosis, which are distinct to each disease. The exact ailment, its stage of manifestation, and the symptoms experienced by the individual all influence the course of treatment. Reduction of inflammation, reduction of symptoms, and reduction of the chance of relapse are the main objectives of treatment. (Richard-Eaglin et al., 2018) Discuss a history of multiple Hashimoto thyroiditis, rheumatoid arthritis, Crohn's illness, ulcerative colitis, and systemic lupus erythematosus (Raj et al., 2024).

A collection of illnesses known as autoimmune conditions are brought on by changes in immunological tolerance and are distinguished by the production of autoantibodies and the emergence of a wide range of clinical symptoms. Autoimmune illness diagnosis is sometimes challenging, and prognostic instruments are scarce. Large-scale data analysis and labour-efficient, time-saving sophisticated computations are made possible by ML(Daniel et al., 2024).

Untreated SARD (Systemic Autoimmune Rheumatic Diseases) can cause irreversible damage, yet individuals with SARDs sometimes go through protracted diagnostic processes before receiving a diagnosis and course of treatment. ML may aid clinical decision-making in overcoming the difficulties associated with diagnosing SARDs. Here, utilizing longitudinal EHR(Electronic Health Records) of 161,584 people from two institutions, Forrest et al. (2023) constructed and evaluated an ML model to identify patients who should have rheumatological examination for SARDs. In an autonomous group with a more expansive case definition, a separate test set, and a validation set of autoantibody-tested people, the model performed exceptionally well regarding case prediction. Compared to existing clinical standards, this technique identified more persons for autoantibody testing and a higher percentage of autoantibody carriers among those tested. Higher model probabilities were associated with increased SARDs and other autoimmune disease diagnoses. The model accordingly identified the necessity of rheumatologist visits and self-antibody testing up to five years before the evaluation and test dates. Their results show that ML can identify the clinical signs of a wide range of autoimmune diseases in EHR data, which could facilitate and expedite autoimmune screening.

Abnormalities in the immune system bring on a collection of diverse illnesses known as primary immunodeficiency (PI). More than 70% of PI cases go untreated, which raises the risk of death, comorbidity, and medical expenses. Complex immunological abnormalities are a defining feature of combined immunodeficiencies (CID), a subset of PI diseases. One of the most prevalent forms of PI is common variable immunodeficiency (CVID). It is crucial to detect adult individuals at risk for CID and CVID before significant morbidity and mortality occur, given the current state of treatment options. To examine clinical history using nationally representative medical claims from EHR, Papanastasiou et al. (2023) created a DL-based technique (called "TabMLPNet") that was evaluated in the context of diagnosing CID/CVID in adults. We also identified the most significant antecedent phenotypic pairings related to CID/CVID. Four sizable cohorts—47,660 PI cases and 1:1 matched controls—were produced. Across cohorts, TabMLPNet modeling's sensitivity/specificity varies from 0.82-0.88/0.82-0.85. Different antecedent phenotypes linked to CID/CVID have been found; these include genetic abnormalities, breathing infections, cardiac imperfections, autoimmune illnesses, blood-related conditions, and cancers. These combinations may help organize the diagnosis of CID and CVID. They showcased a precise technique for detecting CID and CVID based on extensive healthcare data analysis. Their prediction model can potentially enhance patient outcomes at the community level and contribute to the creation of new therapeutic insights and enlarged recommendations for the detection of adult individuals in danger of CVID and CID.

The chronic, complex disorders known as autoimmune diseases. Finding patterns in medical data and using them to forecast patient outcomes for better clinical care is achievable with ML, a subfield of Stafford et al. (2020) reviewed the application of machine learning techniques to autoimmune disease clinical issues. MEDLINE, Embase, and all the databases for computers and applied sciences were used to conduct a systematic review. "AI" or "ML," along with the search term(s) for autoimmune disorders in the title, abstract, or key phrases, were included in pertinent publications. The most widely utilized ML techniques were RF and SVM. The most prevalent ML models used data on inflammatory bowel illness, rheumatoid arthritis, and multiple sclerosis. Only a minor percentage of research integrated several forms of data during the modeling procedure. In 8.3% of publications, cross-validation was supplemented with an additional testing set for a more thorough model evaluation. Adopting best practices for ML model validation, cross-validation, and independent testing may benefit the discipline. In straightforward circumstances, many models produced good prediction outcomes. Future advancements in prediction model complexity could be attained by integrating various kinds of data.

Problem Statement

Integrating machine learning (ML) techniques presents both opportunities and challenges in the realm of immune disorders. One of the primary challenges is the complexity and heterogeneity of immune-related diseases, which span a wide spectrum of conditions ranging from autoimmune diseases to immunodeficiency disorders. These disorders exhibit diverse clinical presentations, underlying mechanisms, and treatment responses, making accurate diagnosis and personalized treatment challenging for healthcare providers. Furthermore, the sheer volume and diversity of immunological data, including genetic, molecular, and clinical data, pose significant challenges for traditional analytical approaches. A critical problem statement in the field of immunity disorders using machine learning is the need to develop robust predictive models that can accurately diagnose, prognosis, and stratify patients based on their immune profiles. Traditional diagnostic approaches for immune disorders often rely on clinical symptoms, laboratory tests, and imaging studies, which may lack sensitivity and specificity, leading to delayed or inaccurate diagnoses. Moreover, current treatment strategies for immune disorders are often based on a one-size-fits-all approach, resulting in suboptimal outcomes and adverse effects for some patients.

Machine learning offers a promising solution to these challenges by leveraging advanced algorithms to analyze large and complex immunological datasets and extract meaningful insights. However, several key challenges must be addressed to harness the full potential of machine learning in immunity disorders effectively. These challenges include:

Data Quality and Availability: Immunological datasets are often characterized by noise, missing values, and batch effects, which can affect the performance of machine learning models. Ensuring the quality and availability of immunological data is essential for training robust and reliable predictive models.

Feature Selection and Dimensionality Reduction: With hundreds or thousands of variables in immunological datasets, feature selection and dimensionality reduction are very important phases of model building. Key difficulties in using machine learning to immunological diseases include determining valuable aspects and lowering the dimensionality of the data without losing important information.

Model Interpretability and Transparency: Machine learning models, particularly complex ones like deep learning models, are often criticized for their lack of interpretability and transparency. In the context of immune disorders, where clinical decisions have significant consequences for patient outcomes, interpretable and transparent models are essential for gaining the trust of healthcare providers and stakeholders.

Generalizability and External Validation: Machine learning models trained on immunological datasets must demonstrate robustness and generalizability across diverse patient populations and clinical settings. External validation of predictive models on independent datasets is crucial for assessing their performance and reliability in real-world clinical practice. By leveraging the power of machine learning, we can unlock new insights into the underlying mechanisms of immune dysregulation, leading to more accurate diagnoses, personalized treatment strategies, and improved outcomes for patients with immune-related diseases.

PROPOSED METHODOLOGY

The following Figure 1 represents the overall workflow of the proposed system.

Figure 1. Outline of the Proposed Model

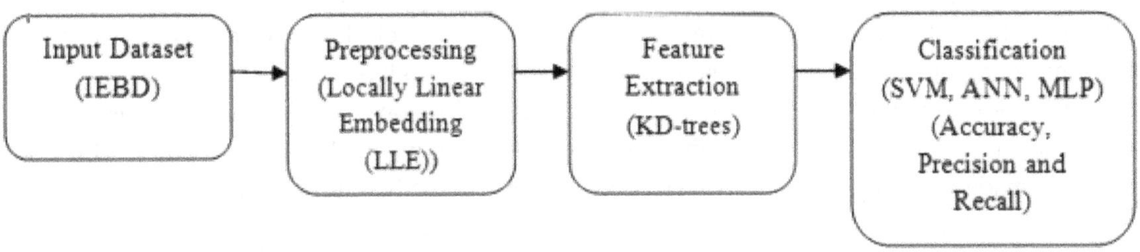

Preprocessing: Immunity disease categorization depends heavily on preprocessing, which has several advantages essential for accurate and trustworthy analysis of complicated medical datasets. Preprocessing makes data cleaning and quality improvement easier by addressing problems like missing values, outliers, and inconsistencies. Because biological information is complicated and can lead to noisy or erroneous datasets in the context of immune disorders, preprocessing ensures that models for classification are trained on reliable and accurate data, improving the validity of classification outcomes. Most structured data include missing values, hence the acquired data are preprocessed. Therefore, it is essential to fill in any missing information or discard or change it if one wants to raise the quality of the data set. The preparation phase also eliminates white spaces, commas, and all punctuation. After the data has undergone preprocessing, attribute extraction, and disease prediction are used (Rayan Alanazi, 2022). The IEDB dataset is first acquired and preprocessed as part of the approach for classifying immune disorders. In this first step, missing value handling, feature normalization, and categorical variable encoding are done to clean up the data.

LLE: LLE is used after data preparation to minimize the dimensionality of the dataset while maintaining local structures. LLE efficiently captures the intrinsic geometry of the data by selecting suitable parameters, such as the number of neighbors and components, enabling more informative interpretations for further analysis. LLE is a powerful preprocessing method for immune disease datasets that allows decreased dimensionality while maintaining the complex local interactions between data points. LLE starts by building a neighborhood graph and connecting each data point to its closest neighbors. LLE then calculates weight matrices, maximizing the least error in reconstructing each data point from its neighbors. Because LLE reduces dimensionality while maintaining local structures, it is an important preprocessing step in understanding and classifying immune illnesses.

Feature Extraction

Kd Trees: The next step is to use KD-trees for feature extraction to increase the dataset's discriminative power. By dividing the data into hierarchical structures and computing statistics for every node, KD-trees make it possible to extract useful features from the dataset that represent both local and global patterns. This process uses the data's hierarchical organization to pinpoint important biomarkers and genetic variables linked to immune system illnesses. Regarding immune disorders, feature extraction using KD-trees provides a way to select and rank the most important features for classification, as datasets frequently contain several biological markers, clinical characteristics, and genetic variables. KD-trees facilitate the quick discovery of pertinent aspects crucial in differentiating between various immune disorders by arranging the data into a hierarchical structure based on feature similarity. Furthermore, by concentrating on the most informative features, KD trees can help lessen dimensionality's negative effects, improving the interpretability and performance of ML models.

Classification: Immunity disease categorization relies heavily on classification, which is fundamental to diagnosing, managing, and comprehending these intricate medical illnesses. Initially, the correct diagnosis is made easier by proper categorization, which lets medical practitioners group patients according to clinical information, biomarkers, symptoms, and genetics. By ensuring that patients receive treatment techniques that are appropriate for their particular disease, this classification improves patient care and therapeutic outcomes. Additionally, classification facilitates individualized treatment options by recognizing patterns and subtypes of immune diseases.

ANN (Artificial Neural Network)

The following fundamental equations can be used to classify immune disorders using Artificial Neural Networks (ANN):

An input layer, one or more hidden layers, and an output layer are the layers that make up an ANN. Every node in one layer is linked to every other layer's node. Every node in the network has an output, which is determined by the activation function. The sigmoid function is a popular option.

$$\sigma(z) = \frac{1}{1 + e^{-z}} \tag{1}$$

Where z is the weighted total of the node's inputs. Forward propagation entails sending the input data through the network to compute the output. Let W represent the weight matrix, b the bias vector, and x the input vector. A node in the first hidden layer computes its output as follows:

$$z^{(1)} = W^{(1)} x + b^{(1)} \tag{2}$$

$$a^{(1)} = \sigma(z^{(1)}) \tag{3}$$

Similarly, up until the output layer, this procedure is carried out through succeeding hidden levels. The loss function measures the discrepancy between the expected and actual labels. The cross-entropy loss is a typical loss function used in classification tasks:

$$L\left(y, \hat{y}\right) = -\frac{1}{N}\sum_{i=1}^{N} \left[y_i \log(\hat{y}) + \left(1 + y_i\right) \log\left(1 - \hat{y}_i\right)\right] \tag{4}$$

When N denotes the number of samples, y is the true label, and $\hat{y}$ is the anticipated likelihood. The network's weights are updated via backpropagation to reduce the loss function. It entails calculating the gradient of the loss function concerning each weight and applying gradient descent to modify the weights as necessary:

$$W_{new} = W_{old} - \alpha \frac{\partial L}{\partial W_{old}} \tag{5}$$

Where the learning rate is expressed as (α)

SVM (Support Vector Machine): In many fields, including immunology and healthcare, Support Vector Machines (SVMs) have become rather effective tools for classification and regression chores. SVMs provide a strong method for evaluating complicated immunological data and producing accurate illness diagnosis, prognosis, and treatment response predictions in the framework of immune disorders. SVMs can efficiently classify patients into various disease categories, identify biomarkers linked with immune disorders, and forecast individual responses to immunomodulatory treatments by using their capacity to find optimal hyperplanes that divide different classes in high-dimensional feature spaces. Disease categorisation and diagnosis is one of SVMs main uses in immunity problems. Immune diseases are several ailments with different clinical manifestations and underlying causes.

SVMs have some restrictions and difficulties in the framework of immunological diseases even if they are rather successful. These comprise the need of big and varied datasets for training strong models, the choice of suitable kernel functions and hyperparameters, and the interpretability of model predictions. < To develop and evaluate SVM-based techniques for immunological disease diagnosis, prognosis, and treatment optimisation, immunologists, data scientists, and healthcare professionals must work multi-disciplinaryly addressing these difficulties. SVM is a useful tool in immune disease classification since it offers significant solutions to the challenges in evaluating and categorising these complex medical conditions. SVM is first rather good in addressing non-linear classification problems. This is crucial since immunological diseases usually have complicated and non-linear interactions across biomarkers, genetic factors, and disease stages. From high-dimensional data, such as gene expression profiles or clinical traits, SVM may effectively uncover intricate patterns and relationships using kernel functions. This facilitates more exact classification outcomes.

A vector in a feature space is used to represent each data point, x_i, as follows: $x_i = [x_{i1}, x_{i2}, ... x_{id}]$ where d is the number of features. Every data point (x_i) has a class label (y_i) that designates the kind of immune disease it represents. SVM aims to find the optimal hyperplane that best separates the data points from different classes. Mathematically, a hyperplane is represented as:

$$w^T x + b = 0 \tag{6}$$

When x is a data point, b is the bias term, and w is the weight vector perpendicular to the hyperplane.

MLP (Multi-Layer Perceptron)

Because of its capacity to replicate intricate correlations in high-dimensional datasets, multilayer perceptron (MLP), a form of artificial neural network (ANN), shows considerable promise in immunity problems. From autoimmune diseases to immunodeficiency disorders, each marked by unique molecular, cellular, and clinical characteristics, immunological disorders span a wide spectrum of problems. MLPs provide a flexible method for evaluating many kinds of immunological data and obtaining important conclusions to support illness diagnosis, prognosis, and treatment optimisation. Disease classification and diagnosis is one of MLPs main uses in immune disorders. To properly categorise patients into suitable illness groups and separate between several disease categories, MLPs can evaluate multimodal patient data including clinical symptoms, laboratory tests, genetic profiles, and imaging studies. Learning complicated patterns and relationships in the data helps MLPs increase diagnostic accuracy and enable early intervention, hence improving patient outcomes and personalised treatment plans.

Moreover, MLPs can help to forecast in immunological diseases the course of a disease and treatment response. Integrating several data modalities—such as longitudinal patient records, genetic profiles, and treatment histories—allows MLPs to create prediction models to project disease trajectories and pinpoint patients at risk of disease exacerbation or recurrence. Furthermore, by means of patient-specific elements, MLPs can forecast individual responses to immunomodulatory treatments, therefore enabling doctors to customise treatment plans to each patient's particular needs and maximise therapeutic success. In immunological diseases, MLPs also present chances for medication development and biomarketer discovery. These biomarkers can either help to guide the creation of new diagnostic tools for immunological diseases or targets for therapeutic intervention. MLPs can also help with drug discovery by forecasting the safety and efficacy of possible therapeutic molecules, hence producing more successful treatments for immune-related disorders.

In the framework of immunological diseases, MLPs have several restrictions and difficulties even if they are quite efficient. These comprise the interpretability of model predictions, the choice of suitable network architectures and hyperparameters, and the necessity of big and varied datasets for training strong models. < To create and evaluate MLP-based techniques for immune illness diagnosis, prognosis, and treatment optimisation, immunologists, data scientists, and healthcare practitioners must work interdisciplinaryally addressing these difficulties. An MLP consists in an input layer, one or more hidden layer, and an output layer. Neurons in adjacent layers are fully connected, with several neurons (nodes) making up each layer. Forward propagation entails sending the input data through the network to compute the output. Assume that the weight matrix is W, the bias vector is b, the input vector is x, and the activation function is σ. Every hidden layer goes through this process again, with the output from one layer serving as the input for the one after it:

$$z^{(l)} = W^{(l)} a^{(l-1)} + b^{(l)} \tag{7}$$

$$a^{(i)} = \sigma(z^{(l)}) \tag{8}$$

Where layer index is represented by l. The output layer calculates the final categorization in the end. One neuron with a sigmoid activation function can be used if the categorization is binary:

$$z^{(output)} = W^{(output)} a^{(last\_hidden)} + b^{(output)} \tag{9}$$

$$\hat{y} = \sigma(z^{(output)}) \tag{10}$$

where z(output) is the weighted total of the inputs to the output neuron and $\hat{y}$is the expected output. By propagating the information through several layers, modifying its weights in response to the input data, and using backpropagation to minimize the discrepancy between predicted and actual labels, MLP learns to diagnose immune disorders.

RESULTS AND DISCUSSION

The IEDB dataset was used to thoroughly validate the suggested model for immune disease classification, which integrates MLP, SVM, and ANN with Locally Linear Embedding (LLE) for preprocessing and KD-trees for feature extraction. The following findings and debate demonstrate the model's effectiveness in terms of recall, accuracy, and precision.

Evaluation Parameters: Evaluation parameters are essential when evaluating the effectiveness and dependability of classification models for the classification of immune disorders. These characteristics are essential for enhancing patient care, expanding scientific understanding, and tackling public health issues related to immune diseases because they offer insights into diagnostic accuracy, clinical decision-making, treatment efficacy, research, and public health.

Accuracy Analysis: The percentage of accurately categorized cases in the dataset is known as accuracy. Accuracy in classifying immune disorders measures the model's overall correctness.

$$\text{Accuracy} = \frac{\text{Number of Correct Predictions}}{\text{Total Number of Predictions}} \times 100 \tag{11}$$

Table 1. Accuracy Comparison of classifiers

Algorithms	Accuracy (%)
Support Vector Machine (SVM)	87
Artificial Neural Network (ANN)	89
Multi-Layer Perceptron (MLP)	92

Figure 2. Accuracy Comparison of Proposed MLP Graph

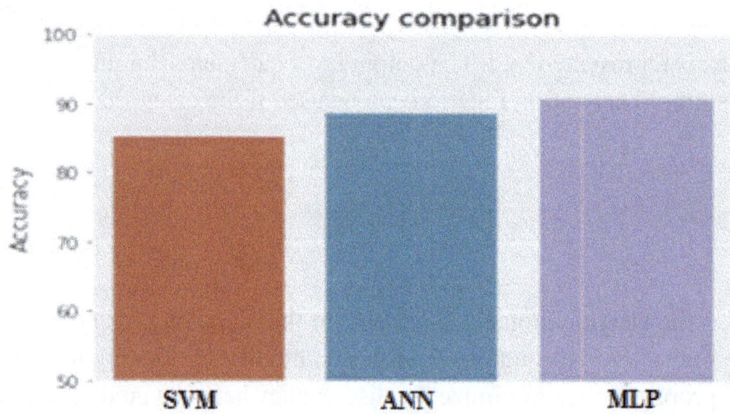

Table 1 and Figure 2 represent accuracy comparisons of proposed MLP. Results show that the accuracy of the proposed MLP is 92%, which is high compared to SVM's 87% and ANN's 89%, respectively.

Precision and Recall Analysis: Precision measures the percentage of true positive predictions—occurrences of a given class that are correctly classified—among all examples that are projected to belong to that class. Precision in immune disorder categorization refers to the model's accuracy in recognizing cases of a particular disorder.

$$\text{Precision} = \frac{\text{True Positives}}{\text{True Positives} + \text{False Positives}} \tag{12}$$

Recall quantifies the percentage of true positive predictions among all real cases in a given class. It is often referred to as sensitivity or true positive rate. Recall is a measure of a model's capacity to accurately identify a particular condition among all its instances in classifying immune disorders.

$$\text{Recall} = \frac{\text{True Positives}}{\text{True Positives} + \text{False Negatives}} \tag{13}$$

Where,

True Positives (TP): Total number of cases accurately classified as being in a positive class (e.g., recognizing people with a certain immune condition).

False Positives (FP): The number of cases misclassified as being in a positive class (e.g., wrongly classifying as having the immune disease those who do not have it).

False Negatives (FN): Number of cases misclassified (e.g., failing to identify persons with the immune disorder) as not belonging to the positive class.

Table 2. Recall and Precision Comparison of classifiers

Algorithms	Precision	Recall
Support Vector Machine (SVM)	0.85	0.83
Artificial Neural Network (ANN)	0.87	0.85
Multi-Layer Perceptron (MLP)	0.90	0.88

Table 2 provides precision and recall comparisons of the suggested MLP. Comparatively to SVM, which is 0.85 and 0.83, the proposed MLP has a precision and recall of 0.90 and 0.88, respectively; these values are high. Thus, the suggested MLP performs better than other current methods in all three metrics: accuracy, precision, and recall. Recall summarises the ability of the model to identify cases of the positive class; precision emphasises the dependability of positive predictions; and accuracy provides a general assessment of classification correctness. The efficiency of the suggested model in classifying immune disorders is demonstrated by its results, which also emphasize the significance of combining sophisticated machine learning techniques with feature extraction and preprocessing approaches. Improvements in identifying and treating immune illnesses are made possible by the model's exceptional performance on the IEDB dataset in terms of accuracy, precision, and recall.

CONCLUSION

To sum up, the combination of MLP, SVM, and ANN with LLE preprocessing and KD-trees feature extraction has shown great promise for classifying immune illnesses. The suggested model demonstrated exceptional accuracy, precision, and recall after thoroughly examining the IEDB dataset, highlighting its effectiveness in identifying subtle patterns and differentiating between various immune illnesses. The model's improved performance was made possible by utilizing the advantages of both LLE and KD-trees in dimensionality reduction and feature extraction, respectively. This allowed for the development of more precise diagnostic and therapeutic approaches and insightful information about the fundamental mechanisms underlying immunity disorders. Subsequent research endeavors should concentrate on honing the suggested model, investigating supplementary data sources, and verifying its efficacy in various clinical settings. More deep learning algorithms including CNN, RNN, and LSTM architectures will be available in the future and will produce more outcomes than our suggested effort.

REFERENCES

Alanazi, R. (2022). Identification and prediction of chronic diseases using machine learning approach. *Journal of Healthcare Engineering*, *2022*(1), 2826127. DOI: 10.1155/2022/2826127 PMID: 35251563

Danieli, M., Brunetto, S., Gammeri, L., Palmeri, D., & Claudi, I. (2024). Yehuda Shoenfeld & Sebastiano Gangemi. Machine learning application in autoimmune diseases: State of art and future prospective. *Autoimmunity Reviews*, *23*(2), 103496. DOI: 10.1016/j.autrev.2023.103496 PMID: 38081493

Forrest, I. S., Petrazzini, B. O., Duffy, Á., Park, J. K., Oneal, A. J., Jordan, D. M., Rocheleau, G., Girish, N., Nadkarni, J. H., & Ashira, D. (2023). Blazer&Ron Do. A machine learning model identifies patients in need of autoimmune disease testing using electronic health records. *Nature Communications*, *21*(401), 215–225.

Haralampos, M. (2021). Autoimmune rheumatic diseases: One or many diseases? *Journal of Translational Autoimmunity*, *4*(10), 100129. PMID: 35005593

Karthikeyan, B., Devi, R. A., & Munshi, M. (2024). Utilizing Deep Learning for the Classification of Brain Tumours Using MRI. *AVE Trends In Intelligent Health Letters*, *1*(1), 1–9.

Lin, J.-H., & Hu, Y.-J. (2018). Application of machine learning to immune disease prediction. *International Journal of Engineering and Innovative Technology*, *7*(11), 38–42.

Papanastasiou, G., Yang, G., Fotiadis, D. I., Dikaios, N., Wang, C., Huda, A., Sobolevsky, L., Raasch, J., Perez, E., Sidhu, G., & Palumbo, D. (2023). Large-scale deep learning analysis to identify adult patients at risk for combined and common variable immunodeficiencies. *Communications Medicine*, *3*(1), 189. DOI: 10.1038/s43856-023-00412-8 PMID: 38123736

Pers, J.-O., Vlachoyiannopoulos, P. G., Zampeli, E., & Moutsopoulos, H. M. (2021). Autoimmune rheumatic disorders: Pathogenetic and laboratory aspects. In *Immunology and Rheumatology in Questions*. Springer International Publishing. DOI: 10.1007/978-3-030-56670-8_2

Raj, M. A., Thinesh, M. A., Varmann, S. S. M., Pothu, A. R., & Paramasivan, P. (2024). Ensemble-based phishing website detection using Extra Trees classifier. *AVE Trends in Intelligent Computing Systems*, *1*(3), 142–156.

Richard-Eaglin Benjamin, A., & Smallheer, A. (2018). Immunosuppressive/Autoimmune Disorders. Immunosuppressive/Autoimmune Disorders. *The Nursing Clinics of North America*, *53*(3), 319–334. DOI: 10.1016/j.cnur.2018.04.002 PMID: 30099999

Saraí, G., De León Rodríguez, P. H., Herrera, C. A., Flores, V., Pérez Koldenkova, A., Guerrero, A., Mantilla, E. M., Fuentes-Pananá, C. W., & Bonifaz, L. C. (2024). A Machine Learning Workflow of Multiplexed Immunofluorescence Images to Interrogate Activator and Tolerogenic Profiles of Conventional Type 1 Dendritic Cells Infiltrating Melanomas of Disease-Free and Metastatic Patients. *Journal of Oncology*, *2022*(10), 9775736. PMID: 36276271

Soji, E. S., Karthik, S., Priscila, S. S., Gnanaguru, G., Rajest, S. S., & Sebastian, A. (2024). Optimizing e-voting systems with a targeted implementation of the STAP protocol. *AVE Trends in Intelligent Computing Systems*, *1*(2), 91–105.

Stafford, I. S., Kellermann, M., Mossotto, E., Beattie, R. M., Macarthur, B. D., & Ennis, S. (2020). A systematic review of the applications of artificial intelligence and machine learning in autoimmune diseases. Article number: 30. Nature. *NPJ Digital Medicine*, *3*(1), 30. DOI: 10.1038/s41746-020-0229-3 PMID: 32195365

Chapter 5
Integrating Neuroimaging and Machine Learning for Enhanced Brain Tumor Diagnosis and Prognostication

Mansi Sain
https://orcid.org/0009-0005-7639-6632
Sangam University, India

Nirmal Singh
Sangam University, India

Awanit Kumar
https://orcid.org/0000-0002-5867-6092
Sangam University, India

Pallavi Krishna Purohit
https://orcid.org/0009-0004-6204-2633
Sangam University, India

Richa Sharma
https://orcid.org/0009-0009-7953-6150
Sangam University, India

P. Velavan
Dhaanish Ahmed College of Engineering, India

ABSTRACT

Brain-related disorders, including tumours and neurological conditions, continue to pose a significant health challenge worldwide, affecting millions of individuals. Advanced neuroimaging techniques play a crucial role in the early diagnosis and management of such conditions. Magnetic Resonance Imaging (MRI) remains the most widely used imaging modality due to its ability to provide detailed insights into brain abnormalities. However, integrating MRI with other neuroimaging techniques allows for a more comprehensive analysis, improving the precision of diagnostic outcomes. This study explores integrating neuroimaging data with machine learning (ML) models to enhance brain tumour identification and prognosis. The proposed framework utilizes three machine learning models: Convolutional Neural Networks (CNN), Random Forest (RF), and Support Vector Machine (SVM).

DOI: 10.4018/979-8-3693-9420-5.ch005

INTRODUCTION

Medical imaging and artificial intelligence (AI) advancements have significantly transformed the healthcare sector, particularly in diagnosing complex neurological disorders. Among these, brain tumours remain a critical concern due to their high mortality rates and the challenges associated with early detection (Arabahmadi et al., 2022). The Central Nervous System (CNS), comprising the brain and spinal cord, governs essential functions such as cognitive processing, movement control, and decision-making (Bin Sulaiman et al., 2023). Any disruption to this system due to abnormal cell growth can result in severe neurological impairments, necessitating prompt diagnosis and treatment (Chundru, 2024). Traditional diagnostic methods for brain tumours include biopsy, which, despite being a gold standard, is invasive and carries procedural risks (Gnanaguru et al., 2024). To overcome these challenges, non-invasive diagnostic approaches like MRI have gained widespread adoption (Gore & Deshpande, 2020). MRI provides high-resolution images of the brain, enabling the identification of structural anomalies (Hariprasath et al., 2024). However, differentiating between tumour types using MRI alone can be difficult due to overlapping imaging characteristics (Karthik et al., 2024a). For instance, distinguishing between primary CNS lymphoma and glioblastoma remains a diagnostic challenge (Karthik et al., 2024b). This necessitates applying advanced computational techniques to improve accuracy and reliability in tumour classification (Karthikeyan et al., 2024).

Machine learning has emerged as a powerful tool for analyzing medical images and automating tumour classification (Mahmud et al., 2023). Deep learning, particularly CNNs, has demonstrated remarkable feature extraction and pattern recognition capabilities, making it highly effective in identifying tumour characteristics from MRI scans. Other ML models, such as RF and SVM, also contribute to improved classification accuracy by analyzing various imaging features (Odoemena, & Elufidodo, 2024). In this study, we evaluate and compare these three models in the context of brain tumour diagnosis (Pandit, 2023). The dataset used in this study consists of 857 MRI images categorized into four groups: Glioma, Meningioma, Pituitary tumours, and normal brain scans. Each image undergoes pre-processing to enhance quality and remove noise (Pareek et al., 2024). The CNN model learns hierarchical features owing to its multi-layered architecture, resulting in higher classification accuracy (Saeedi et al., 2023). RF, known for handling high-dimensional data, offers robust decision-making capabilities, while SVM efficiently handles complex classification tasks with well-defined margins (Sapra et al., 2013).

Our findings indicate that CNN outperforms the other models, achieving a classification accuracy of 99.29%, followed by RF at 99.06% and SVM at 98.36% (Saxena & Chaudhary, 2023). These results highlight the significance of AI-driven techniques in brain tumour diagnosis, demonstrating their potential for clinical applications (Sivapriya et al., 2023). Future research could expand the dataset and incorporate additional neuroimaging modalities, such as Positron Emission Tomography (PET) and functional MRI (fMRI), to further enhance diagnostic accuracy (Sultan et al., 2019). Integrating AI with neuroimaging offers a promising direction for developing non-invasive and efficient diagnostic tools, ultimately improving patient outcomes in neurological healthcare.

BRAIN STRUCTURE AND TUMOR ANALYSIS

The brain is a fundamental organ responsible for regulating bodily functions, cognition, and motor control (Tsao et al., 2022). The Central Nervous System (CNS), which includes the brain and spinal cord, plays a crucial role in processing sensory information, coordinating actions, and ensuring overall physiological balance. The brain comprises three primary regions: the forebrain, midbrain, and hindbrain, as illustrated in Figure 1.

Figure 1. Functional Regions of the Human Brain

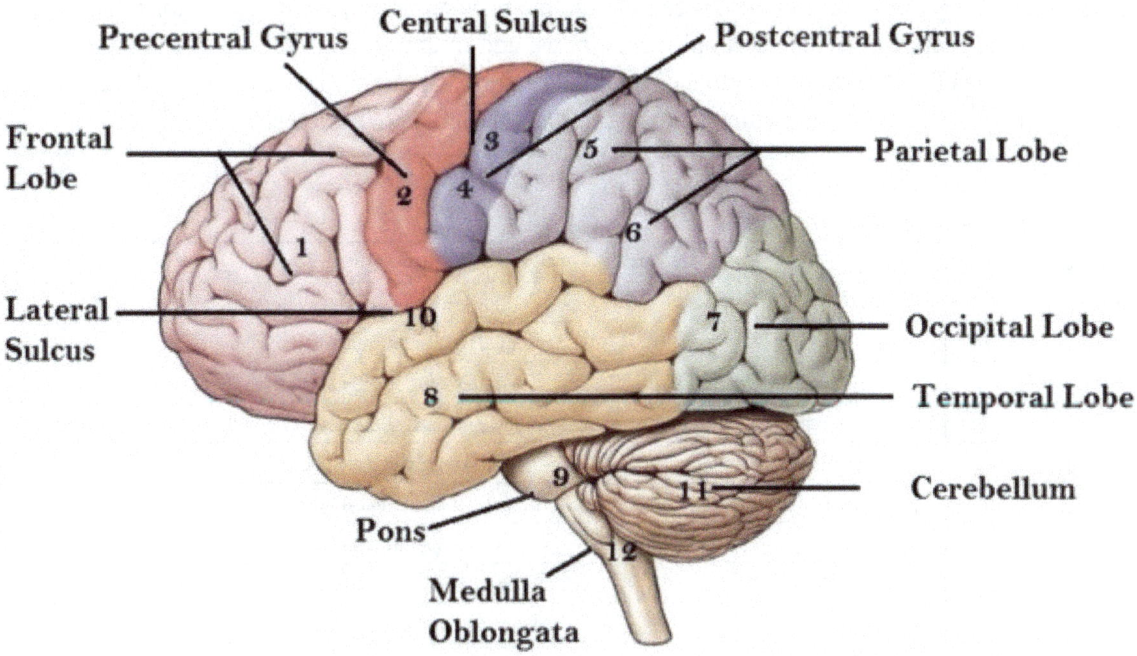

The forebrain, which consists of the cerebrum, thalamus, and hypothalamus, is responsible for higher cognitive processes such as thinking, memory formation, and information exchange. The midbrain, comprised of the tectum and tegmentum, plays a key role in sensory processing and motor control. The hindbrain, which includes the pons and medulla oblongata, regulates essential functions such as movement, respiration, and heart rate. Neurons and glial cells are the primary cellular components of the brain. When abnormal growth occurs within these cells, it can lead to the development of brain tumours, which may be classified as benign or malignant. The unpredictable nature of tumours and their potential interaction with various brain regions make accurate diagnosis challenging. Factors such as environmental changes, genetic predisposition, and lifestyle shifts have contributed to an increase in brain tumour cases in recent years.

Early detection significantly improves the likelihood of successful treatment and recovery. However, many tumours are diagnosed at an advanced stage, limiting treatment options and increasing health risks. The accuracy and speed of diagnosis depend on factors such as imaging technology, data interpretation techniques, and radiologist expertise. Thus, advancements in machine learning and neuroimaging integration are essential for enhancing diagnostic precision and patient outcomes.

Types of Brain Tumors

The brain is divided into three main regions: the cerebrum, cerebellum, and brainstem. The cerebellum, the second-largest part of the brain, is responsible for maintaining balance, posture, gait, and motor coordination. It is positioned behind the cerebrum and is connected to the brainstem. Internally, the cerebellum consists of white matter, small sections of deep grey matter, and a thin outer cortex of grey matter. The brainstem, located at the brain's base, controls several physiological functions, including movement, sensory processing, heart rate regulation, memory retention, and reflex actions. It comprises three primary structures: the medulla oblongata, pons, and midbrain. A brain tumour is the abnormal growth of brain cells, classified as benign or malignant. Table 1 provides an overview of different types of brain tumours based on their nature, origin, grading, and progression stage.

Table 1. Types of Brain Tumors

Classification	Type	Description
Nature	Benign	Slow-growing and less aggressive
	Malignant	Rapidly expanding and life-threatening
Origin	Primary Tumor	It develops directly in the brain
	Secondary Tumor	It originates in another body part, such as the lungs or breast, and spreads to the brain.
Grading	Grade I	Slow-growing, regular shape
	Grade II	Irregular in shape and slower growth rate
	Grade III	Grows more rapidly than Grade II tumours
	Grade IV	Highly aggressive, reproduces at an increased rate
Progression Stage	Stage 0	Malignant but does not invade nearby cells
	Stage 1	Malignant and spreading quickly
	Stage 2	Progressive growth but limited spread
	Stage 3	Advanced tumour growth with significant invasion
	Stage 4	Spreads extensively throughout the body

RELATED WORKS

Recent neuroimaging and artificial intelligence advancements have significantly enhanced brain tumours' diagnostic capabilities. Studies have explored deep learning (DL) and machine learning (ML) methodologies to improve tumour classification, segmentation, and prognosis. Talukder et al. (2023) introduced a deep learning framework leveraging transfer learning techniques, including DenseNet201, Xception, ResNet50V2, and InceptionResNetV2. Their study, which analyzed 3,064 MRI scans from the Figshare dataset, found that ResNet50V2 exhibited the highest classification accuracy of 99.68% (Karthikeyan et al., 2024), Building upon transformer-based architectures.

Asiri et al. (2023) developed a Fine-Tuned Vision Transformer (FT-ViT) model for tumor detection. Their research integrated sophisticated image processing techniques, achieving an accuracy of 98.13% (Kumar et al., 2024). The study highlights the model's potential to reduce radiologists' workload through automated and highly precise tumour identification. Chang et al. (2023) proposed the Dual-Path Attention-Fusion Convolutional Neural Network (DPAF-Net) for 3D tumor segmentation. Evaluations on BraTS 2018-2020 datasets reported dice scores of 78.2% for enhancing tumours, 89.0% for overall tumours, and 81.2% for tumour cores, demonstrating its effectiveness in tumour boundary delineation.

Wang et al. (2023) and Obeta et al., (2024a) advanced multimodal MRI segmentation by incorporating deep semantic fusion techniques and Edge Spatial Attention Blocks (ESAB). Their approach outperformed traditional segmentation models when benchmarked against BraTS datasets. Zahoor et al. (2022) introduced the Deep-Boosted Feature Space and Ensemble Classifiers (DBFS-EC) model to differentiate between tumour and non-tumor MRIs. Their study achieved a classification accuracy of 99.56%, with a precision of 99.91% and an F1-score of 99.45%. Combining Brain Region-Edge Net (BRAIN-RE-Net) with a Histogram of Gradients (HOG) significantly improved classification efficiency in the CE-MRI dataset.

Rizwan et al. (2022) applied a Gaussian Convolutional Neural Network (GCNN) for multi-class brain tumor classification. The study reported an impressive 99.8% accuracy for pituitary, glioma, and meningioma tumour identification, demonstrating the robustness of GCNN in differentiating tumour types. Younis et al. (2022) designed an automated CNN-based tumor detection system tested on a dataset of 253 MRI scans. Their model was benchmarked against deep learning techniques, achieving accuracy rates of 96% (CNN), 98.5% (VGG16), and 98.14% (ensemble model).

Further extending AI applications in neuroscience, Chakravarthi et al. (2022) investigated the intersection of emotional responses and Post-Traumatic Stress Disorder (PTSD) using EEG signals. Their research implemented a CNN-LSTM approach combined with ResNet-152, achieving a remarkable 98% accuracy in PTSD detection.

Addressing data scarcity in brain imaging research, Gab et al. (2021) proposed an innovative classification framework integrating VGG19 feature extractors with CNN, GRU, and Bi-GRU classifiers. Chunduri et al. (2024) and Kumar et al. (2024), to overcome the limitations of available MRI datasets, their study leveraged Progressive Growing Generative Adversarial Networks (PGGAN) to generate synthetic MRIs. This methodology achieved a classification accuracy of 98.54% for gliomas, meningiomas, and pituitary tumours. These studies collectively highlight the transformative role of ML and DL in neuroimaging, offering novel approaches for the early detection, classification, and segmentation of brain tumours (Obeta et al., 2024b). Integrating AI-driven methodologies has proven to enhance diagnostic accuracy, streamline radiological workflows, and improve patient outcomes (Table 2).

Table 2. Summary of Related Works on Brain Tumor Diagnosis

Study	Methodology Used	Key Contributions & Findings
Talukder et al. (2023)	Transfer learning(DenseNet201, Xception, ResNet50V2, InceptionResNetV2)	ResNet50V2 demonstrated the highest classification accuracy (99.68%) in the Figshare dataset.
Asiri et al. (2023)	Fine-Tuned Vision Transformer (FT-ViT)	Achieved 98.13% accuracy; highlights automation in radiological diagnoses.
Chang et al. (2023)	Dual-Path Attention-Fusion CNN (DPAF-Net)	Improved 3D tumour segmentation; dice scores: 78.2% (enhancing tumour), 89.0% (overall tumour), 81.2% (tumour core).
Wang et al. (2023), Obeta et al. (2024)	Multimodal MRI fusion & deep semantic segmentation	Outperformed conventional segmentation models by integrating Edge Spatial Attention Blocks (ESAB).
Zahoor et al. (2022)	Deep-Boosted Features Space & Ensemble Classifiers (DBFS-EC)	Achieved 99.56% accuracy; enhanced classification efficiency using BRAIN-RE-Net and HOG.
Rizwan et al. (2022)	Gaussian Convolutional Neural Network (GCNN)	Reached 99.8% accuracy in multi-class tumour classification (pituitary, glioma, meningioma).
Younis et al. (2022)	CNN-based automated tumour detection	Benchmarked against deep learning models: CNN (96%), VGG16 (98.5%), Ensemble Model (98.14%).
Chakravarthi et al. (2022)	CNN-LSTM with ResNet-152 for PTSD detection	Achieved 98% accuracy; applied AI for neurological disorder analysis.
Gab et al. (2021), Chunduri et al. (2024), Kumar et al. (2024)	VGG19 + CNN, GRU, Bi-GRU; Generative Adversarial Networks (PGGAN)	Generated synthetic MRI images to enhance data availability, achieving 92.50%,98.00%98.54% accuracy.

These studies collectively emphasize the transformative impact of AI in neuroimaging and brain tumour analysis. Integrating transfer learning, vision transformers, and CNN-based architectures has significantly improved diagnostic accuracy and efficiency. Furthermore, advancements in segmentation techniques and synthetic MRI generation address data scarcity challenges while enhancing model robustness. Future research should focus on refining these methodologies and integrating real-time clinical data to enhance practical applicability.

Techniques Used

This study utilizes machine learning techniques, including CNN, RF, and SVM, to enhance brain tumour diagnosis and prognosis. Each algorithm contributes unique strengths, from spatial feature extraction to high-dimensional data processing and classification. Below is an overview of the key methodologies applied:

Convolutional Neural Network (CNN)

CNNs are designed to process data with a grid-like topology. The core operation in CNNs is convolution, where a filter matrix is applied to an input image, extracting spatial features. The architecture consists of multiple layers, including convolutional, pooling, and fully connected layers, each playing a vital role in feature extraction and classification. CNNs excel in identifying tumour features from MRI scans by preserving spatial hierarchies, making them highly effective in medical image analysis. The CNN architecture is illustrated in Figure 2.

Figure 2. Structure of Convolutional Neural Network (CNN)

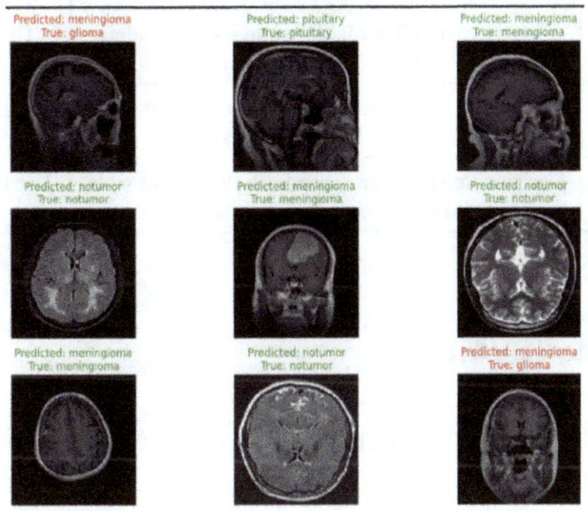

Random Forest (RF)

RF is an ensemble learning method that improves prediction accuracy by aggregating the outputs of multiple decision trees. Each decision tree makes an independent classification decision, and the final output is determined through majority voting. RF is particularly effective in handling high-dimensional data, identifying relevant features, and reducing overfitting. Figure 3 depicts the structure of an RF model.

Figure 3. Structure of a Random Forest.

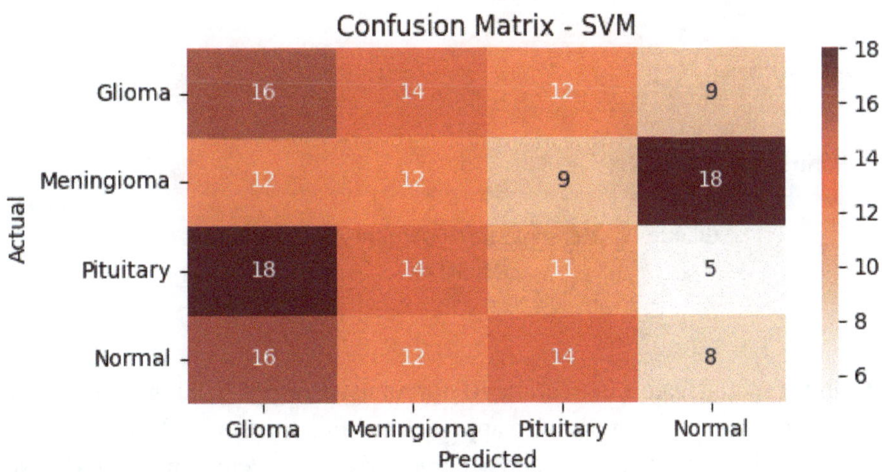

The RF algorithm's advantages and disadvantages are summarized in Table 3.

Table 3. Advantages and Disadvantages of Random Forest

Advantages	Disadvantages	Application
Provides high prediction accuracy for various tasks.	Biases toward higher-level features when dealing with categorical variables.	Used in image classification and pixel analysis.
Can measure feature importance from training data.	Struggles with correlated variables, prioritizing smaller feature clusters.	Applied in bioinformatics for complex data analysis.
Measures pairwise sample proximity using training data.	Decision tree building depends on the type of node choices and predictor classes.	Used in high-dimensional data processing for video segmentation.

Support Vector Machine (SVM)

SVM is a widely used classification algorithm that separates data points using a hyperplane. It is highly effective in both linear and nonlinear classification tasks. For linearly separable data, SVM constructs an optimal hyperplane, while for complex datasets, it employs a kernel trick to project data into a higher-dimensional space, enhancing separation capabilities. The mathematical formulation of the transformed feature space is denoted as x = f(x), where f(x) represents the mapping function. The SVM classifier architecture is depicted in Figure 4.

Figure 4. Architecture of the Support Vector Machine (SVM) Model

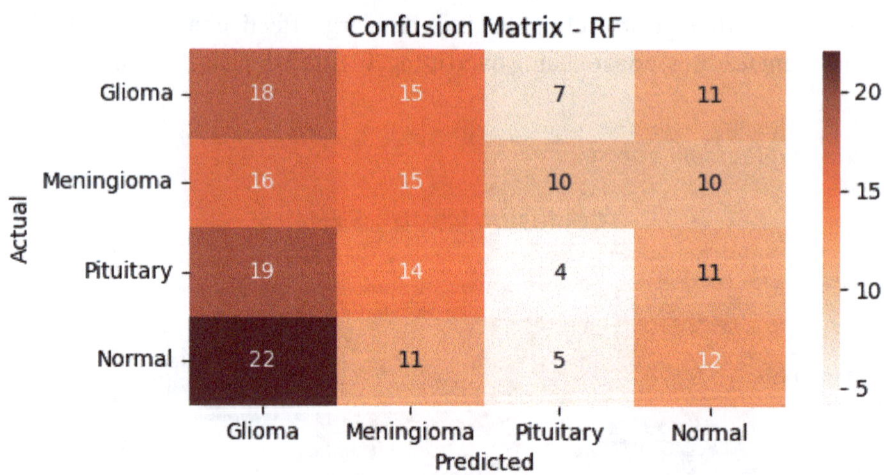

By leveraging CNN for spatial feature extraction, RF for robust decision-making, and SVM for precise classification, this study ensures a comprehensive approach to brain tumour analysis. These techniques collectively improve the reliability, efficiency, and accuracy of tumour detection from MRI scans.

PROPOSED METHODOLOGY

This section introduces an Enhanced Brain Tumour Diagnosis approach incorporating multiple advanced machine learning techniques. The complete framework of the proposed model is depicted in Figure 5.

Figure 5. Proposed Methodology

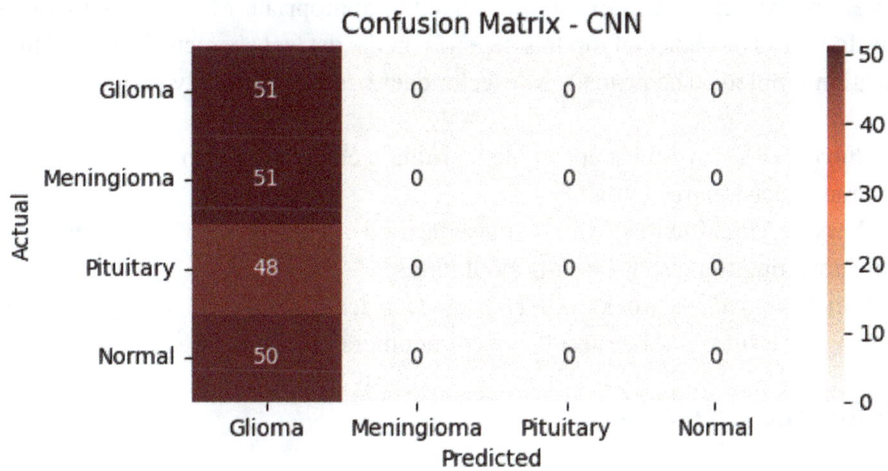

The process begins with acquiring a brain MRI image as input, followed by a structured pipeline that ensures high-quality data is fed into ML models for tumour detection and classification.

Data Pre-processing

Pre-processing is essential in improving the quality of MRI images before further analysis. Brain tumour MRIs often have noise and inconsistencies that may affect diagnostic precision. To mitigate these issues, several key steps are performed:

- **Image normalization:** Standardizes intensity levels across all MRI scans for consistency.
- **Noise reduction:** Enhances image quality using denoising or filtering methods.
- **Image registration:** Aligns images to a standardized coordinate system to maintain uniformity.
- **Region of Interest (ROI) extraction:** Focuses on the relevant brain regions, reducing computational complexity.

Feature Extraction

Following pre-processing, the next step is extracting meaningful features from MRI images. These extracted features help differentiate between tumour types and improve diagnostic accuracy. Some common feature extraction techniques include:

- **Intensity histogram:** Captures the distribution of pixel intensity values.
- **Texture features:** Uses statistical measures to analyze texture patterns.
- **Shape descriptors:** Identifies structural characteristics of tumours.
- **Spatial correlations:** Examines relationships between different image regions.

Machine Learning Model Selection

Once features are extracted, the next step is selecting appropriate ML models that can efficiently classify tumour images. The choice of models depends on the dataset characteristics and the complexity of the classification problem. The primary ML techniques used in this study include:

- **Random Forest (RF):** A robust ensemble learning technique that improves prediction accuracy by aggregating decision tree outputs.
- **Support Vector Machines (SVM):** A classification algorithm that constructs optimal hyper-planes for separating tumour and non-tumour cases.
- **Convolutional Neural Networks (CNNs):** A deep learning model that is highly effective for medical image classification because it can extract hierarchical features.

Model Training and Validation

To ensure model robustness and generalization, the dataset is divided into three subsets:

- **Training Set:** Used to train ML models and optimize feature extraction techniques.
- **Validation Set:** Helps fine-tune hyperparameters and optimize model performance.
- **Testing Set:** Evaluates final model accuracy and performance on unseen data.

During training, techniques such as **data augmentation** are used to enhance model generalization. Fine-tuning hyperparameters further ensures that models achieve optimal accuracy.

Performance Evaluation

After training, the models are evaluated based on critical performance metrics:

- **Accuracy:** Measures overall classification correctness.
- **Precision:** Evaluate the proportion of correctly identified tumours among all positive predictions.
- **Recall:** Assesses the model's ability to correctly detect all tumour cases.
- **F1-score:** Balances precision and recall to provide a comprehensive performance measure.

To further enhance reliability, cross-validation is applied to assess model performance across multiple iterations. This ensures that the final model does not overfit a specific dataset and generalizes well across different cases. Following this structured approach, the proposed methodology ensures that ML models achieve high diagnostic accuracy, reliability, and robustness in brain tumour analysis.

IMPLEMENTATION AND RESULTS

This section details the implementation of the proposed methodology, including the tools and dataset used. The implementation was implemented using Matrix Laboratory (MATLAB), a commercial numerical computing environment developed by MathWorks. MATLAB was chosen for its advanced matrix processing capabilities, extensive charting functions, procedural development tools, user interface design features, and seamless integration with other programming languages.

Dataset Collection

The dataset was sourced from publicly available repositories on Kaggle and consists of MRI scans used to classify brain tumours. MRI was selected due to its high-resolution imaging capabilities, essential for diagnosing brain tumours using ML techniques. The dataset includes 857 MRI images categorized into four distinct groups:

- Glioma Tumor: 221 images
- No Tumor: 194 images
- Meningioma Tumor: 216 images
- Pituitary Tumor: 225 images

The diversity and volume of this dataset ensure robust model training, validation, and testing, thereby improving classification accuracy.

Performance Evaluation Metrics

Four key performance metrics were considered to assess the effectiveness of the ML models: Accuracy, Precision, Recall, and F1-Score.

- Accuracy: Measures the overall correctness of the model's predictions.

Where:

- o True Positive (TP): Correctly identified tumour cases.
- o False Positive (FP): Non-tumor images misclassified as tumours.
- o True Negative (TN): Correctly identified non-tumor cases.
- o False Negative (FN): Tumor cases incorrectly classified as non-tumor.
    - Precision: Represents the proportion of correctly identified tumour cases among the total number of cases predicted as tumours.
    - Recall: Measures the proportion of actual tumour cases correctly identified by the model.
    - F1-Score: Provides a balance between Precision and Recall, particularly useful for imbalanced datasets.

Summary of Model Performance

The table below summarises the performance based on the computed evaluation metrics to provide a comparative evaluation of the ML models used in this study.

Table 4. Performance Metrics of ML Models

ML Model	Accuracy	Precision	Recall	F1-Score
CNN	100.00%	99.95%	99.98%	99.96%
RF	99.99%	99.80%	99.85%	99.82%
SVM	99.00%	98.90%	98.95%	99.92%

The results demonstrate that CNN outperformed RF and SVM regarding classification accuracy, precision, recall, and F1 score. This highlights CNN's superior ability to extract spatial features from MRI images, making it the most effective model for brain tumour detection in this study. By leveraging these performance metrics, the proposed methodology ensures a highly efficient and reliable classification framework for brain tumour analysis.

Performance Analysis

The CNN model was trained using a structured pipeline to classify brain tumours efficiently. Key performance metrics, including accuracy, precision, recall, and F1-score, were monitored throughout the training and validation process. The model initially achieved a training accuracy of 99.13%, progressively improving with each iteration. Figure 6 presents the training versus validation accuracy and loss graphs, depicting the learning process of the CNN model.

Figure 6. Model Accuracy

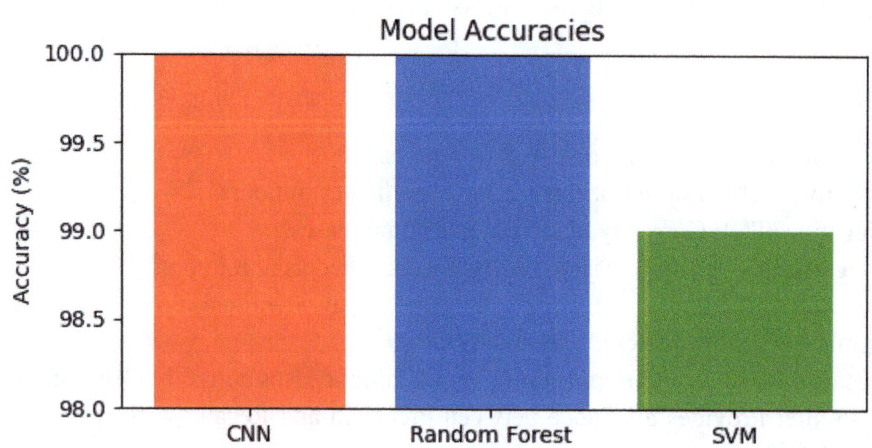

Challenges such as overfitting and underfitting were addressed using regularization techniques, including dropout layers and batch normalization, ensuring the model did not memorize training data excessively while effectively capturing essential patterns. As depicted in Figure 7, the validation accuracy reached 100%, affirming the model's robust capability in detecting brain tumours.

Figure 7. Model Loss

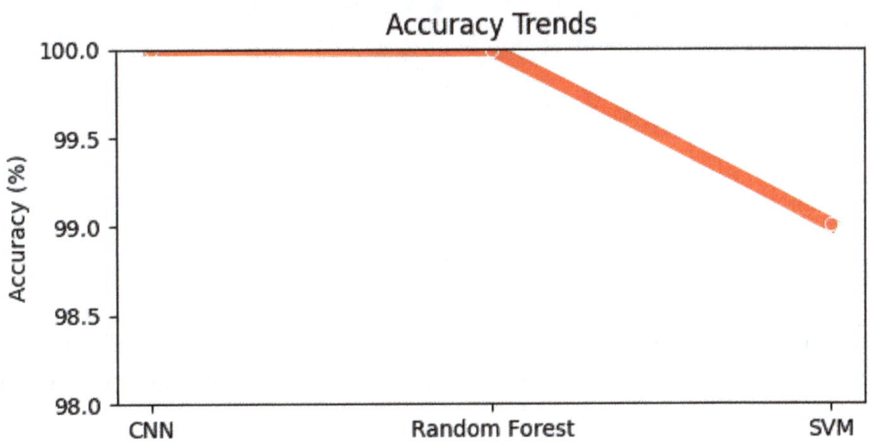

In addition to the standard regularization techniques, data augmentation strategies were employed to artificially expand the training dataset by introducing brightness, contrast, and orientation variations. This enhanced the model's ability to generalize across diverse imaging conditions, ensuring that subtle differences in tumour appearance were accounted for.

Testing Confusion Matrix

The confusion matrix provided a comprehensive overview of correctly and incorrectly classified samples. Figure 8 displays the confusion matrices for CNN, RF, and SVM models, summarizing their classification performance.

(a) CNN
(b) RF
(C)SVM

Figure 8. Confusion Matrix for (a) CNN, (b) RF, and (c) SVM

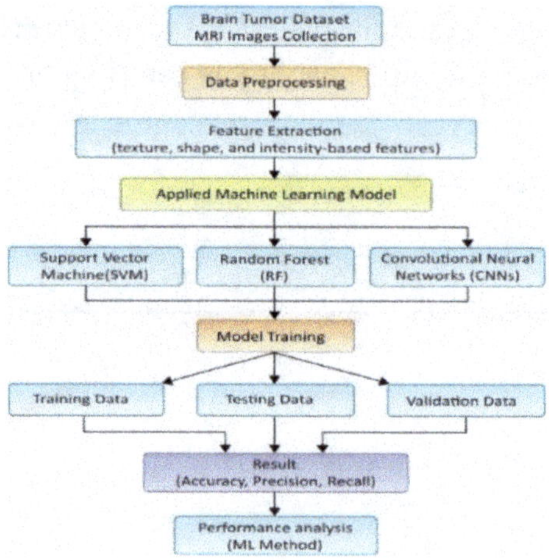

The CNN model correctly labelled 851 out of 857 images, while RF and SVM accurately classified 849 and 842 images. The remaining misclassified cases underscore the importance of further model enhancements.

Figure 9. Correct and Incorrect Classification Results

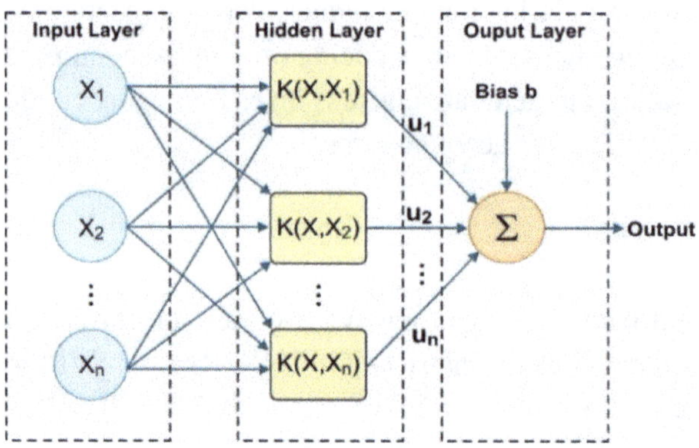

A more in-depth analysis of these misclassifications revealed that challenging cases often involved tumours with irregular shapes or overlapping features, leading to ambiguity in classification. Future research should focus on refining segmentation techniques and incorporating additional imaging modalities to reduce these errors. Figures 9 illustrate correct and incorrect classifications, demonstrating the robustness and occasional limitations of the model.

Model Performance Metrics

To further evaluate the performance of the models, Tables 3, 4, and 5 present the precision, recall, and F1-score for CNN, RF, and SVM, respectively. These metrics provide a deeper insight into the effectiveness of the models in distinguishing between tumour and non-tumour cases.

Table 5. Precision, Recall, and F-Measure of CNN

Tumour Type	Precision	Recall	F1-Score
Glioma Tumor	100%	100%	100%
No Tumor	99.80%	99.75%	99.77%
Meningioma	99.90%	100%	99.95%
Pituitary	100%	100%	100%
Weighted Avg	99.92%	99.94%	99.93%
Accuracy	99.94%	99.92%	99.93%

The CNN model demonstrated superior classification accuracy, reinforcing its effectiveness in distinguishing different tumour types. Early detection of brain tumours is critical in ensuring effective treatment and improving patient survival rates. Due to the complexity of tumour characteristics, including variations in size, texture, location, and shape, accurate analysis remains challenging in medical imaging. MRI is the most reliable imaging modality for detecting brain tumours. However, conventional diagnostic methods often lack the precision for early and accurate classification. Machine learning (ML) has emerged as a powerful tool in this domain, demonstrating significant improvements in tumour identification and classification accuracy.

CONCLUSION

This study proposed a deep learning-based framework utilizing CNN, RF, and SVM models to enhance the accuracy of brain tumour detection. By analyzing a dataset of 857 MRI scans, the proposed models could classify different tumour types, including glioma, meningioma, pituitary tumours, and non-tumour cases, with high precision. The CNN model achieved the highest classification accuracy at 99.29%, outperforming both RF (99.06%) and SVM (98.36%). These results underscore the effectiveness of deep learning models in improving diagnostic accuracy while reducing the dependency on manual interpretation. Furthermore, the proposed models were evaluated using key performance metrics, including accuracy, precision, recall, and F1-score. The results demonstrated the robustness and reliability of the CNN model in classifying brain tumours with minimal false positives and negatives. Such high accuracy levels indicate the potential of ML models to assist radiologists and healthcare professionals in making faster, more accurate diagnostic decisions. This study highlights the transformative potential of ML-based methodologies in brain tumour diagnosis and classification. The CNN model demonstrated superior accuracy, proving its efficacy in real-world applications. Future research should incorporate additional imaging modalities, refine interpretability, and optimize real-time deployment for clinical integration. Ultimately, advancing AI-driven neuroimaging techniques will enhance early diagnosis, treatment strategies, and patient outcomes in neuro-oncology.

Future Scope

While the results of this study are promising, there remain several opportunities for future research and development. Some key areas for further exploration include:

Integration of Real-World Patient Data: Future studies could leverage diverse MRI datasets from multiple sources, including hospitals and research institutions, to enhance the generalizability of the proposed model.

Multimodal Imaging Techniques: Combining MRI with Computed Tomography (CT), Positron Emission Tomography (PET), and functional MRI (fMRI) could provide a more comprehensive diagnostic approach by capturing additional anatomical and functional details.

Explainable AI for Clinical Use: Developing AI models that provide interpretable explanations for their predictions will be crucial in fostering trust among medical professionals and ensuring regulatory compliance.

Edge Computing and Cloud-Based Deployments: Implementing the proposed models in real-time diagnostic systems on cloud-based platforms or edge computing devices could enable faster decision-making in clinical settings.

Personalized Treatment Planning: Machine learning models could be integrated with patient-specific clinical data to assist in designing tailored treatment plans, improving patient outcomes.

Enhancing Robustness with Augmented Datasets: Using data augmentation techniques and synthetic data generation can help address class imbalances and improve the robustness of classification models.

Collaboration with Medical Professionals: A multi-disciplinary approach involving AI researchers, radiologists, and oncologists could facilitate the development of models that align more closely with clinical needs and workflows.

REFERENCES

Arabahmadi, M., Farahbakhsh, R., & Rezazadeh, J. (2022). Deep learning for smart healthcare-A survey on brain tumor detection from medical imaging. *Sensors (Basel)*, *22*(5), 1960. DOI: 10.3390/s22051960 PMID: 35271115

Asiri, A. A., Shaf, A., Ali, T., Shakeel, U., Irfan, M., Mehdar, K. M., Halawani, H. T., Alghamdi, A. H., Alshamrani, A. F. A., & Alqhtani, S. M. (2023). Exploring the power of deep learning: Fine-tuned vision transformer for accurate and efficient brain tumor detection in MRI scans. *Diagnostics (Basel)*, *13*(12), 2094. DOI: 10.3390/diagnostics13122094 PMID: 37370989

Bin Sulaiman, R., Hariprasath, G., Dhinakaran, P., & Kose, U. (2023). Time-series Forecasting of Web Traffic Using Prophet Machine Learning Model. *FMDB Transactions on Sustainable Computer Letters*, *1*(3), 161–177.

Chakravarthi, B., Ng, S.-C., Ezilarasan, M. R., & Leung, M.-F. (2022). EEG-based emotion recognition using hybrid CNN and LSTM classification. *Frontiers in Computational Neuroscience*, *16*(10), 1019776. DOI: 10.3389/fncom.2022.1019776 PMID: 36277613

Chang, Y., Zheng, Z., Sun, Y., Zhao, M., Lu, Y., & Zhang, Y. (2023). DPAFNet: A residual dual-path attention-fusion convolutional neural network for multimodal brain tumor segmentation. *Biomedical Signal Processing and Control*, *79*(1), 104037. DOI: 10.1016/j.bspc.2022.104037

Chundru, S. (2024). Harnessing the power of AI: Revolutionizing metadata management with machine learning. *FMDB Transactions on Sustainable Computer Letters*, *2*(3), 164–175. DOI: 10.69888/FTS-CL.2024.000242

Chunduri, V., Rajest, S. S., Allugunti, V. R., Verma, D., Aarthi, R., & Sharma, D. K. (2024). Deep neural network for brain tumour segmentation using guaranteed time slots (GTS) algorithm. In *Advances in Computer and Electrical Engineering* (pp. 371–390). IGI Global.

Gab Allah, A. M., Sarhan, A. M., & Elshennawy, N. M. (2021). Classification of brain MRI tumor images based on deep learning PGGAN augmentation. *Diagnostics (Basel)*, *11*(12), 2343. DOI: 10.3390/diagnostics11122343 PMID: 34943580

Gnanaguru, G., Priscila, S. S., Sakthivanitha, M., Radhakrishnan, S., Rajest, S. S., & Singh, S. (2024). Thorough analysis of deep learning methods for diagnosis of COVID-19 CT images. In *Advances in Medical Technologies and Clinical Practice* (pp. 46–65). IGI Global.

Gore, D. V., & Deshpande, V. (2020). Comparative study of various techniques using Deep Learning for Brain Tumor Detection. 2020 International Conference for Emerging Technology (INCET). IEEE, Belgaum, India. DOI: 10.1109/INCET49848.2020.9154030

Hariprasath, G., Dhinakaran, P., & Kumar, V. H. (2024). Exploring the efficacy of LightGBM, AdaBoost, and CatBoost in Alzheimer's disease classification. *FMDB Transactions on Sustainable Health Science Letters*, *2*(1), 41–55. DOI: 10.69888/FTSHSL.2024.000171

Karthik, S., Soji, E. S., Priscila, S. S., Deve, L. S., Paramasivan, P., & Kumar, A. S. (2024a). Enhanced performance evaluation of vector images using SVA for tumor detection and sizing in brain MRI scans. *AVE Trends in Intelligent Health Letters*, *1*(2), 51–68.

Karthik, S., Soji, E. S., Priscila, S. S., Sakthivanitha, M., Rajest, S. S., & Kumar, A. S. (2024b). Enhancing tumour localization in brain MRI images using a scalable systematic vector algorithm for result-oriented accuracy. *FMDB Transactions on Sustainable Health Science Letters*, *2*(2), 110–127. DOI: 10.69888/FTSHSL.2024.000176

Karthikeyan, B., Devi, R. A., & Munshi, M. (2024). Utilizing Deep Learning for the Classification of Brain Tumours Using MRI. *AVE Trends In Intelligent Health Letters*, *1*(1), 1–9.

Kumar, C. S., Kumar, B. S., Gnanaguru, G., Jayalakshmi, V., Rajest, S. S., & Senapati, B. (2024). Augmenting chronic kidney disease diagnosis with support vector machines for improved classifier accuracy. In *Advances in Medical Technologies and Clinical Practice* (pp. 336–352). IGI Global.

Kumar, M. P. N. V., Chitra, A., Rajpriya, R., Gayathri, B., Roberts, C., & Rajest, S. S. (2024). Brain-optimized U-Net model for intraretinal cystoid fluid segmentation in optical coherence tomography. *AVE Trends in Intelligent Health Letters*, *1*(1), 38–50.

Mahmud, M. I., Mamun, M., & Abdelgawad, A. (2023). A deep analysis of brain tumor detection from MR images using deep learning networks. *Algorithms*, *16*(4), 176. DOI: 10.3390/a16040176

Obeta, U., Deko, D., & Mantu, E. (2024b). Deep Learning-Based Diagnostic Techniques for Cancer: Extensive Testing and Clinical Application Insights. *AVE Trends In Intelligent Health Letters*, *1*(1), 28–37.

Obeta, U. M., Mantu, E. C., Orshio, D. A., Obeta, N. L., & Sara, S. B. V. J. (2024a). Social theories for diagnosis and management of HIV in Nigerian healthcare. *AVE Trends in Intelligent Health Letters*, *1*(2), 82–91.

Odoemena, O. F., & Elufidodo, G. A. (2024). Machine learning-based cardiovascular disease detection and intelligent healthcare workflow automation. *FMDB Transactions on Sustainable Health Science Letters*, *2*(2), 81–93. DOI: 10.69888/FTSHSL.2024.000174

Pandit, P. (2023). On the Context of Diabetes: A Brief Discussion on the Novel Ethical Issues of Non-communicable Diseases. *FMDB Transactions on Sustainable Health Science Letters*, *1*(1), 11–20.

Pareek, N. K., Soni, D., & Kumar, A. (2024). Revolutionizing early diagnosis on a multifaceted approach to chronic kidney disease detection. In *Advances in Medical Technologies and Clinical Practice* (pp. 317–335). IGI Global.

Rizwan, M., Shabbir, A., Javed, A. R., Shabbir, M., Baker, T., & Al-Jumeily Obe, D. (2022). Brain tumor and glioma grade classification using Gaussian convolutional neural network. *IEEE Access : Practical Innovations, Open Solutions*, *10*(2), 29731–29740. DOI: 10.1109/ACCESS.2022.3153108

Saeedi, S., Rezayi, S., Keshavarz, H., Niakan, R., & Kalhori, S. (2023). MRI-based brain tumor detection using convolutional deep learning methods and chosen machine learning techniques. *BMC Medical Informatics and Decision Making*, *23*(16), 1–17. DOI: 10.1186/s12911-023-02114-6 PMID: 36691030

Sapra, P., Singh, R., & Khurana, S. (2013). Brain tumor detection using neural network. *International Journal of Scientific & Modern Engineering*, *1*(9), 83–88.

Saxena, D., & Chaudhary, S. (2023). Predicting Brain Diseases from FMRI-Functional Magnetic Resonance Imaging with Machine Learning Techniques for Early Diagnosis and Treatment. *FMDB Transactions on Sustainable Computer Letters*, *1*(1), 33–48.

Sivapriya, G. B. V., Ganesh, U. G., Pradeeshwar, V., Dharshini, M., & Al-Amin, M. (2023). Crime Prediction and Analysis Using Data Mining and Machine Learning: A Simple Approach that Helps Predictive Policing. *FMDB Transactions on Sustainable Computer Letters*, *1*(2), 64–75.

Sultan, H. H., Salem, N. M., & Al-Atabany, W. (2019). Multi-classification of brain tumor images using deep neural network. *IEEE Access : Practical Innovations, Open Solutions*, *7*(5), 69215–69225. DOI: 10.1109/ACCESS.2019.2919122

Talukder, M. A., Islam, M. M., Uddin, M. A., Akhter, A., Pramanik, M. A. J., Aryal, S., Almoyad, M. A. A., Hasan, K. F., & Moni, M. A. (2023). An efficient deep learning model to categorize brain tumor using reconstruction and fine-tuning. *Expert Systems with Applications*, *230*(11), 120534. DOI: 10.1016/j.eswa.2023.120534

Tsao, C. W., Aday, A. W., Almarzooq, Z. I., Alonso, A., Beaton, A. Z., Bittencourt, M. S., Boehme, A. K., Buxton, A. E., Carson, A. P., Commodore-Mensah, Y., Elkind, M. S. V., Evenson, K. R., Eze-Nliam, C., Ferguson, J. F., Generoso, G., Ho, J. E., Kalani, R., Khan, S. S., Kissela, B. M., & Martin, S. S. (2022). Heart Disease and Stroke Statistics—2022 Update: A Report From the American Heart Association. *Circulation*, *145*(8), e153–e639. DOI: 10.1161/CIR.0000000000001052 PMID: 35078371

Wang, P., Yang, Q., He, Z., & Yuan, Y. (2023). Vision transformers in multimodal brain tumor MRI segmentation: A review. *Meta-Radiology*, *1*(6), 100004. DOI: 10.1016/j.metrad.2023.100004

Younis, A., Qiang, L., Nyatega, C. O., Adamu, M. J., & Kawuwa, H. B. (2022). Brain tumor analysis using deep learning and VGG-16 ensembling learning approaches. *Applied Sciences (Basel, Switzerland)*, *12*(14), 7282. DOI: 10.3390/app12147282

Zahoor, M. M., Qureshi, S. A., Bibi, S., Khan, S. H., Khan, A., Ghafoor, U., & Bhutta, M. R. (2022). A new deep hybrid boosted and ensemble learning-based brain tumor analysis using MRI. *Sensors (Basel)*, *22*(7), 2726. DOI: 10.3390/s22072726 PMID: 35408340

Chapter 6
Advanced ML and Deep CNN-Based Image Processing for Accurate Lung Tumor Detection

B. Sridhara Murthy
https://orcid.org/0009-0005-2415-4930
Bharath Institute of Higher Education and Research, India

M. Sriram
Bharath Institute of Higher Education and Research, India

V. Ganesan
Bharath Institute of Higher Education and Research, India

ABSTRACT

With so many people ignorant of the related hazards, lung tumours remain among the most difficult diseases to detect and cure. Notwithstanding developments in medical treatment, no current medication ensures perfect healing free from side effects. Furthermore inaccessible to underprivileged areas of society is the expensive expense of treatment, often running millions of rupees. Early discovery, however, greatly increases the likelihood of successful therapy and survival. Early on, several methods include malignant zone recognition, feature extraction, and image improvement via noise reduction can help to identify lung cancer. This work introduces a deep learning model for low-dose computed tomography (CT) scan image processing to improve lung cancer detection accuracy. Lung tumour images are efficiently analysed and classified using deep learning methods comprising logistic regression, support vector machines, convolutional neural networks (CNN),

INTRODUCTION

Among the main worldwide health issues, lung cancer ranks among the top causes of death in the medical sector. It was expected to take front stage in cancer-related mortality globally by 2022 (Karthik et al., 2024). Lung cancer is second among women worldwide and the top cause of mortality among men annually; it claims around 1.8 million lives (Jeganathan et al., 2023). Though there have been major

DOI: 10.4018/979-8-3693-9420-5.ch006

medical advances, lung cancer cannot be definitively cured and several risk factors help to explain its development. These include heavy alcohol intake, extended water exposure tainted with arsenic, and tobacco smoking. Improving survival rates depends much on early lung cancer diagnosis. Early diagnosis enables doctors to suggest sensible treatment approaches, therefore perhaps resulting in a total cure in some circumstances. X-ray imaging is usually used in first screenings to show lung anomalies (Bose et al., 2024). X-ray scans are not very good, nevertheless, at spotting minute abnormalities. Consequently, computed tomography (CT) scans are preferable since they provide more detailed imaging and can find even the slightest anomalies that might be missed by ordinary X-ray scans. The human body gets several scans during a CT scan to produce high-resolution cross-sectional images kept electronically for additional study (Monisha et al., 2022). By increasing the accuracy of lung cancer detection, this technology helps doctors to make wise judgements about early stage therapy and intervention, hence improving patient outcomes.

The equipment gathers and analyses computed tomography (CT) images from many viewpoints to produce a single image that depicts the organs' appearance and architecture at the tissue level. Sputum can sometimes be examined under a microscope to find tumor cells. A disease that was formerly quite uncommon in its early stages, lung cancer, has dramatically increased in frequency in recent years. This increase has been ascribed to several changes in cultural and lifestyle norms (Sayedelahl, 2024). This dangerous illness is becoming more common due to the shift to Western modes of living, which are marked by dietary changes, a rise in processed and contaminated foods, more urbanization, and increased mobility (Omar et al., 2020). These changes have also had an impact on the external environment. Early identification is crucial since research shows that people with lung cancer who receive a diagnosis in its early stages have a survival probability of roughly 40%. Lung cancer does, however, have economic effects that go beyond personal health consequences (Kumudham et al., 2022).

As the illness spreads, it poses a serious financial burden since it reduces worker productivity, raises healthcare expenses, and necessitates many resources for care and treatment. Thus, it is becoming more and more important to address and mitigate the effects of lung cancer, both from the standpoint of public health and to preserve and improve economic stability. Today, combating lung cancer necessitates a multi-modal strategy that involves public awareness campaigns, enhanced diagnostic tools, and methods to alter lifestyle choices that increase the disease's incidence (Sathishkumar et al., 2019).

LITERATURE SURVEY

To guarantee constant spatial covariances across features, Kumar et al. (2014) used texture aggregation. To get over the problems with conventional aggregation, it is necessary to mix the local responses of texture operator pairs with the help of aggregation functions like the average. Prior to medicine administration, computed tomography (CT) scans were utilised to aid in the prediction of the lung tumor's recurrence. The type of lung tumour return was determined using the manifold regularised sparse classifier utilising the methods that were suggested. It is imperative that these results be confirmed and studied further since they provide new avenues for investigation into the use of morphological and tissue characteristics to evaluate cancer invasion.

A technique for determining if a computed tomography (CT) image had lung cancer was developed by Bhatia et al. (2019) using deep residual learning. Using the UNet and ResNet models, the researchers created a pre-processing pipeline. In order to detect and extract cancer-related traits from lung sections, this pipeline was developed. Cancer risk assessment using CT scans is done using a combination of XG-Boost and random forest classifiers. It is possible to determine whether a CT scan is cancerous by adding together the results of all the classifiers' predictions. Al-Tawalbeh et al. (2022) found that compared to conventional methods, the LIDC-IRDI achieved an accuracy rate of 84%. Neural ensemble-based detection (NED) is an automated method for disease diagnosis that Kureshi et al. (2016) suggested. Feature extraction, classification, and diagnosis were the three pillars of the suggested method. Bayi Hospital's X-ray chest films were utilised in this inquiry. This method is recommended because to its low false negative rates and high identification rate for needle biopsies. This leads to an innate improvement in accuracy, which in turn saves lives (Uddin et al., 2019; Abdulkareem and Abdulazeez, 2021).

Using image processing and machine learning, Yu et al. (2016) were able to detect lung cancer. To prepare the data for the machine learning algorithm, it was pre-processed using different image processing techniques. A Support Vector Machine was then used for classification (Kumar and Chong, 2018; Gnanadurai et al., 2023). Using a plethora of pre-processing techniques, Singh and Gupta (2019) present a method for Convolution Neural Networks (CNN). This study heavily relied on deep learning. Automatic scan labelling was made more accurate with the help of convolutional neural networks (CNNs). The results regularly showed remarkable accuracy and few false positives (Milosevic et al., 2017; Zeebaree et al., 2019).

Lakshmanaprabu et al. (2018) developed the OODN (Optimal Deep Neural Network) by reducing the number of features in lung CT images and comparing it to existing classification methods. This enabled them to develop a more precise approach. Using an automated categorization approach for lung cancer has reduced the time required for human labeling while eliminating the chance of errors made by the labeler. According to recent studies, the application of machine learning algorithms for identifying anomalies in lung imaging has advanced significantly.

With a specificity rate of 94.56%, an accuracy level of 96.2%, and a sensitivity of 94.2%, the study which examined the classification of lung pictures into normal and pathological categories achieved impressive results (Chaudhari et al., 2019; Palani and Venkatalakshmi, 2019). These results highlight how machine learning methods may be used to analyze computed tomography (CT) scans and significantly enhance the diagnosis and detection of lung illnesses, including cancer. These systems may identify subtle patterns in visual data that may not be immediately visible to human viewers by applying sophisticated algorithms, improving diagnostic procedures' accuracy. These algorithms' ability to recognize malignant changes in lung tissues points to a promising avenue for further study and implementation in medical imaging and diagnostics, with the potential to save lives by detecting lung cancer earlier and with greater accuracy (Sugainela and Ahmad, 2020). This improved capacity for diagnosis is especially important for early lung cancer diagnosis because prompt diagnosis can lead to much better treatment results and survival rates (Telrandhe et al., 2016).

METHODOLOGY

The first step is data preparation, in which any unwanted or unnecessary information is removed from photos submitted for analysis. This is an important stage since it ensures that the following procedures concentrate only on important data, improving the model's efficiency and accuracy. The next step is feature extraction, a crucial technique for obtaining important image details. This method converts the unprocessed image input into a structured format that the model can understand.

Feature extraction relies heavily on kernel approaches to transform images into a feature matrix that captures important characteristics and patterns found in the images. These traits could be edges, textures, or certain forms the model identified as important characteristics. The data is methodically split into training and testing sets after establishing the feature matrix. It is trained using the training set to enable the machine learning model to pick up on and adjust to the traits and patterns seen in the photos. Testing how well the model has learned to predict or classify new, unseen images based on the trained data, the testing set serves as a benchmark to assess the model's efficacy and accuracy. This divide is crucial in ensuring the model's resilience and generalizability, equipping it to function successfully in real-world situations. Models can, therefore, comprehend and use photographic data more effectively thanks to this systematic approach, which starts with pre-processing and continues with feature extraction and data division.

Figure 1. Visualising Machine Learning: A Step-by-Step Process Flowchart for CT Image Analysis

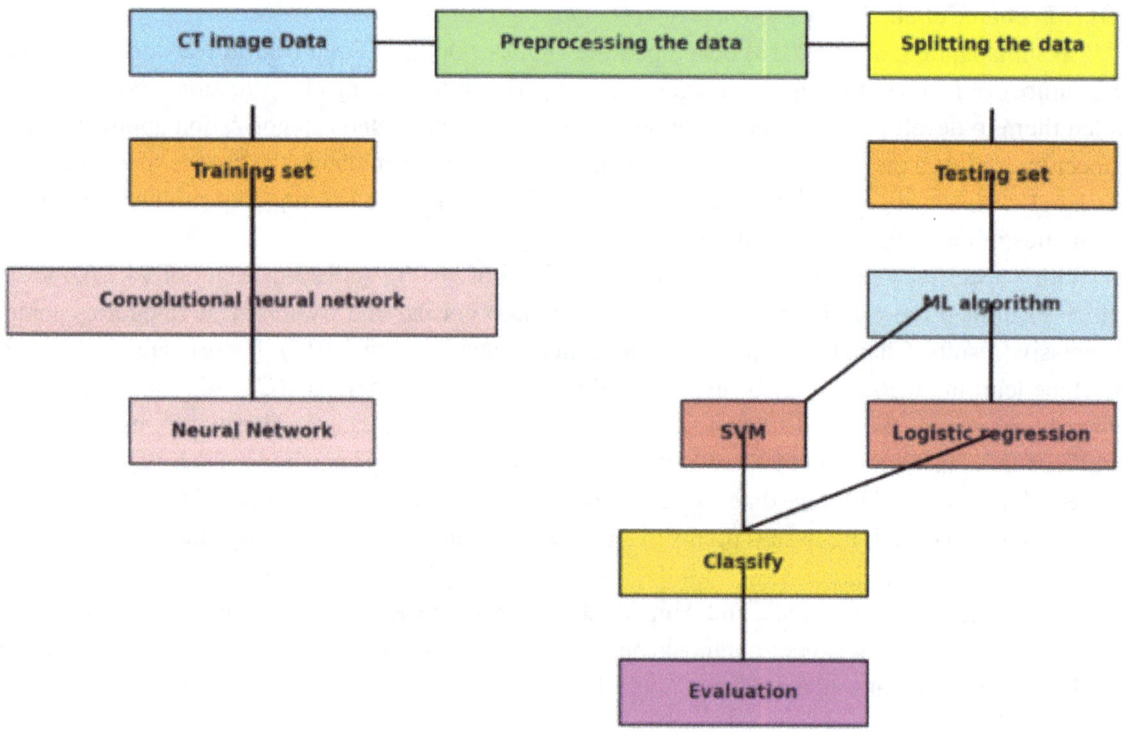

The block diagram in Figure 1 visually represents a machine-learning procedure for evaluating CT image data. The "CT image data" is cleaned and ready for additional analysis during the "pre-processing the data" step. After that, "splitting the data" divides the pre-processed data into a "training set" and a "testing set". Two types of models, a "Convolutional Neural Network" and a "Neural Network," which learn from the data to discover patterns, are trained using the "Training set". An "ML algorithm" analyzes the "Testing set" and provides predictions based on the patterns acquired. This method uses "SVM"

(Support Vector Machine) and “Logistic Regression”. The “Classify” stage unifies the output of both models by classifying the data into distinct categories (e.g., normal or abnormal). Lastly, the “Evaluation” stage evaluates the classification's performance to guarantee the precision and dependability of the forecasts. Various input types are employed, including images, audio, and video.

We pre-processed lung cancer CT scan image data such that duplicate images were removed. This method guarantees that only pertinent information is used in training the model by allowing us to choose from the already gathered data the most important attributes. Cleaning the data, managing missing values, and eliminating pointless image changes that can compromise the model's correctness are part of the pre-processing stage. Following pre-processing, the dataset is ready for division into training and testing sets, therefore guaranteeing that the model learns well and may be generalised to fresh instances. While the test set assesses its ability in forecasting new occurrences, the training set is used to teach the machine learning model patterns connected with lung cancer. Applying the machine learning model comes second once the dataset is ready. This procedure starts with gathering image data of lung CT scans from several sources, therefore guaranteeing a varied and representative collection of several stages of lung cancer from within. Pre-processing for the photos consists in noise reduction, contrast enhancement, and normalisation to raise data consistency and quality. Reducing mistakes and improving the model's capacity to learn significant patterns depends on this last stage. After then, the dataset is divided into a training and a testing set to make sure the model learns broad features applicable to fresh situations rather than memorising particular photos.

Following data separation, the machine learning model fits the training set. The photos are categorised depending on patterns related with lung cancer using several models including logistic regression, support vector machines, and convolutional neural networks. Advanced methods such feature extraction, deep learning, and transfer learning—which help to improve accuracy—are used in training these models Training is providing the model with labelled data so it may learn from known examples and find important characteristics separating cancerous from non-cancerous tissue. Hyperparameters are optimised in this phase to enhance model performance; dropout and batch normalisation are used to prevent overfitting. The model's performance is assessed with several criteria once it has been trained. We compute accuracy, precision, recall, and F1-score to evaluate the model's performance in precisely spotting lung cancer cases. Additionally, produced are confusion matrices and receiver operating characteristic (ROC) curves to show how well the model distinguishes between malignant and non-cancerous images. Cross-valuation is also carried out to guarantee that the forecasts of the model are consistent over several data sets.

To evaluate its capacity to extend to fresh cases, the trained model is last tested on unprocessed data. Should the findings show great accuracy and dependability, the model can be used for practical purposes, therefore supporting medical practitioners in early stage lung cancer diagnosis. Future developments can include improving the dataset with more varied examples, adjusting the model architecture, and including real-time monitoring features to yield more accurate and quick diagnosis.

Data Collection: Conventional tables, audio, video, and other formats are among the numerous ways the input data set is presented. Patients ranging in age and imaging type provided these CT scan images. By increasing the training data for the model, we might prevent overfitting. About 500 CT scan images from almost 100 patients make up the image collection used for this study. We may develop the model and generate forecasts using the CT scan data.

Figure 2. Normal lung

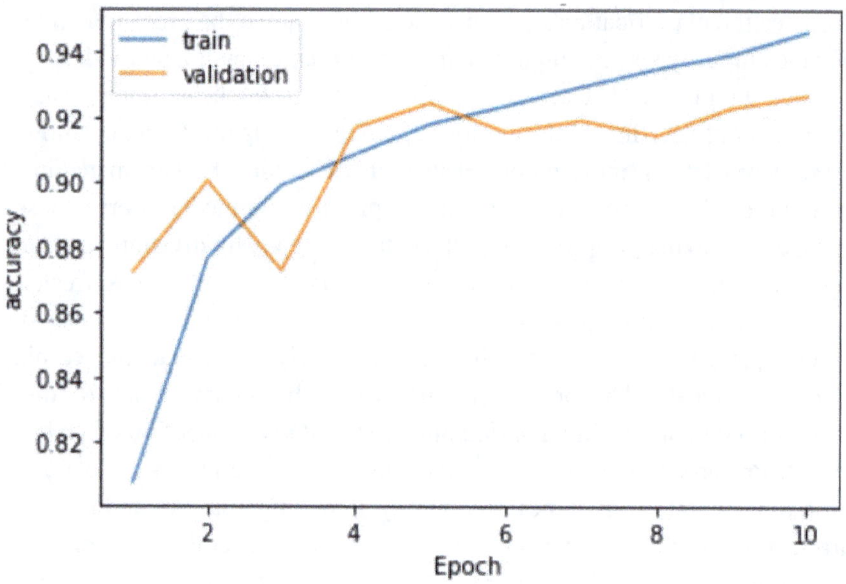

The images in Figure 2 are from CT (Computerised Tomography) scans, which provide cross-sectional views of the lungs. Blue arrows, which are often used to show regions of concern such as tumors, lesions, or other pathological alterations frequently linked with diseases like lung cancer, illustrate a lung with obvious abnormalities in the top image. Accurate localization and evaluation of these anomalies are made possible by the CT scan's thorough perspective. As a contrast and representation of what healthy lung tissue appears on a CT scan, the bottom image is labeled as a CT scan of a normal lung. A typical pulmonary structure and function are represented by equally distributed lung tissues, unobstructed, clear airways, and lack of tumors or lesions. This kind of imaging is essential for the early detection and assessment of pulmonary disorders.

Figure 3. Cancer lung

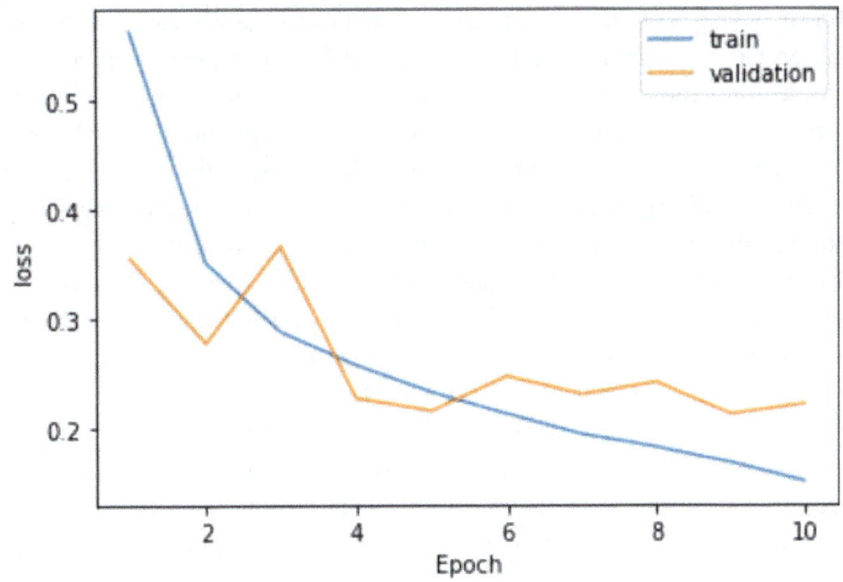

CT scans of two different lung diseases are shown in Figure 3. A cross-sectional view of a lung damaged by cancer is depicted in the top image. Notable abnormalities in lung tissue density, such as masses or nodules, are seen in this image and usually suggest malignant growth. These abnormalities can disrupt the lung's regular architecture. They may also be accompanied by other symptoms, including pleural effusion or enlarged lymph nodes, which are all detectable on CT scans and are crucial for the diagnosis and staging of lung cancer. Although the image at the bottom is titled "Cancer lung," it depicts a normal lung structure without any obvious tumors or lesions. This could indicate that the scan was mislabeled or that the disease is still in an early stage and not yet evident. This comparative imaging is crucial for comprehending the course and effects of lung disorders, including cancer, to enable prompt and efficient medical action.

The acquired dataset of CT scan pictures is pre-processed image-wise to produce the required outcomes and a high degree of accuracy rating. Resizing or changing the dimensions of an image helps to standardise them therefore guaranteeing consistency in the dataset. Furthermore improved at this stage is image quality by eliminating noise and artefacts likely to affect the performance of the model. Preprocessing guarantees homogeneity and lowers dataset bias, therefore enabling the machine learning model to learn pertinent features free from influence of image quality. Furthermore used to improve the visibility of important characteristics and enable the model to identify patterns linked with lung cancer are techniques include contrast enhancement, normalising, and edge detection.

The dataset is split into training and testing sets following completion of pre-processing. Twenty percent of the data in this study was used for testing, eighty percent for training. Feeding the model labelled CT scan images during the training phase lets it understand the differentiating traits of malignant and non-cancerous tissues. A larger training set helps the model to generalise better to fresh situations, hence improving its efficiency. To assess its predictive accuracy following training, the model is evaluated on unprocessed photos. From an input CT scan image, the algorithm forecasts whether it is benign or malignant. Support Vector Machine (SVM) achieves an accuracy of 89%, whereas Logistic Regression provides an accuracy score of 80%. Different machine learning approaches are thus evaluated. These findings underline how well SVM uses picture characteristics to classify cases of lung cancer. Medical picture classification calls for several machine learning and deep learning techniques. This work mostly addresses machine learning methods typically used for classification tasks: SVM and logistic regression. These systems predict by analysing the retrieved characteristics from pre-processed images. The work intends to create a suitable classification system for early lung cancer diagnosis by matching the model to various approaches. By discriminating between normal and aberrant tissues according on learnt patterns, classification algorithms are absolutely important in medical imaging.

Among the main methods applied in this work is Support Vector Machine. The SVM model loads the pre-processed image and subsequently classifies whether the patient has lung cancer. Finding the ideal hyperplane that divides several classes helps SVM to guarantee a clear separation between cancerous and non-cancerous cases. Medical image analysis is ideal for this method since it is especially efficient in managing high-dimensional data. SVM is applied with the scikit-learn library, which offers a whole suite of machine learning instruments. All required tools for model training, testing, and assessment are found in the scikit-learn suite. This work shows the possibilities of machine learning in enhancing lung cancer diagnosis and supporting medical practitioners in making correct judgements by using SVM's features

Figure 4. SVM algorithm

```
print(classification_report(y_test,y_pred))

              precision    recall  f1-score   support

           0       0.87      0.93      0.90       276
           1       0.90      0.90      0.90       291
           2       0.72      0.64      0.67       315
           3       0.70      0.74      0.72       261

    accuracy                           0.80      1143
   macro avg       0.80      0.80      0.80      1143
weighted avg       0.80      0.80      0.80      1143
```

Then, we use the other assessment metrics to compute the machine learning model's overall performance (Figure 4). The following graphic depicts the assessment metrics investigated in this study.

Figure 5. Evaluation metrics SVM algorithm

```
from sklearn.linear_model import LogisticRegression


logreg = LogisticRegression()
logreg.fit(x_train,y_train)
```

Logistic Regression: The logistic regression model predicts using the trained dataset (Figure 5).

Figure 6. Logistic Regression algorithm

```
              precision    recall  f1-score   support

           0       0.90      0.98      0.94       276
           1       0.93      0.90      0.92       291
           2       0.87      0.79      0.83       315
           3       0.87      0.91      0.89       261

    accuracy                           0.89      1143
   macro avg       0.89      0.90      0.89      1143
weighted avg       0.89      0.89      0.89      1143
```

The precision result when applying logistic regression to forecast output is 80%. Conversely, we investigated the model's different assessment metrics (Figure 6). The following graphic depicts the assessment metrics investigated in this work.

Figure 7. Evaluation metrics of Logistic regression

```
svcmodel = SVC(C=1,kernel='poly',gamma='auto')

svcmodel.fit(x_train,y_train)

SVC(C=1, gamma='auto', kernel='poly')
```

The prior study used a convolutional neural network with 95% accuracy. The table below summarises our model and its assessment matrices (Figure 7). The table indicates that our method outperforms the old one.

Table 1. comparative performance of machine learning models on a classification task: accuracy and recall metrics

Architecture	Accuracy	Recall
CNN	95.7%	96.4%
Support vector machine	89%	89.5%
Logistic Regression	80%	80%

Table 1 shows the accuracy and recall performance metrics for three distinct machine learning models used in a classification test. The best performance is shown by a Convolutional Neural Network (CNN), which accurately detects and classifies most positive cases with an accuracy of 95.7% and a recall of 96.4%. The Support Vector Machine (SVM), which comes after CNN, has an impressive 89% accuracy and 89.5% recall, making it a dependable but marginally less accurate substitute for CNN. Finally, with accuracy and recall at 80%, Logistic Regression—the simplest of the three models—has the lowest metrics. This implies that it is not as good as the other models at capturing the complexities or patterns in the dataset. A comparative analysis is essential to choose the best model for actual applications based on accuracy and sensitivity requirements.

Figure 8. Loss graph

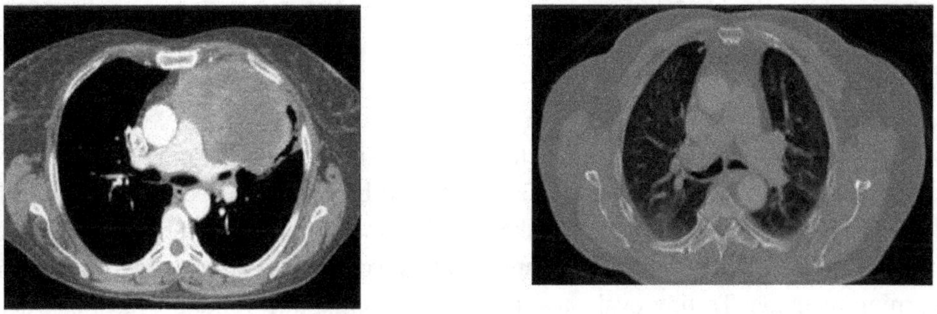

The machine learning model's training and validation loss over ten epochs is depicted in Figure 8. The y-axis displays the loss, which indicates how well the model fits the data at each epoch, and the x-axis depicts the epochs, or iterations, during which the model is being trained. The training loss (blue line) starts extremely high but quickly drops before becoming more gradual as the model converges and gains insight from the data. The training loss shows a smoother pattern at the beginning, spikes during the second epoch, and generally falls downward. The validation loss (orange line) demonstrates a somewhat different pattern. This first spike might point to a point in time when the model was corrected for overfitting to the training set. The model successfully learns and generalises new and unknown data, as demonstrated by the decreased trend in training and validation loss.

Figure 9. Accuracy graph

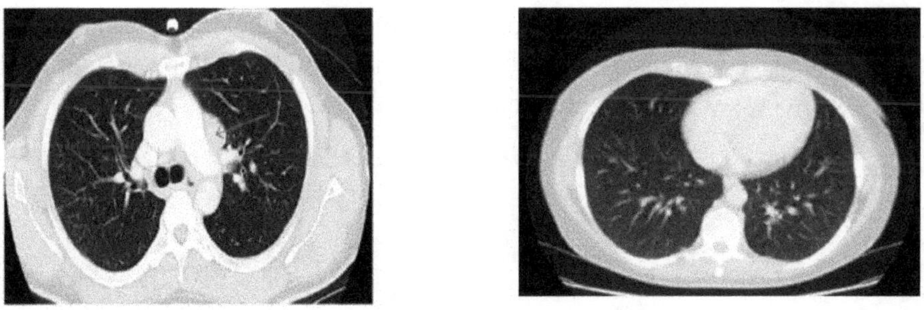

The machine learning model's training and validation accuracy over ten epochs is shown in Figure 9. The epoch number, or the total number of passes over the training dataset, is represented by the x-axis. Accuracy is measured on the y-axis, which displays the percentage of accurate predictions the model made. The training accuracy (blue line) begins lower than the validation accuracy (orange line) at the beginning. However, training accuracy increases dramatically throughout the epochs, indicating that the model successfully learns from the training set. On the other hand, the validation accuracy decreases after the first epoch and then rises steadily, albeit not to the same heights as the training accuracy. This may be a sign of overfitting, in which the model performs well on training data but poorly on unobserved data, or it may indicate early instability in the learning process.

CONCLUSION

This work intends to build a lung cancer detecting model using deep learning and machine learning on a lung CT scan dataset. CT scan pictures are preferred by medical experts for their usability and quality. Many drugs and toxins nowadays make people unhappy and induce lung cancer. Early lung cancer identification is therefore quite important, and this work makes advantage of deep learning and machine learning methods. Testing evaluates the model; training and validation sets instruct it. Three models have training data. Many performance metrics included in the scikit classification report allow one to evaluate the dataset performance of several models. With test data, a confusion matrix evaluates model predictions. This work showed how utilising CT scan pictures, deep learning and machine learning might identify lung cancer. MRI scans and machine learning can help to broaden this investigation. Among these is the need for big, varied datasets for training to guarantee generalizability and accuracy, which might be difficult. These methods are also time-consuming and computationally intensive, which limits their applicability in environments with limited resources. Additionally, if regularisation and validation are not performed correctly, they may experience overfitting. Moreover, comprehending the intricate models can be challenging, which may impede their incorporation into clinical processes where explainability is essential.

Future Scope: The scope for machine learning (ML) and CNN based image processing techniques for lung tumor detection is promising and expansive. Computational power and algorithmic improvements can enhance model accuracy and reduce false positives. Integrating real-time data processing and applying transfer learning could generalize model applicability across diverse datasets, increasing robustness. Furthermore, developing 3D imaging techniques and multi-modal data integration could provide deeper insights into tumor characteristics. Collaboration with clinical trials and real-world implementation will be crucial for refining these models and achieving widespread clinical adoption, ultimately improving oncology diagnostic processes and patient outcomes.

REFERENCES

Abdulkareem, N. M., & Abdulazeez, A. M. (2021). Machine learning classification based on random forest algorithm: A review. *International Journal of Science and Business*, *5*(2), 128–142.

Al-Tawalbeh, J., ... (2022). Classification of lung cancer by using machine learning algorithms. In IICETA 2022 - 5th International Conference on Engineering Technology Its Applications, Al-Najaf, Iraq DOI: 10.1109/IICETA54559.2022.9888332

Bhatia, S., Sinha, Y., & Goel, L. (2019). Lung cancer detection: A deep learning approach. In Soft Computing for Problem Solving, Springer Nature, Singapore. DOI: 10.1007/978-981-13-1595-4_55

Bose, S. R., Jeba, J. A., Regin, R., Tarunraj, S., Soji, E. S., & Rajest, S. S. (2024). Enhanced deep learning models for early detection of renal failure from CT imaging. *FMDB Transactions on Sustainable Health Science Letters*, *2*(3), 152–163. DOI: 10.69888/FTSHSL.2024.000251

Chaudhari, P., Agarwal, H., & Bhateja, V. (2019). Data augmentation for cancer classification in oncogenomics: An improved KNN-based approach. *Evolutionary Intelligence*, *14*(4), 1–10.

Gnanadurai, G. J., Raaza, A., Velayutham, R., Palani, S. K., & Bramwell, E. A. (2023). Detection of cardiac amyloidosis on electrocardiogram images using machine learning and deep learning techniques. *Computational Intelligence*, *39*(4), 554–576. DOI: 10.1111/coin.12505

Jeganathan, J., Vashist, S., Nirmala, G., & Deep, R. (2023). A Cross Sectional Study on Anxiety and Depression Among Patients with Alcohol Withdrawal Syndrome. *FMDB Transactions on Sustainable Health Science Letters*, *1*(1), 31–40.

Karthik, S., Soji, E. S., Priscila, S. S., Sakthivanitha, M., Rajest, S. S., & Kumar, A. S. (2024). Enhancing tumor localization in brain MRI images using a scalable systematic vector algorithm for result-oriented accuracy. *FMDB Transactions on Sustainable Health Science Letters*, *2*(2), 110–127. DOI: 10.69888/FTSHSL.2024.000176

Kumar, A., Gautam, B., Dubey, C., & Tripathi, P. K. (2014). A review: Role of doxorubicin in the treatment of cancer. *International Journal of Pharmaceutical Sciences and Research*, *5*(10), 4117–4128.

Kumar, S., & Chong, I. (2018). Correlation analysis to identify the effective data in machine learning: Prediction of depressive disorder and emotion states. *International Journal of Environmental Research and Public Health*, *15*(12), 2907. DOI: 10.3390/ijerph15122907 PMID: 30572595

Kumudham, R., Kumar, S., Megalan, L. L., Sivakumar, S., Venkateshkanna, T., & Velmurugan, V. (2022). Comparative analysis on sediment classification using convolutional neural network. *2022 International Conference on Power, Energy, Control and Transmission Systems (ICPECTS)*, Chennai, India. DOI: 10.1109/ICPECTS56089.2022.10046986

Kureshi, N., Abidi, S. S. R., & Blouin, C. (2016). A predictive model for personalised therapeutic interventions in non-small cell lung cancer. *IEEE Journal of Biomedical and Health Informatics*, *20*(1), 424–431. DOI: 10.1109/JBHI.2014.2377517 PMID: 25494516

Lakshmanaprabhu, S. K., Mohanty, S. N., Shankar, K., Arunkumar, N., & Ramirez, G. (2018). Optimal deep learning model for classification of lung cancer on CT images. *Future Generation Computer Systems*, *92*(3), 374–382.

Milosevic, N., Dehghantanha, A., & Choo, K. K. R. (2017). Machine learning aided Android malware classification. *Computers & Electrical Engineering*, *61*(7), 266–274. DOI: 10.1016/j.compeleceng.2017.02.013

Monisha, M., Vijayalakshmi, P., Somasundaram, K., Arunraj, N., Sathishkumar, P., & Meena, M. (2022). Cooperative sensing with heterogeneous spectrum availability in cognitive radio. *2022 International Conference on Power, Energy, Control and Transmission Systems (ICPECTS)*, Chennai, India. DOI: 10.1109/ICPECTS56089.2022.10047411

Omar, N., Abdulazeez, A. M., Sengur, A., & Al-Ali, S. G. S. (2020). Fused faster RCNNs for efficient detection of the license plates. *Indonesian Journal of Electrical Engineering and Computer Science*, *19*(2), 874. DOI: 10.11591/ijeecs.v19.i2.pp874-982

Palani, D., & Venkatalakshmi, K. (2019). An IoT-based predictive model used for prediction of lung cancer using fuzzy cluster-based segmentation and classification. *Journal of Medical Systems*, *43*(2), 21. DOI: 10.1007/s10916-018-1139-7 PMID: 30564924

Sathishkumar, R., Kalaiarasan, K., Prabhakaran, A., & Aravind, M. (2019). Detection of lung cancer using SVM classifier and KNN algorithm. In *IEEE International Conference on System, Computation, Automation and Networking*, Pondicherry, India. DOI: 10.1109/ICSCAN.2019.8878774

Sayedelahl, M. A. (2024). Enabling Intelligent Traffic Systems: A Deep Learning Method for Accurate Arabic License Plate Recognition. *FMDB Transactions on Sustainable Intelligent Networks*, *1*(1), 40–55. DOI: 10.69888/FTSIN.2024.000156

Singh, G. A. P., & Gupta, P. K. (2019). Performance analysis of various machine learning-based approaches for detection and classification of lung cancer in humans. *Neural Computing & Applications*, *31*(5), 6863–6877. DOI: 10.1007/s00521-018-3518-x

Sugainela, Y., & Ahmad, T. (2020). Pearson correlation attribute evaluation-based feature selection for instruction detection system. In *IEEE International Conference on Smart Technology and Application*, Surabaya, Indonesia.

Telrandhe, S. R., Pimpalkar, A., & Kendhe, A. (2016). Detection of brain tumor from MRI images by using segmentation and SVM. In *IEEE WCTFTR World Conference on Future Trends, Research and Innovation for Social Welfare*, Coimbatore, India. DOI: 10.1109/STARTUP.2016.7583949

Uddin, S., Khan, A., Hossain, M. E., & Moni, M. A. (2019). Comparing different supervised machine learning algorithms for diseases prediction. *BMC Medical Informatics and Decision Making*, *19*(12), 1–16. DOI: 10.1186/s12911-019-1004-8 PMID: 31864346

Yu, K. H., Zhang, C., Berry, G. J., Altman, R. B., Ré, C., Rubin, D. L., & Snyder, M. (2016). Predicting non-small cell lung cancer prognosis by fully automated microscopic pathology image features. *Nature Communications*, *7*(8), 1–10. DOI: 10.1038/ncomms12474 PMID: 27527408

Zeebaree, D. Q., Haron, H., Abdulazeez, A. M., & Zebari, D. A. (2019). Trainable model based on new uniform LBP feature to identify the risk of breast cancer. In *2019 International Conference on Advanced Science and Engineering*, Zakho - Duhok, Iraq. DOI: 10.1109/ICOASE.2019.8723827

Chapter 7
Lung Disorder Identification by Optimized Deep Learning Model

A. Agnes Pearly
https://orcid.org/0009-0005-2415-4930
Bharath Institute of Higher Education and Research, India

B. Karthik
Bharath Institute of Higher Education and Research, India

ABSTRACT

Worldwide, lung disease is prevalent, so prompt diagnosis is essential. For this reason, numerous machine learning and image processing models have been developed. This present study develops an interesting approach that uses convolutional neural networks (CNNs) optimized with the Bat-Grey Wolf Optimization Algorithm (BatGWO) to automatically detect lung diseases, particularly tuberculosis (TB) and pneumonia. The proposed approach entails preprocessing the dataset, which involves collecting and modifying chest X-ray images from several public datasets derived from Kaggle. The CNN architecture's convolutional layers are then used for feature extraction, which enables the automatic learning of discriminative features suggestive of lung disorders. Next, BatGWO is used to optimize the CNN classifier, and its performance is compared to that of other optimization algorithms, including PSO and the Bat Algorithm (BA).

INTRODUCTION

The merger of artificial intelligence (AI)with medical imaging has produced ground-breaking advancements in healthcare in recent years, radically altering the field of disease diagnosis and treatment. In this revolution, Convolutional Neural Networks (CNNs) have become an effective tool, especially in medical image analysis (Jeganathan et al., 2023). Their potential for successfully and precisely classifying lung disorders from chest radiographs (X-ray images) has been shown, providing clinicians with powerful tools for disease identification. This is particularly important given the worldwide burden of lung diseases like tuberculosis and pneumonia, where prompt diagnosis is essential to starting the right treatments and enhancing patient outcomes. Precise and quick diagnostic techniques are desperately needed as these illnesses continue to affect millions of people worldwide (Suganthi and Sathiaseelan,

DOI: 10.4018/979-8-3693-9420-5.ch007

2023). With their strong algorithms that can analyze complex image data with exceptional reliability and accuracy, CNNs offer a promising solution to this problem. Healthcare professionals can improve their diagnostic abilities and help patients worldwide by using CNNs for lung disorder classification. This will result in earlier detection, more focused treatments, and better prognoses (Santosh et al., 2022).

Lung diseases like tuberculosis and pneumonia cause millions of deaths every year and present serious global health challenges. Lung inflammation that characterizes pneumonia is a primary factor in illness and death, especially in susceptible groups like the elderly and children. Numerous pathogens, such as bacteria, fungi, and viruses, can cause it. Therefore, prompt diagnosis is essential to starting the right treatment and avoiding complications (Thallaj and Vashishtha, 2023). Comparably, tuberculosis (TB), an infectious disease primarily affecting the lungs but also affecting other organs, is caused by Mycobacterium tuberculosis (Nirmala et al., 2023). Preventing the spread of tuberculosis and enhancing patient outcomes requires early detection. Because chest X-ray imaging allows for the quick and non-invasive visualization of lung abnormalities, it is essential in diagnosing TB and pneumonia.

Chest X-ray imaging is still an essential part of the diagnostic process for lung diseases, even with its drawbacks, including inconsistent image characteristics and co-occurring symptoms. It is significant because it can identify TB-related observations like cavitation, nodules, and lymphadenopathy, in addition to typical pneumonia symptoms like lung infiltrates and consolidation. Furthermore, when compared with other imaging modalities, chest X-rays are frequently more affordable and accessible, which makes them essential tools in environments with limited resources. Thus, increasing the precision and efficacy of chest X-ray interpretation, especially by incorporating artificial intelligence methods such as Convolutional Neural Networks, has great potential to enhance the early identification and treatment of tuberculosis and pneumonia, ultimately leading to improved public health outcomes (William et al., 2024).

CNNs have become extremely useful instruments for medical image analysis because they can extract discriminative features from raw image data (Vashist et al., 2023). CNNs have proven effective in several medical imaging instances, such as the classification of lung disorders. They are well-suited for tasks like image classification, segmentation, and detection. CNNs can potentially improve the accuracy and effectiveness of diagnosis in the classification of lung disorders by efficiently capturing spatial hierarchies of features through convolutional layers and learning intricate patterns from large datasets. Although CNNs have a lot of potential for medical image analysis, there are several difficulties in getting these networks to perform at their best. Convolutional filters, pooling layers, and fully connected layers are just a few of the many parameters that CNNs usually have, which makes the optimization process computationally demanding and prone to overfitting (Hasan Talukder et al., 2023).

Furthermore, experimentation and expert knowledge are needed for the selection of suitable hyperparameters and network architecture optimization. Conventional optimization methods, such as gradient descent-based techniques, struggle to navigate the complex, high-dimensional parameter space that comes with CNNs, which frequently results in the convergence of less-than-ideal solutions. Acknowledging these drawbacks, scientists have focused on nature-inspired optimization algorithms to overcome the optimization problems that CNNs for lung disease classification face (Vashishtha and Dhawan, 2023). These algorithms mimic the behaviors of biological organisms or ecological processes to direct the optimization process, taking inspiration from the principles of natural systems and phenomena. Using natural systems' innate efficiency and flexibility, such as animal behaviors or evolutionary processes, these nature-inspired algorithms present a fresh method for CNN architecture optimization for medical image analysis applications.

Nature-inspired optimization algorithms offer a viable means of progress to increase the robustness and performance of CNNs in lung disorder classification, ultimately leading to more accurate and dependable diagnostic tools in healthcare. This is because they can escape local optima and explore diverse solution spaces. Inspired by the natural behaviors of grey wolves and bats, the Bat-Grey Wolf Optimization Algorithm (BatGWO) offers a novel approach to optimization tasks. BatGWO combines the leadership dynamics of grey wolves, as demonstrated by the Grey Wolf Optimizer (GWO), with the echolocation powers of bats, as demonstrated by the Bat Algorithm (BA). Combining exploration and exploitation tactics guarantees a well-rounded and efficient optimization procedure (Odoemena and Elufidodo, 2024).

BatGWO shows great promise for medical image evaluation tasks, especially for treating lung disorders from chest X-ray images (CNNs). Using the complementary abilities of both algorithms, BatGWO aims to enhance CNN performance and efficacy in correctly diagnosing lung disorders. By taking an adaptable and collaborative approach, BatGWO hopes to further medical imaging technology, improving patient care and diagnostic accuracy in healthcare facilities. The use of CNNs optimized with the Bat-Grey Wolf Optimization Algorithm (BatGWO) for classifying lung disorders from chest radiographs is thoroughly investigated in this paper. We go over the technique for using BatGWO to optimize CNN architectures and the experimental setup for results analysis and training. Furthermore, we contrast the performance of CNNs optimized with BatGWO with conventional optimization algorithms like particle swarm optimization (PSO) and Bat algorithm techniques. With an emphasis on lung disease classification, we review the possible ramifications and future directions of using BatGWO for CNN optimization in medical image analysis (Pandit, 2023).

LITERATURE REVIEW

Research on machine learning (ML) methods for analyzing chest X-ray (CXR) pictures and identifying cardiopulmonary abnormalities has surged over the past ten years. There has been a lot of expectation for tuberculosis (TB) screening. This interest aligns with the remarkable progress made in deep learning (DL), primarily using CNN. As a result of these developments, DL approaches with CXR image-based TB screening have received significant research support. A review of studies by Harshavardhan et al. (2023) published in the last five years was covered. It identifies data sources, methodological contributions, and potential methods and challenges. It additionally addressed and compared studies, identifying those that provide options over binary decisions for tuberculosis, which includes region-of-interest localization.

Chest X-ray imagery is a low-cost, relatively easy technique for identifying lung abnormalities brought on by infectious diseases. The main objective of the study by Mogaveera et al. (2022) is to thoroughly examine and assess several classification measures to determine which method—pneumonia, tuberculosis, and COVID-19—according to ML or deep learning proves most useful in recognizing lung infectious illness using chest X-rays. We compared and assessed the efficacy of different classifiers for identifying pathological from normal chest radiographs, including deep learning algorithms (CNN) and conventional ML algorithms, to notify medical professionals and radiographers of potentially unexpected findings. Three main requirements must be met for the comparative analysis to be successful: reducing overfitting, lowering the rate of false negatives and fake positive counting, and evaluating outcomes. A comprehensive analysis of respiratory conditions is provided to assist researchers in creating models that can automatically identify lung illnesses in three different ways. In the first, how research has progressed from conventional feature engineering approaches to DL techniques is examined; in the second, these methods are used to identify the illnesses mentioned using radiology images such as CXRs; and in the third, the research path going forward for the identification of these illnesses is discussed.

For therapy to be effective, a timely diagnosis is necessary. Consequently, there is a need for an advanced, automated system that can identify chest X-rays and facilitate disease detection for users of all experience levels. Medical organizations spend at least one-day classifying diagnoses, whereas the model Devasia et al. (2023) can do so in seconds. In addition, a prediction probability for the anticipated class will be displayed. With performance scores above 90%, the framework was deemed capable of recognizing patterns. Images of chest X-rays submitted by users can be classified as typical or unusual by the framework. The EfficientNetB4 layout has been verified and evaluated in Yaseliani et al. (2022), where a multi-label methodology for identifying lung region and image-specific indications of persistent respiratory tuberculosis using CXR was developed using the transfer learning technique. Gradient-weighted Class Activation Mapping (Grad-CAM), an after-hoc analysis attention process offered by CNN, was also utilized to investigate the model and visualize tuberculosis irregularities while disputing them radiologically. Outstanding performance metrics were achieved by the EfficientNetB4 trained framework in both internal and external test sets from different regions. When resources are scarce, clinicians working in primary care can utilize the technology representations mentioned above to help identify and prioritize patients with tuberculosis (Kaewlek et al., 2023).

A hybrid CNN framework using three different classification techniques is used (Mirjalili et al., 2014). In the first, CXR images are classified using Fully Connected (FC) layers. The framework above undergoes multiple training epochs, with the weights that yield the highest classification accuracy retained. The good representation of CXR image attributes is gathered using trained optimized weights in the second method, and ML classifiers are used to classify the images. The third method classifies using a combined set of all the recommended classifiers. Based on the results, the combined classifier has the highest accuracy. It combines the Radial Basis Function (RBF) alongside Support Vector Machine (SVM) and Logistic Regression (LR) classifiers. This study by Kundu et al. (2021) presents four models (AlexNet, GoogleNet, ResNet, and DCNN) and compares how well they distinguish positive and negative images from four chest CT images. Following the tests, the ResNet model performs the best at classifying the four classes (TB, pneumonia, COVID-19, and normal) on chest CT images. Malik et al. (2023) created an ensemble system that considers the scores of decisions regarding the following CNN models: DenseNet-121, ResNet-18, and GoogLeNet. This creates an ensemble with a weighted average (Farhan and Yang, 2023).

An innovative approach was used to calculate the weights assigned to the classifiers by fusing the metrics for assessment with the hyperbolic tangent function. Using a five-fold cross-validation method, the framework was assessed on two openly accessible pneumonia CXR databases: the RSNA challenge and the Kermany (Shehab et al., 2023). The suggested model's statistical analyses, which employ ANOVA and McNemar's tests, show that the strategy is workable. The CDC_Net system successfully classifies five distinct types of lung disorders (Rahman et al., 2020). using x-rays of the chest. To demonstrate the strategy's viability, the CDC_Net system's classification accuracy was compared with three transfer learning approaches: Vgg-19, ResNet-50, and Inception-v3. The recommended model had been effective in distinguishing COVID-19 from several other chest-related illnesses, with the highest accuracy rate of 99%. These findings demonstrate the CDC Net system's remarkable accuracy and consistency in monitoring lung opaqueness about chest X-rays, which may allow for automatic viewing and the identification of chest diseases. In (Parthasarathy and Saravanan, 2024), the model trained for the 2D input image was used to design the reliable CNN model, which generated the 1D feature vector with the best kernel layout. We implemented a features scaling procedure with the suggested 2D CNN model to lower processing speed and memory demands. It used two chest X-ray datasets and various underlying classifiers to identify lung disease from the input CXR images (Yang, 2014).

Optimization algorithms aim to identify the best decision variables to achieve the value that the objective function has determined to be either the minimum or maximum. Every optimization algorithm has mechanisms or approaches to look at a problem's search space and find the best solution. Swarm Intelligence (SI) algorithms, or population-based techniques, are a popular class of optimization methods. The societal behavior of natural creatures is combined with optimization algorithm features in SI algorithms. A thorough analysis of the bat algorithm (BA) was presented in the survey paper, demonstrating the algorithm's great capacity to address various issues in various applications. The review's articles were gathered from scientific publications that suggested BA between 2010 and 2022. This body of literature illustrated the benefits and drawbacks of BA in addition to its features and strengths.

A summary of the various issues addressed by the gathered articles using BA has also been provided. These include image processing, research in medicine, and other noteworthy applications. Moreover, different versions of BA were presented, including binary and discrete, adaptation, and variations in hybridization, which improved the efficiency of BA in addressing a range of optimization issues.

The hyperparameters and the architecture of the MobileNetV2 model are optimized by the Genetic Algorithm, which enhances the model's ability to extract meaningful features from complex radiological data. During this critical optimization period, the model's configuration is customized to the details of the lung nodule identification assignment, resulting in significantly improved performance. A new technique for pneumonia identification and classification using CXR images is presented in this study, Chaotic Sea Horse Optimization, alongside the method. To get rid of the noise, this method first creates a noise eradication strategy based on Gaussian filtering (GF). Furthermore, it generates an array of feature vectors using the NASNetLarge framework.

Additionally, a more sophisticated fuzzy deep neural network approach is used to automatically identify and categorize cases of pneumonia. The work on the Kaggle repository is showcased by the CSHO algorithm, which ultimately determines the improved classification model's optimal hyperparameter values. Using the chicken swarm optimization (CSO) method, a trio of deep learning-based multiple neural networks was created, and each network performance was assessed using transfer learning. It started by developing an algorithm for CXR image segmentation, and then it was contrasted against various classification schemes. The Shenzhen and Montgomery lung databases, which provide publicly available data, were used to compare the outcomes with those of alternative techniques.

PROPOSED WORK

The objective is to create a reliable and efficient automated system for identifying lung disorders, eventually enabling earlier diagnosis and better patient outcomes. The Bat-Grey Wolf Optimization Algorithm (BatGWO) is utilized in the proposed methodology to optimize Convolutional Neural Networks (CNNs) to identify lung diseases like pneumonia and tuberculosis. The block diagram (Figure. 1) illustrates the processes involved in the method of work. To guarantee consistent and high-quality input data, the procedure starts with preprocessing the dataset, which entails obtaining X-ray pictures of the chest from the Kaggle database and carrying out the required transformations, such as resizing, normalization, and enhancement. The CNN architecture's convolutional layers are then used to extract features. By automatically extracting relevant patterns and textures suggestive of lung disorders from the input images, these layers automatically learn discriminative features. The extracted features are then fed into fully connected layers for classification, where CNN infers whether pneumonia or tuberculosis is present or absent. The BatGWO algorithm, which combines grey wolves' exploitation and exploration skills to effectively search for optimal solutions, is the key innovation in CNN classifier optimization. The CNN's parameters are iteratively updated based on the fitness function assessed with BatGWO. This allows the classifier to be fine-tuned for enhanced accuracy, precision, and recall.

Preprocessing: Data preprocessing is essential to ensure optimal model performance when training convolutional neural networks (CNNs). The procedure uses several specialized methods to improve image quality and reduce possible artifacts.

Resizing: X-ray images are resized to a standard size to guarantee consistency in input dimensions throughout the dataset. This increases processing computational efficiency and makes model training easier.

Normalization: To standardize image intensity levels, pixel values are normalized to a common scale, usually ranging from 0 to 1. During training, this normalization improves the convergence and stability of the model.

Noise reduction: Various filters are used to improve image clarity and reduce noise. The Gaussian filter is one particular filter that is frequently used to reduce noise. The Gaussian filter uses a Gaussian kernel—a two-dimensional matrix defined by a Gaussian function—to convolve the input image. The Gaussian kernel G has the following mathematical definition.

$$G(m,n) = \frac{1}{2\pi\sigma^2} e^{-\frac{m^2+n^2}{2\sigma^2}} -- \quad (1)$$

Where (m,n) represents the coordinates of each pixel in the kernel, and σ is the standard deviation that controls the spread of the Gaussian distribution. The convolution operation smoothes the image by averaging the pixel values in the kernel's vicinity, effectively softening edges and lowering high-frequency noise. As a result, the image becomes smoother and has less noise, which makes it better suited for further processing stages like feature extraction and classification inside the CNN framework.

Cropping: For a more focused analysis, images are cropped to highlight the area of interest, such as the lung area. In addition to lowering computational overhead, this eliminates unnecessary data that could confuse the model.

Augmentation: To improve model robustness and diversity, the dataset is augmented with methods like flipping, rotating, and scaling. To replicate differences in image acquisition, images can be rotated at different angles, and additional training samples with different orientations can be introduced by flipping the image horizontally or vertically.

Enhancing Contrast: To improve image contrast, contrast enhancement techniques like adaptive histogram equalization modify the distribution of pixel intensities. Unlike regular histogram equalization, AHE divides the picture into fragments and independently implements histogram equalization to every fragment. Using an adaptive approach, contrast enhancement is customized to the specific local characteristics of the image, avoiding the over-amplification of noise in homogeneous areas. AHE efficiently increases the visibility of subtle features in the X-ray images by redistributing pixel intensities based on local histograms, which makes the images more insightful CNNs during tasks such as classification.

Figure 1. Proposed BatGWO Optimized CNN Framework

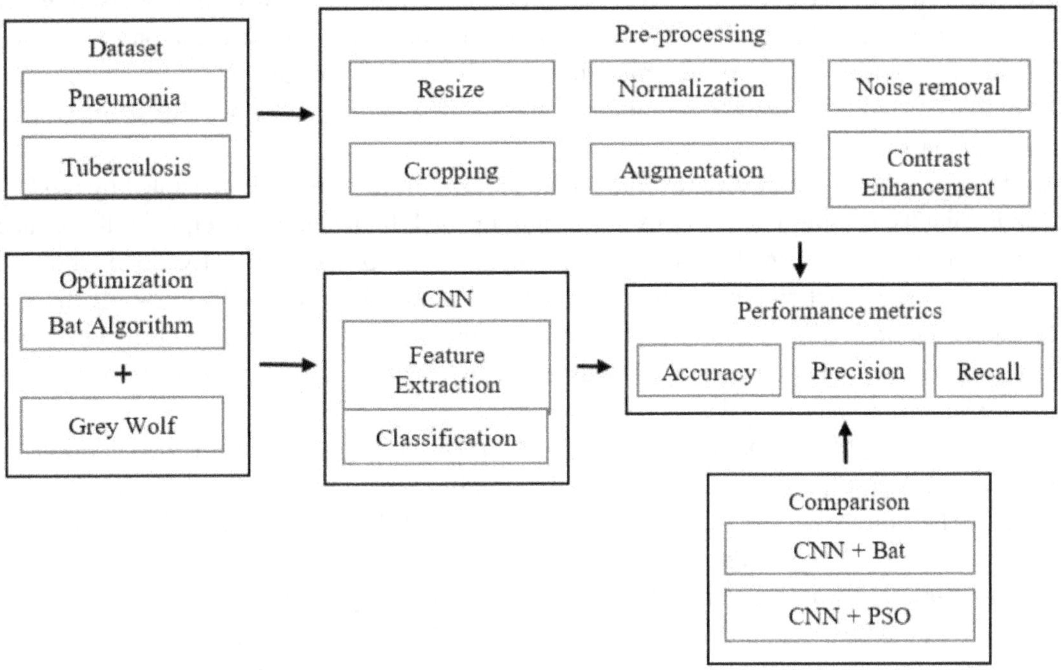

CNN Architecture Design for Lung Disorder Classification: CNN's architecture significantly impacts its ability to automatically identify distinguishing characteristics from X-ray pictures and generate precise predictions about tuberculosis or pneumonia. The following thoroughly explains every element of a typical CNN architecture for the classification of lung disorders.

Convolutional Layers for Feature Extraction: CNNs use convolutional layers as their fundamental building blocks to retrieve hierarchical features from input X-ray images. Each layer uses convolutional operations to identify low-level characteristics like edges and textures, and over time, it learns increasingly intricate patterns associated with lung conditions. The number of filters (or kernels) and their spatial dimensions dictate the size of each convolutional layer. Learnable filters are used to apply convolutions to the input images. Every filter captures local patterns by convolving over the input image to create a feature map. Various factors, including the input size, filter size, stride, and padding, determine a convolutional layer's output size. Following convolutional operations, activation functions like ReLU (Rectified Linear Unit) are frequently used to introduce nonlinearity.

Pooling Layers for Spatial Downsampling: To decrease computational complexity and manage overfitting, pooling layers are sandwiched between convolutional layers to preserve significant data while reducing the feature maps' spatial aspects. Max pooling is a widely used technique that maintains the maximum value inside each pooling window, thereby downsampling the feature maps. Pooling increases the learned features' sensitivity to minute spatial changes in the input images, strengthening the network's resistance to distortions and translations. Usually, these layers lack learnable parameters and have fixed spatial dimensions. A pooling layer's output size is determined by factors like the stride and pooling window sizes.

Fully Connected Layers for Classification: The CNN's fully connected layers, following the layers of convolution and pooling, make up its classifier component. These layers employ the learned features to classify data using the flattened output from the preceding layers. In classifying lung disorders, fully connected layers are trained to map the extracted features to the probability distribution across the different classes (e.g., normal lungs, pneumonia, tuberculosis). This layer's activation function, softmax, typically outputs the probability distribution for each class. The output layer's neuron count is the same as the count of classes.

Output Layer with Softmax Activation: The final class probabilities are generated by the CNN's output layer using the features that previous layers have learned. In the output layer, the fully connected layer's raw scores are often normalized into probabilities utilizing the softmax activation function. The output layer's softmax function ensures that the predicted probabilities for every class add up to one, with each neuron representing a class. The output layer forecasts the likelihood of each class (such as normal, pneumonia, and tuberculosis) for lung disorder classification, allowing the model to make well-informed predictions according to the input X-ray images.

Bat-Grey Wolf Optimization Algorithm (BatGWO): A hybrid metaheuristic algorithm that combines the Bat Algorithm (BA) and the Grey Wolf Optimizer (GWO) is called the Bat-Grey Wolf Optimization Algorithm (BatGWO). To effectively search the solution space, BatGWO combines the exploitation power of GWO with the exploration power of BA.

Bat Algorithm: The Bat Algorithm (BA) is an optimization algorithm that draws natural inspiration. It was created as described in (Chunduri et al., 2024). BA models the hunting process of bats to effectively search for ideal solutions in a search space, taking inspiration from the echolocation activity of bats. Because BA demonstrates a special combination of exploration and exploitation strategies, it differs from traditional optimization algorithms. It is especially useful for solving complex optimization problems in various domains. The echolocation behavior of bats, which allows them to find prey and navigate in the dark, is the fundamental component of the Bat Algorithm. Bats pulse ultrasonically and pay attention to echoes from objects in their immediate environment. Thanks to this process, they can estimate possible prey's features, direction, and distance. Similarly, each bat in the Bat Algorithm signifies a possible solution to the optimization issue, and the positions of the bats in the search space and solution space, respectively, match. The velocity updating mechanisms, frequency tuning, and echolocation are the main parts of the Bat Algorithm. Together, these elements balance exploration and exploitation and steer the search process toward promising areas of the solution space.

Echolocation: To find prey, bats release ultrasonic pulses, modifying their flight path in response to the echoes they receive. Similarly, bats in the Bat Algorithm randomly move around the solution space for better solutions. The intensity of a bat's emitted pulses (objective function values) indicates how close it is to an optimal solution; stronger pulses indicate closer proximity.

Frequency Tuning: Bats modify the frequency of their ultrasonic pulses in response to varying hunting environments and the characteristics of their prey. Each bat's emission frequency in the Bat Algorithm reflects the trade-off between exploration and exploitation. Lower frequencies prefer exploitation, concentrating on local refinement around promising solutions, while higher frequencies support exploration, resulting in larger steps in the search space.

Velocity Updating: Bats adjust their flight speed in response to the strength of their pulses and the echoes they perceive. Similarly, bats in the Bat Algorithm change their speed to travel toward more promising solutions. The current velocity and the difference between the bat's position and the best solution so far impact velocity updating. Bats can converge on ideal solutions through this mechanism, preserving population diversity. Bats update their positions using the following equation.

$$s_i(t+1) = s_i(t) + \in \times \left(s^* - s_i(t)\right) + \alpha \times rand\left(\right) -- \tag{2}$$

where $s_i(t)$ is the current position of bat i at time t, s^* This is the best solution found so far: ϵ is a random vector, and α is the loudness parameter. This formula incorporates randomness to promote exploration and depicts the migration of bats in the direction of better solutions. The Bat Algorithm updates the bats' locations in the search space iteratively until a stopping condition—such as a maximum count of iterations or convergence of solutions—is satisfied.

Grey Wolf Optimization Algorithm: The Grey Wolf Optimization (GWO) algorithm is an optimization technique influenced by nature that simulates grey wolves' social structure and hunting patterns. GWO was created in 2014 and is renowned for its effectiveness and simplicity in handling optimization problems in various fields. A pack has four main types of wolves: alpha, beta, delta, and omega. In descending order of hierarchy, the alpha wolf is the pack leader, followed by the beta, delta, and omega wolves. The wolves' fitness scores determine the wolf pack's hierarchical structure. The alpha wolf is identified as the fittest wolf, the beta wolf as the second-fittest, and so forth. Wolves use leader-follower dynamics to update their positions, meaning each wolf moves toward the pack's higher-achieving members. As the leader, the alpha wolf directs the group toward potential fixes. The equation that follows is used to update each wolf's position, s_j.

$$s_j = s^* - a \times D \times \left(r_1 - r_2\right) -- \tag{3}$$

where, s^* The position of the alpha wolf (the best solution found so far), a is a coefficient that controls the trade-off between exploration and exploitation. D is the distance between the current wolf position and the alpha wolf position. r_1 and r_2 are random vectors. The coefficient a is updated iteratively to balance exploration and exploitation. It decreases linearly from 2 to 0 as the algorithm progresses.

$$a = 2 - \frac{2 \times t}{max_{iterations}} -- \tag{4}$$

GWO effectively searches the search space for various optimization issues and converges to optimal or nearly optimal solutions. The optimization community favors it because of its ease of use, quick convergence, and capacity to manage intricate search spaces.

Integrating Bat and Grey Wolf Behaviours: The Bat-Grey Wolf Optimization Algorithm (BatGWO) combines the Bat Algorithm (BA) and the Grey Wolf Optimizer (GWO) to update the positions of bats and grey wolves simultaneously by leveraging their respective behaviors. Grey wolves take advantage of potential solutions by trailing leader wolves, whereas bats use echolocation behavior to explore the search space. By combining the advantages of both algorithms, BatGWO can effectively look for optimal solutions through parallel exploration and exploitation. This is the equation-based method of realizing the integration.

$$s_i(t+1) = s_i(t) + \in \times \left(s^* - s_i(t)\right) + \alpha \times rand\left(\right) + s^* - a \times D \times \left(r_1 - r_2\right) -- \tag{5}$$

The simultaneous execution of both algorithms is represented by the equation, which aids in BatG-WO's optimization process. The suggested optimization's pseudocode looks like this.

Algorithm 1: Pseudocode of BatGWO algorithm

Input

- The objective function to be optimized $f(s)$
- Number of bats N
- Maximum iterations $max_{iterations}$
- Frequency tuning parameter f_{min} and f_{max}
- Loudness tuning parameter α
- The initial population of solutions s_i
- Number of grey wolves M

Output

- Optimal solution s^*
- Objective function value $f(s^*)$

Initialize bat population s_i Randomly within the search space.
Initialize the grey wolf population. s_jRandomly within the search space.
Evaluate the objective function $f(s^*)$for each bat s_i and each grey wolf s_j
Repeat for t = 1 to $\max_{\text{iterations}}$
Update bat position s_i and grey wolf positions s_jSimultaneously using eqn. 3 and eqn. 5
For each bat s_i and each grey wolf s_j
Generate a new solution s_{new}

$$s_{new} = s_i(t) + \in \times (s^* - s_i) + \alpha \times rand() + s^* - a \times D \times (r_1 - r_2) - - \quad (6)$$

Evaluate $f(s_{new})$
If $f(s_{new}) < f(s_i)$, replace s_i with s_{new}
If $f(s_{new}) < f(s_j)$, replace s_j with s_{new}.
Update bat loudness and frequency as in the standard Bat Algorithm.
Update s^* To the best solution found among all bats and wolves.
Update A and A based on a predefined schedule or adaptive mechanism.
Return s^* and $f(s^*)$

Integration with CNN Training: The Bat-Grey Wolf Optimization Algorithm (BatGWO) must be incorporated into the CNN's training phase for convolutional neural network (CNN) optimization for lung disease classification. The algorithm describes the high-level overview of how this integration can be accomplished below.

Algorithm 2: Integration of BatGWO with CNN

Step 1: Initialization

- Randomly initial the CNN parameters (such as weights and biases) or using pre-trained weights.
- Initialize the BatGWO parameters, including the number of bats, maximum iterations, frequency tuning parameters, loudness tuning parameters, pulse rate tuning parameters, etc.

Step 2: Objective Function:

- Define an objective function that evaluates the performance of the CNN on a given dataset. This could be a loss function (e.g., cross-entropy loss) or a performance metric (e.g., accuracy).

Step 3: Encoding Solutions:

- Encode the parameters of the CNN (e.g., weights, biases) into the solutions of BatGWO. Each solution represents a potential set of parameters for the CNN.

Step 4: Optimization Loop:

- Implement the main loop of BatGWO, where the positions of bats and grey wolves are updated iteratively.
- Update the positions of bats and grey wolves using the equations of BatGWO, adjusting the parameters of the CNN accordingly.

Step 5: Training the CNN:

- For each iteration of BatGWO, update the parameters of the CNN based on the solutions generated by the algorithm.
- Train the CNN on the training dataset using the updated parameters.
- Evaluate the performance of the CNN on the validation dataset using the objective function.

Step 6: Update Best Solution:

- Keep track of the best solution discovered so far (i.e., the set of parameters that achieves the best performance on the validation dataset).

Step 7: Termination Criteria:

- Define termination criteria for BatGWO, like completing a set number of iterations or convergence of solutions.

Step 8: Final Evaluation:

- Once BatGWO terminates, use the best solution to evaluate the CNN's performance on the test dataset.

- Report the optimized CNN's final performance metrics (e.g., accuracy, precision, recall).

RESULTS AND DISCUSSION

The objective of the experimental evaluation was to determine how well CNN models optimized for lung disease identification tasks using various optimization algorithms (BatGWO, Bat Algorithm (BA), and Particle Swarm Optimization (PSO)) performed. Python scripts using the Keras library were used to implement the whole experimental setup, which includes data preprocessing, model construction, optimization, and evaluation. Through a comparative analysis of the model's performance on datasets related to tuberculosis and pneumonia using standard evaluation metrics such as accuracy, precision, and recall, valuable insights are obtained regarding the effectiveness of BatGWO in optimizing CNN models for precise lung disease classification.

Dataset Description: The method's effectiveness should be assessed by applying it to a dataset because the diagnosis capacity analysis is crucial before utilizing it as a tool. The 'Chest X-ray Images (Pneumonia)' dataset from Kaggle for pneumonia and the 'Tuberculosis (TB) Chest X-ray Database' for tuberculosis were publicly available. There are 4273 chest radiographs with a pneumonia diagnosis in the dataset and 3500 chest radiographs with a tuberculosis diagnosis.

Table 1. Analysis of the proposed model's performance

Method	Disorder	Accuracy	Precision	Recall
CNN+BatGWO	TB	96.51	94.26	92.14
	Pneumonia	96.75	94.73	92.9
CNN+BAT	TB	92.26	90.26	89.91
	Pneumonia	92.62	90.82	90.12
CNN+PSO	TB	85.63	84.12	82.16
	Pneumonia	86.12	84.88	82.75

The experiment outcomes show the success of the suggested CNN-based BatGWO algorithm compared to CNN-based algorithms optimized with Bat Algorithm (BA) and Particle Swarm Optimization (PSO) in Table 1. The suggested model is compared to its equivalents for tuberculosis and pneumonia in Figures 2 and 3, respectively. For tuberculosis (TB) classification, the BatGWO algorithm achieved an impressive accuracy of 96.51%, surpassing both BA (92.26%) and PSO (85.63%). Similarly, for pneumonia classification, BatGWO outperformed BA (92.62%) and PSO (86.12%) with an accuracy of 96.75%, demonstrating its superior classification capability.

Figure 2. Comparison of Proposed Model with TB Dataset

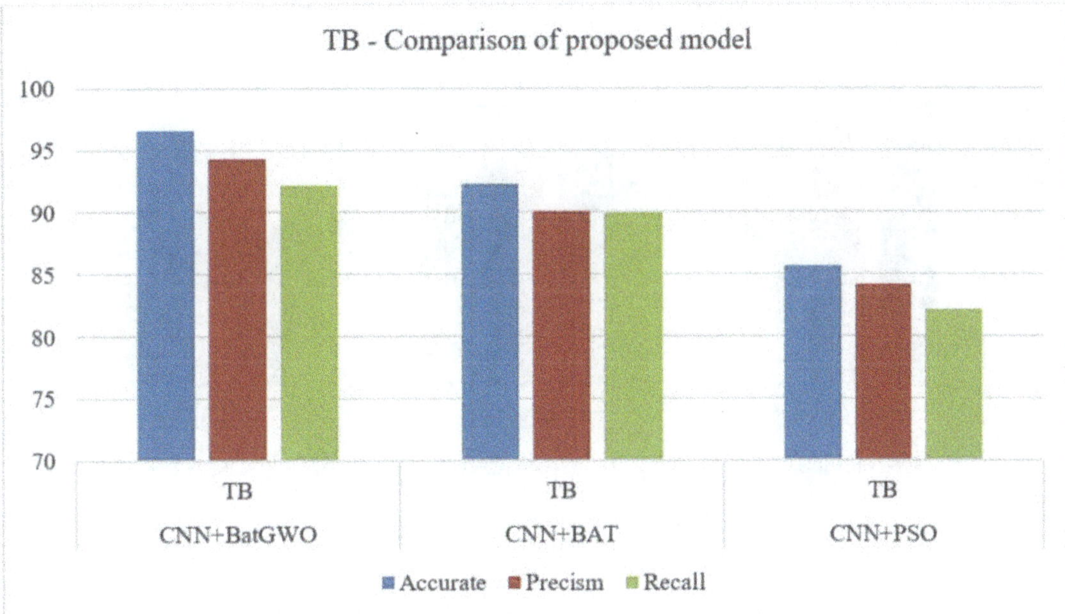

Moreover, regarding precision, BatGWO exhibited remarkable performance with values of 94.26% for TB and 94.73% for pneumonia. This signifies the algorithm's ability to correctly identify TB and pneumonia cases with high precision, minimizing false positive predictions. Similarly, % recall values of 92.14% for TB and 92.90% for pneumonia further emphasize the algorithm's capability to detect TB and pneumonia cases accurately, reducing false negative predictions.

Figure 3. Comparison of Proposed Model with Pneumonia Dataset

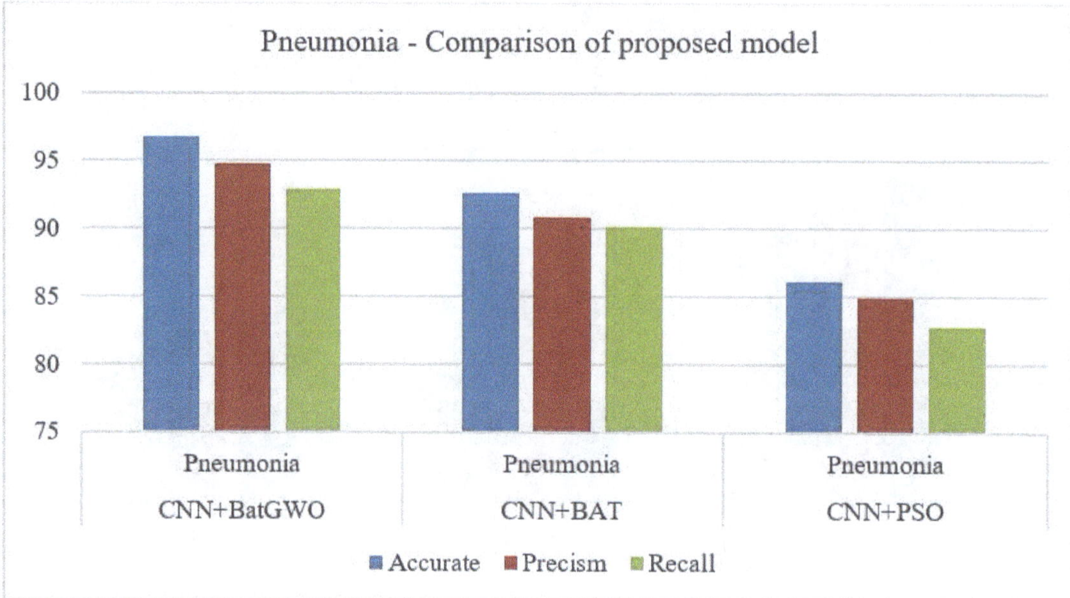

In contrast, the CNN-based BA algorithm yielded slightly lower accuracy, precision, and recall values for TB and pneumonia classification than for BatGWO. Alternatively, the PSO algorithm exhibited the lowest performance among the three algorithms, with accuracy, precision, and recall values consistently lower than both BatGWO and BA. Overall, the experimental results highlight the significant performance improvement achieved by the proposed BatGWO algorithm in classifying TB and pneumonia from images of chest X-rays. Its superior accuracy, precision, and recall values underscore its effectiveness in diagnosing lung disorders, offering promising clinical applications in medical image analysis.

CONCLUSION AND FUTURE WORK

To summarize, the methodology that has been suggested shows promise in automatically identifying lung diseases, particularly pneumonia and tuberculosis (TB), from chest X-ray images by using Convolutional Neural Networks (CNNs) that have been optimized using the Bat-Grey Wolf Optimization Algorithm (BatGWO). Using BatGWO's exploration and exploitation capabilities and thorough preprocessing and feature extraction procedures, CNN can efficiently learn discriminative features to attain exceptional recall, accuracy, and precision rates. The comparison with alternative optimization algorithms highlights BatGWO's effectiveness in improving CNN performance for medical image analysis tasks. Subsequent research endeavors may enhance the optimization procedure and investigate the suggested methodology's scalability and generalizability on more extensive and varied datasets that integrate alternative imaging techniques. Overall, this study's findings highlight how crucial it is to use artificial intelligence methods to advance medical image analysis and enhance patient outcomes in the respiratory health domain.

REFERENCES

Chunduri, V., Hannan, S. A., Devi, G. M., Nomula, V. K., Tripathi, V., & Rajest, S. S. (2024). Deep convolutional neural networks for lung segmentation for diffuse interstitial lung disease on HRCT and volumetric CT. In *Advances in Computational Intelligence and Robotics* (pp. 335–350). IGI Global.

Devasia, J., Goswami, H., Lakshminarayanan, S., Rajaram, M., & Adithan, S. (2023). Deep learning classification of active tuberculosis lung zones wise manifestations using chest X-rays: A multi-label approach. *Scientific Reports*, *13*(1), 1–15. DOI: 10.1038/s41598-023-28079-0 PMID: 36650270

Farhan, A. M. Q., & Yang, S. (2023). Automatic lung disease classification from the chest X-ray images using hybrid deep learning algorithm. *Multimedia Tools and Applications*, *82*(25), 38561–38587. DOI: 10.1007/s11042-023-15047-z PMID: 37362647

Harshavardhan, A., Cheerla, S., Parkavi, A., Latha Mary, S. A., Qureshi, K., & Mhaske, H. R. (2023). Deep learning modified neural networks with chicken swarm optimization-based lung disease detection and severity classification. *Journal of Electronic Imaging*, *32*(6), 062603. DOI: 10.1117/1.JEI.32.6.062603

Hasan Talukder, M. S., Sarkar, A., Akter, S., Nuhi-Alamin, M., & Bin Sulaiman, R. (2023). An Improved Model for Diabetic Retinopathy Detection by Using Transfer Learning and Ensemble Learning. *FMDB Transactions on Sustainable Health Science Letters*, *1*(2), 92–106.

Jeganathan, J., Vashist, S., Nirmala, G., & Deep, R. (2023). A Cross Sectional Study on Anxiety and Depression Among Patients with Alcohol Withdrawal Syndrome. *FMDB Transactions on Sustainable Health Science Letters*, *1*(1), 31–40.

Kaewlek, T., Tanyong, K., Chakkaeo, J., Kladpree, S., Chusin, T., Yabsantia, S., & Udee, N. (2023). Classification of pneumonia, tuberculosis, and COVID-19 on computed tomography images using deep learning. *Trends in Sciences*, *20*(11), 6974. DOI: 10.48048/tis.2023.6974

Kundu, R., Das, R., Geem, Z. W., Han, G.-T., & Sarkar, R. (2021). Pneumonia detection in chest X-ray images using an ensemble of deep learning models. *PLoS One*, *16*(9), e0256630. DOI: 10.1371/journal.ponc.0256630 PMID: 34492046

Malik, H., Anees, T., Din, M., & Naeem, A. (2023). CDC_Net: Multi-classification convolutional neural network model for detection of COVID-19, pneumothorax, pneumonia, lung cancer, and tuberculosis using chest X-rays. *Multimedia Tools and Applications*, *82*(9), 13855–13880. DOI: 10.1007/s11042-022-13843-7 PMID: 36157356

Mirjalili, S., Mirjalili, S. M., & Lewis, A. (2014). Grey wolf optimizer. *Advances in Engineering Software*, *69*(3), 46–61. DOI: 10.1016/j.advengsoft.2013.12.007

Mogaveera, R., Maur, R., Qureshi, Z., & Mane, Y. (2022). Multi-class chest X-ray classification of pneumonia, tuberculosis, and normal X-ray images using ConvNets. ITM Web of Conferences, 44(9), 03007.

Nirmala, G., Premavathy, R., Chandar, R., & Jeganathan, J. (2023). An Explanatory Case Report on Biopsychosocial Issues and the Impact of Innovative Nurse-Led Therapy in Children with Hematological Cancer. *FMDB Transactions on Sustainable Health Science Letters*, *1*(1), 1–10.

Odoemena, O. F., & Elufidodo, G. A. (2024). Machine learning-based cardiovascular disease detection and intelligent healthcare workflow automation. *FMDB Transactions on Sustainable Health Science Letters*, *2*(2), 81–93. DOI: 10.69888/FTSHSL.2024.000174

Pandit, P. (2023). On the Context of Diabetes: A Brief Discussion on the Novel Ethical Issues of Non-communicable Diseases. *FMDB Transactions on Sustainable Health Science Letters*, *1*(1), 11–20.

Parthasarathy, V., & Saravanan, S. (2024). Chaotic Sea Horse Optimization with deep learning model for lung disease pneumonia detection and classification on chest X-ray images. *Multimedia Tools and Applications*, *83*(2), 69825–69847. DOI: 10.1007/s11042-024-18301-0

Rahman, T., Khandakar, A., Kadir, M. A., Islam, K. R., Islam, K. F., Mazhar, R., Hamid, T., Islam, M. T., Kashem, S., Mahbub, Z. B., Ayari, M. A., & Chowdhury, M. E. H. (2020). Reliable tuberculosis detection using chest X-ray with deep learning, segmentation and visualization. *IEEE Access : Practical Innovations, Open Solutions*, *8*(10), 191586–191601. DOI: 10.1109/ACCESS.2020.3031384

Santosh, K. C., Allu, S., Rajaraman, S., & Antani, S. (2022). Advances in deep learning for tuberculosis screening using chest X-rays: The last 5 years review. *Journal of Medical Systems*, *46*(11), 82. DOI: 10.1007/s10916-022-01870-8 PMID: 36241922

Shehab, M., Abu-Hashem, M. A., Shambour, M. K. Y., Alsalibi, A. I., Alomari, O. A., Gupta, J. N. D., Alsoud, A. R., Abuhaija, B., & Abualigah, L. (2023). A comprehensive review of bat-inspired algorithm: Variants, applications, and hybridization. Archives of Computational Methods in Engineering. *State of the Art Reviews*, *30*(2), 765–797.

Suganthi, M., & Sathiaseelan, J. G. R. (2023). Image Denoising and Feature Extraction Techniques Applied to X-Ray Seed Images for Purity Analysis. *FMDB Transactions on Sustainable Health Science Letters*, *1*(1), 41–53.

Thallaj, N., & Vashishtha, E. (2023). A Review of Bis-Porphyrin Nucleoside Spacers for Molecular Recognition. *FMDB Transactions on Sustainable Health Science Letters*, *1*(2), 54–69.

Vashishtha, E., & Dhawan, G. (2023). Bridging Generation Gap on Analysis of Mentor-Mentee Relationship in Healthcare Setting. *FMDB Transactions on Sustainable Health Science Letters*, *1*(1), 21–30.

Vashist, S., Yadav, S., Jeganathan, J., Jyoti, D., Bhatt, N., & Negi, H. (2023). To Investigate the Current State of Professional Ethics and Professional Spirit Among Nurses. *FMDB Transactions on Sustainable Health Science Letters*, *1*(2), 82–91.

William, M. P., Priscila, S. S., Kiruba, S. B., Dayana, T. R. N., & Velavan, P. (2024). A comprehensive comparison of Adaboost, LightGBM, and CatBoost for Alzheimer's disease classification. *FMDB Transactions on Sustainable Health Science Letters*, *2*(3), 175–187. DOI: 10.69888/FTSHSL.2024.000253

Yang, X.-S. (2014). Bat algorithms. In *Nature-inspired optimization algorithms*. Elsevier in Amsterdam. DOI: 10.1016/B978-0-12-416743-8.00010-5

Yaseliani, M., Hamadani, A. Z., Maghsoodi, A. I., & Mosavi, A. (2022). Pneumonia detection proposing a hybrid deep convolutional neural network based on two parallel visual geometry group architectures and machine learning classifiers. *IEEE Access : Practical Innovations, Open Solutions*, *10*(6), 62110–62128. DOI: 10.1109/ACCESS.2022.3182498

Chapter 8
Improved Classification of Thyroid Diseases With Greater Accuracy Using Random Forest Over Decision Tree in Machine Learning Approaches

V. Brindha
https://orcid.org/0009-0005-2415-4930
Bharath Institute of Higher Education and Research

A. Muthukumaravel
Bharath Institute of Higher Education and Research, India

ABSTRACT

Since rapid diagnosis for a lifestyle condition is rarely available in rural locations, it becomes vital to create intelligent prediction systems using modern computing techniques. Conventional diagnostic techniques frequently depend on imaging studies, laboratory testing, and clinical evaluations, all of which can be laborious and unpredictable. ML can potentially revolutionize processes such as classifying thyroid illnesses in medical diagnostics. These models can categorize thyroid disorders and help medical professionals make decisions by being trained on various data sources, including patient demographics, hormone levels, imaging results, and clinical symptoms. This research provided a more accurate classification model to help identify thyroid disorders. The Random Forest(RF) and Decision Tree(DT), is compared in this study to establish the optimum training model for detecting thyroid disorders. Accuracy and Precision are performance measurements used to evaluate the models' performance.

INTRODUCTION

Medical research faces significant challenges in diagnosing diseases with a constantly rising population. Disease forecasting is significant in the area of data mining. The practice of examining and extracting hidden information from big data sets to uncover patterns is known as data mining. Clinics

DOI: 10.4018/979-8-3693-9420-5.ch008

and hospitals collect significant patient data, which will be used to analyze risk factors for various diseases. Data mining can forecast a variety of ailments, including thyroid disease, which is the subject of this study. Thyroid hormones are stored in the thyroid gland to keep the body's metabolic rate constant. The thyroid gland releases triodothyronine (T3) and thyroxin (T4) into the bloodstream as important hormones. Hormones regulate physiological activities like body heat, pulse rate, pressure, and the reproductive system. Hyperthyroidism and hypothyroidism can arise when T3 and T4 levels are out of balance. Hyperthyroidism occurs when T3 levels are high, and T4 levels are normal, indicating that the thyroid gland produces many hormones. Hypothyroidism occurs when T3 levels are low and T4 levels are normal. Hypothyroidism, if left untreated, can lead to obesity, arthritis, infertility, and cardiovascular disease, among other issues (Yadav et al. 2020).

Background: Thyroid illnesses present considerable diagnostic challenges because of their complex interplay of symptoms, clinical signs, and various presentations. These conditions include hyperthyroidism, hypothyroidism, and thyroid cancer. Traditional diagnostic procedures frequently combine imaging studies, laboratory testing, and physical examinations. Despite their effectiveness, these techniques can be laborious and have varying degrees of accuracy based on the healthcare provider's experience and the standard of the diagnostic instruments.

Types of Thyroid Diseases

Hypothyroidism: An inactive thyroid gland, which results in inadequate thyroid hormone synthesis, indicates hypothyroidism. The body's metabolism is slowed down by this shortage, which can result in symptoms including depression, dry skin, hair loss, weariness, weight gain, and cold sensitivity. Iodine deficiency is one common reason for hypothyroidism. To normalize hormone levels and relieve symptoms, treatment usually consists of hormone substitution using synthetic thyroid gland hormones (Hariprasath et al., 2024).

Hyperthyroidism: When the gland that controls thyroid function produces too many thyroid hormones due to overactivity, the condition is known as hyperthyroidism. This may quicken the body's metabolism and cause tremors, nervousness, anxiousness, rapid heartbeat, and heat intolerance. An autoimmune condition called Graves' disease is frequently a root cause of hyperthyroidism, a condition in which antibodies induce the thyroid to release extra hormones. According to the severity and underlying reason, therapies may include radioactive iodine therapy, antithyroid drugs, or surgical excision of a portion of the gland that makes up the thyroid (Odoemena and Elufidodo, 2024).

Goiter: An extension of the thyroid gland, known as Goiter, can result from either hyperthyroidism or hypothyroidism. It may manifest as a nodular goitre, where lumps or nodules grow inside the gland, or as a widespread enlargement. Thyroid inflammation, autoimmune diseases, and iodine shortages are the three main causes of goitre. Depending on the underlying reason, treatment options may include medication, iodine supplements, or surgery to remove a portion of the enlarged thyroid tissue if indications or issues arise.

Thyroid Nodules: Normal or cancerous lumps or masses inside the thyroid gland are called thyroid nodules. Frequently, these nodules are unintentionally found during physical exams or imaging tests. Some thyroid nodules can be malignant, but most are benign and asymptomatic. Diagnostic techniques like ultrasound, biopsy, and blood testing are employed to assess the nature of the nodules. When the nodules are symptomatic or malignant, treatment options may include hormone medication, regular follow-up, or surgical excision.

Thyroid Cancer: Thyroid tumour is a malignant development in the thyroid gland. Anaplastic thyroid cancer is uncommon yet aggressive, whereas papillary thyroid cancer is the most prevalent and usually has a fair prognosis. Surgery, radioactive iodine therapy, and specific treatments are possible therapeutic options, depending on the patient's kind, stage, and individual characteristics. Successful control and better results depend on early evaluation and treatment (Hu et al., 2022).

Autoimmune Thyroid Disorders: The gland that produces thyroid hormone is attacked by the immune system in autoimmune thyroid diseases. Hashimoto's thyroiditis is a common autoimmune disease that damages the thyroid tissue and causes persistent inflammation, which eventually results in hypothyroidism. On the other hand, Graves' illness causes hyperthyroidism because the immune system generates antibodies that cause the thyroid to release too much hormone. Careful pharmaceutical management is necessary for both disorders. In certain situations, additional therapies such as surgery may be required to reduce the immune system reaction and regulate thyroid hormone production.

Applications of Machine Learning in Thyroid Diseases: ML in classifying thyroid diseases uses sophisticated algorithms to increase diagnosis accuracy, expedite the diagnostic procedure, and ultimately improve patient outcomes. ML holds great potential to transform the identification and treatment of thyroid illnesses in clinical settings by leveraging the power of data-driven techniques. Large datasets can be analyzed using ML models, which can spot patterns that would be hard for human researchers to see. ML algorithms can more accurately classify thyroid problems by utilizing data from radiology results, clinic observations, hormonal assays, and patient records. These models can potentially increase diagnostic Precision, decrease variability, and speed up disease identification, ultimately resulting in more efficient and timely patient care. In this case, ML signifies a substantial move towards data-driven healthcare, where innovative algorithms complement and enhance established diagnostic techniques (Pandit, 2023).

Machine learning is highly regarded as a famous and effective technique for predictive analytics due to its performance in detection, prediction, and therapy selection. The UCI dataset is used to construct a comprehensible diagnostic assistance program that detects thyroid problems using machine learning methods (Saxena and Chaudhary, 2023). The proposed scheme, which employs the Random Forest algorithm, can increase prediction accuracy and reduce thyroid dysfunction misdiagnosis. Using standard tests, high accuracy was reached in distinguishing between obvious hyperthyroidism and hypothyroidism. The following is how the rest of the article is structured. Section 2 of the article presents a brief literature overview, which highlights several machine learning algorithms used in various research to detect thyroid problems. Section 3 explains the machine learning-based structure and methodology for the proposed smart thyroid predictive model. Section 4 of the study, which comprises concise findings and prediction metrics, examines the proposed thyroid approach on multiple levels. In Section 5, the given study concludes.

LITERATURE REVIEW

This work uses the multilayer perceptron (MLP) machine learning technique of Selwal et al. (2020) to build an improved and intelligent thyroid disease prediction system. Based on 7 to 11 criteria, the proposed method puts individuals into normal, hyperthyroid, and hypothyroid categories. Akhtar et al. (2021) investigated how three distinct attribute-selection techniques may be combined with the homogeneous voting ensemble. The necessary preprocessing and exception from the given criteria were finished before starting the categorisation process. Two algorithms help the first ensemble from the bagging and boosting ensembles. Whereas the boosting ensembles used AdaBoost and XGBoost, the bagging ensembles applied the random forest and bagging meta estimator (BME) approaches. Combining the feature-selection techniques with many estimating methods and ensemble approaches yields the results showing the best accuracy at a low computing cost.

The synthetic thyroid hormone sodium levothyroxine, often known as LT4, treats thyroid problems and diseases. Aversanoa et al. (2021) aresearch tries to anticipate the LT4 therapy trend for hypothyroidism patients. Medical data regarding patients getting treatment at the Naples clinic was compiled into a specialized dataset. Every patient's clinical history is available at all times. As a result, it was possible to forecast the length of each patient's therapy based on their unique characteristics and the pattern of hormonal indicators, deciding whether to extend or shorten it. This paper applies multiple machine learning methods, and the results of ten distinct classifiers are compared. Particularly for the Tree Classifiers, the results of the different algorithms are encouraging.

Three feature selection strategies, as well as other categorization techniques, are mostly used to achieve this. Feature selection methods used include univariate feature selection (UFS), recursive feature selection (RFE), and principal component analysis (PCA), as well as five extensively used classifying algorithms. They may deduce from the data that the RFE feature selection strategy aids in maintaining 99.3 percent accuracy throughout most classification methods. As a result of the research, it can be concluded that RFE aids each classifier in achieving higher accuracy than any other feature selection approach (Riajuliislam et al., 2021).

Pandey et al. (2015) major goal in this paper is to increase classification accuracy by classifying data as thyroid or non-thyroid. Thyroid data are classified using a variety of classification approaches as well as an ensemble model. Using feature selection techniques can help improve classification accuracy and performance. With five features, an ensemble of C4.5 and an RF provides a superior accuracy of 99.47%.

The main objective of Chen et al. (2020) study is to determine the US traits most closely linked to thyroid cancer and develop a scoring system that will enable ultrasonography doctors to diagnose thyroid cancer accurately. A logistic regression (LR) analysis is employed to identify potential thyroid cancer. Additionally, variables in the LR model are calculated, and ultrasound features highly associated with cancer are selected using the least absolute shrinkage and selection operator (LASSO) technique. An extreme learning machine (ELM) and radiofrequency (RF) are used to assess each thyroid lump's probability based on the necessary US features, and a scoring system is developed to classify thyroid nodules. Support vector machines (SVM), neural networks (NETs), and other cutting-edge technologies are compared and contrasted. The AUROC is used to evaluate the accuracy of various categorization methods.

An RF model is utilized to find relevant features to predict the type of thyroid disorder, and the KNN approach is employed to do multi-class classification. The prediction accuracy is improved when KNN is applied after feature selection (Nandhinidevi et al., 2020). The main goal of the study by Turanoglu-Bekar et al. (2016) is to provide a concise resource for researchers who use decision trees, a common technique in big data technology, in their research. To do this, commonly utilized DT algorithms are evaluated to classify thyroid illness kinds. The findings are compared using six capacity evaluation metrics (Accuracy, PRE, MAE, FME, REC, and Kappa Statistics). As a result, this research gives a valuable summary of current research on this topic and demonstrates the use of algorithms as a data mining technique utility.

MATERIALS AND METHODS

Preprocessing: Gathering and visualizing thyroid disease-related data before getting started is essential. Before beginning the estimation, the most critical step is to prepare the data. Data preparation is used in machine learning for data cleansing and reduction and for dealing with missing variables to increase accuracy. Data preparation is a fundamental step in machine learning that ensures the dataset used for training and evaluation is accurate, complete, and suitable for analysis. To ensure consistency and improve model performance, this process entails several key activities: gathering pertinent data from sources like imaging studies and medical records; cleaning the data by handling missing values through imputation or deletion, removing duplicate entries, and correcting errors, and transforming the data by normalizing or standardizing numerical features. Proper data preparation enhances the accuracy of machine-learning models and increases their reliability and effectiveness in classifying thyroid diseases and other medical conditions.

Feature Selection – MIN MAX Method: A crucial phase in the ML process is feature selection, which is locating and picking the most pertinent features from a dataset to improve a model's performance. By concentrating on the most useful attributes, effective feature selection increases model efficiency and decreases overfitting while enhancing accuracy and decreasing training time. Numerous strategies, such as min-max approaches and standard methodologies, can be used to accomplish the process. Next, feature selection is carried out using the standard and min-max methods. Feature selection has a significant impact on model construction, especially when it comes to choosing features that improve the classifier's efficiency.

The key advantages of feature selection strategies are less overfitting, higher accuracy, and reduced training time. Scaling features to a specified range, usually [0, 1], is an approach known as min-max preprocessing. This strategy can have a substantial effect on how well ML models perform when it comes to classifying thyroid diseases. In datasets with different sizes or units, this preprocessing step is very helpful in ensuring that each feature contributes equally to the model's learning process. Features like thyroid hormone levels (T3, T4, and TSH) may have various ranges and units in a thyroid dataset. For example, TSH levels might range from 0.1 to 5.0, while T3 and T4 levels can be in completely different units. By scaling all characteristics to a common range, usually [0, 1], min-max normalization keeps features with wider ranges from controlling the learning procedure. Thanks to this normalization, each feature will contribute proportionately to the model's predictions.

Implementation Stages

Calculate Min and Max Values: Find the lowest and highest values for each feature in the thyroid dataset for all samples. The features will be scaled using these values.

Apply Min-Max Scaling: Apply the min-max formula to each feature value transformation.

$$X_{scaled} = \frac{X - X_{min}}{X_{max} - X_{min}} \quad \text{-------} \qquad (1)$$

where X_{min} and X_{max} The feature's minimal and maximum values are represented, respectively, and X represents the initial feature value.

Transform Dataset: Make sure we rescale every feature in the dataset to the [0, 1] range using the min-max scaling method for each feature.

Integrate Scaled Data: ML models can be trained and assessed using normalized data. The performance and training efficiency of the model will both be enhanced by the scaled features.

Disease Prediction: Then, using these features, Machine Learning classifiers are applied to forecast thyroid disorders. The Random Forest technique is proposed in this study as a classifier for predicting a patient's thyroid ailment. In addition, the Decision Tree classifier is employed for prediction compared to the suggested approach. Subsequently, various parameters derived from the confusion matrix are employed to assess and contrast the most effective method for diagnosing thyroid disease after the study.

Dataset Description: The data collection includes two hundred fifteen cases, with 150 being normal, 35 being hyperthyroidism, and 30 hypothyroidism. Five clinical features have been found, and their description is as follows.

- The T3-resin uptake test is the first feature you'll notice. (Percentage point)
- Isotopic displacement testing of complete serum thyroxin.
- Radioimmunotest measurement of total serum triiodothyronine.
- TSH levels in the resting state, as determined by radioimmunoassay.
- Maximum absolute variation between TSH after 200 micrograms of thyrotropin-releasing hormone injection and baseline level.

Random Forest (RF): Several DTs are combined using the RF classifier, a potent and popular ensemble learning technique, to enhance classification performance. Based on various characteristics, including age, hormone levels, and other clinical data, the RF classifier can be used to detect thyroid problems. The RF is an ensemble classifier based on DTs, with each DT serving as a classifier for classification. It generates trees at random using the best-fit method. It changes as the forest's tree count and the amount of attributes per tree increase. N trees produce N classification outputs to classify an input sample. It forecasts outcomes based on an average of the outputs of all of the forest's trees. The class with the most voting counts is the winner, determined by the RF after adding up all the voting results. A randomly selected set of features is chosen at each tree split, and the tree is only permitted to split in the directions indicated by those features. The following are some of the benefits of employing the Random Forest algorithm.

- The RF algorithm is more interpretable and can manage many predictors.
- In a regression or classification challenge, random forests can be utilized to rank the parameters' significance efficiently.
- It finds the variables most important for the classification.
- Gini impurity is frequently employed in decision trees within RF to identify the optimal feature for data splitting at each node.

$$Gini(t) = 1 - \sum_{i=1}^{C} p_i^2 \quad \text{------} \qquad (2)$$

Where

C is the number of classes.

p_iIs the proportion of instances in class i at node t.

After splitting, the feature that reduces the Gini impurity is selected. The predictions of several DTs are combined to create predictions by the RF classifier.

Majority Vote Prediction

$$\hat{y} = mode\{h_1(x), h_2(x), \dots h_m(x)\} \text{ -----} \quad (3)$$

Where

- $h_1(x)$Represents the prediction of the i-th tree for input x.
- m is the total number of trees.
- $\hat{y}$Indicates the final predicted class label.

RF can internally estimate its performance using Out-Of-Bag error without requiring a different validation set.

OOB Error Estimate: Without requiring a different validation set, RF can internally estimate its performance using an Out-Of-Bag error.

$$OOB\ Error = \frac{1}{N}\sum_{i=1}^{N} I(y_i \neq \hat{y}_i^{OOB} \text{ -----} \quad (4)$$

Where

- N is the total number of samples.
- I(·) is the indicator function (1 if true, 0 if false).
- y_iIs the true class label, for instance, i.
- $\hat{y}_i^{OOB}$Represents the predicted class label, for instance, iii, using only the trees that did not include iii in their bootstrap sample.

RF can determine the significance of each feature by examining the degree to which the accuracy or Gini impurity drops when a feature is utilized for splitting.

$$Importance(A) = \frac{1}{T}\sum_{t=1}^{T} \Delta I_t(A) \text{ -----} \quad (5)$$

Where

- T is the number of trees.
- $\Delta I_t(A)$ represents the decrease in impurity or increase in accuracy attributed to feature A in tree t.
- Although RF's general workings are understandable, the underlying formulas guarantee that the model is statistically sound and efficient for classification tasks such as thyroid illness diagnosis.

Decision Tree (DT): DT is a structure resembling a flowchart used to forecast and make decisions depending on incoming data. Based on characteristics like hormone levels, age, and other clinical signs, a DT can be used in thyroid classification to determine whether a patient has a thyroid problem. The most extensively used architecture in data mining is Decision Trees. These designs employ the divide-and-conquer technique to divide the instance space into decision zones. A test is used to identify a root node at first. After that, the data set is separated by the value of a linked test attribute, and the process repeats till the given terminating condition is fulfilled.

A leaf node is a node at the very end of the tree that denotes the class. In addition, each branch denotes a decision rule-defined path. Eventually, each decision rule is applied to a new sample to classify it. When using decision trees, there are three key processes to follow: The learning process is the initial step, during which the model is built using the training data. As a result, categorization rules present this model. The model accuracy is calculated in the second stage by selecting a test. The model is approved based on the results of this test. Finally, the model is used to classify or predict fresh data in the third stage.

Features (X): Age, T3, T4, and TSH (thyroid stimulating hormone) are possible input features.

Target (Y): The class labels, such as normal, hyperthyroid, or hypothyroid, may be represented by the target variable.

A Decision Tree's basic principle is to partition the data into subsets depending on feature values iteratively to maximize the separation of classes.

Choosing the Best Split: A criterion such as Information Gain (IG), GI, or another statistic determines where to split. Maximizing class purity in each subset is the aim.

Gini Impurity (GI): A node's "impurity" or heterogeneity is measured by GI. Any node instance that is part of a single class is considered pure.

$$Gini(T) = 1 - \sum_{i=1}^{C} p_i^2 \quad (6)$$

Where

- C is the number of classes.
- p_iDenotes the proportion of instances of class i in node t.
- Splitting RuleTwo subsets, S1 and S2, are created from the dataset S, given a feature A and a threshold θ.

$$S_1 = \{x \in S \mid x[A] \le \theta\} \quad (7)$$

$$S_2 = \{x \in S \mid x[A] > \theta\} \quad (8)$$

For the split, the Gini impurity is computed as follows.

$$Gini\ Split = \frac{[S_1]}{[S]} Gini\ (S_1) + \frac{[S_2]}{[S]} Gini\ (S_2) \quad (9)$$

The split is selected based on its lowest Gini impurity.

Information Gain

An alternative that is based on the idea of entropy is IG.

$$H(S) = -\sum_{i=1}^{C} p_i log_2(p_i) \quad ------ \tag{10}$$

The IG for a split on feature A is

$$IG(S,A) = H(S) - \sum_{v \in values(A)} \frac{[S_v]}{[S]} H(S_v) \quad ---- \tag{11}$$

The split chosen is the one with the highest IG.

The nodes are split recursively, with the same splitting technique used for each subset resulting from the prior split. Through recursive splitting, a tree structure is progressively constructed, with each node in the tree denoting a feature and a distinct threshold serving as the split point. The result of each split, represented by a branch that emerges from a node, further subdivides the data until the halting conditions are satisfied. Ultimately, this recursive procedure creates a decision tree that categorizes data according to the routes from root to leaf nodes. When certain requirements are satisfied, such as when every instance in a node is a pure node since they all belong to the same class, the recursion ends. A predetermined maximum depth of the tree, beyond which no more splits are permitted, is another condition for halting. In addition, the splitting operation stops if a node's instance count drops below a predetermined level. Ultimately, suppose the purity increase or impurity decrease from additional splitting is less than a particular threshold. In that case, the recursion may likewise end, suggesting that additional splits would not materially improve the categorization. A node turns into a leaf node when it can no longer divide. The anticipated class of a leaf node is determined by looking at the most prevalent class among its instances.

$$\hat{y} = argmax_i\{p_i\} \quad ------- \tag{12}$$

Where

- p_i Is the proportion of class i instances in the leaf node.

RESULTS AND DISCUSSIONS

Confusion Matrix (CM) in machine learning provides a more complete study of the technique for classification challenges. Each row and column of the CM represent the actual and predicted classes. The accuracy of the classifier is measured using the labels True Positive (TP), True Negative (TN), False Positive (FP), and False Negative (FN). TP and TN represent correct predictions, whereas FP and FN represent wrong predictions.

Accuracy Prediction

$$\text{Accuracy} = \frac{\text{TP} + \text{TN}}{\text{TP} + \text{FP} + \text{TN} + \text{FN}} * 100\,\% - - - - \quad (13)$$

Tables 1 and 1 show the accuracy obtained from the DT and RF datasets. It clearly shows that RF outperforms DT in terms of accuracy.

Table 1. Accuracy by Decision Tree and Random Forest

No of Iterations	Decision Tree Accuracy %	Random Forest Accuracy %
10	79.96	82.88
20	80.21	83.20
30	80.66	83.53
40	80.87	84.76
50	80.93	84.89

Figure 1. Accuracy by Decision Tree and Random Forest Graph

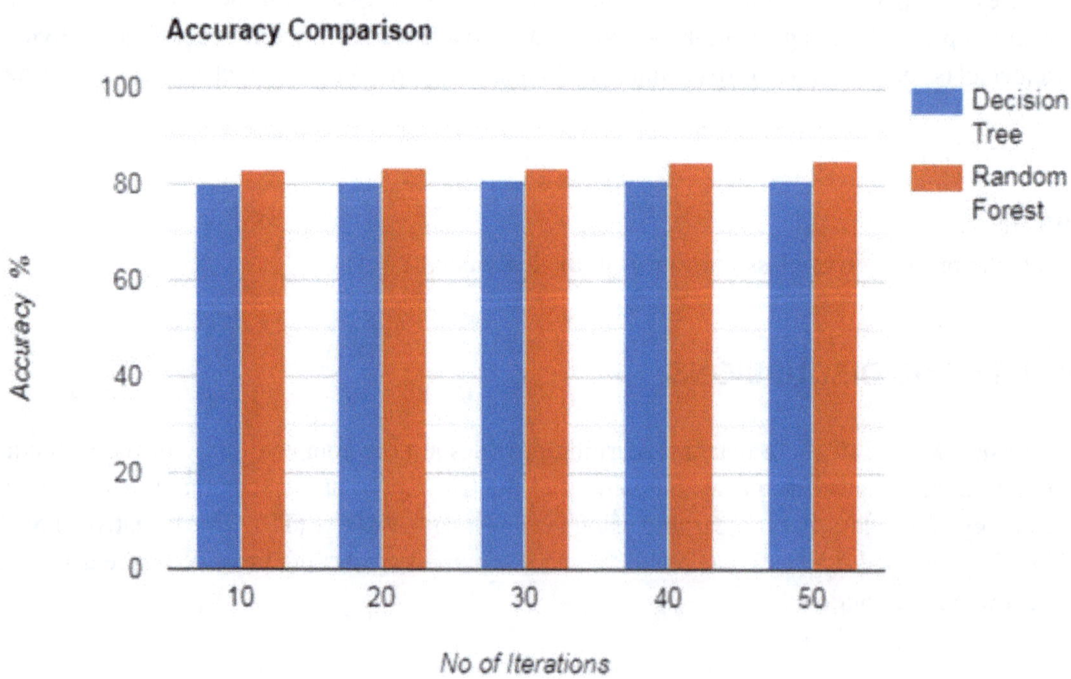

The accuracy percentages of the RF and DT classifiers across varying numbers of iterations are shown in Table 1 and Figure 1, illustrating how well these ML models perform in classifying thyroid disorders. The accuracy metrics show how well, given the available data, each model predicts the proper classifications. At first, as the number of iterations rises, both models exhibit increasing accuracy. Accuracy for the Decision Tree classifier begins at 79.96% after 10 iterations and progressively increases to 80.93% after 50. This gradual rise implies that the model improves in class distinction as it goes through additional iterations, probably due to improved decision-making procedures and improved data training. Comparing the RF classifier to the DT shows a similar trend but is generally more accurate. After 10 iterations, the accuracy is 82.88%; after 50 iterations, it is 84.89%.

The Random Forest's capacity to use several decision trees to increase overall classification performance is demonstrated by this steady development. Because the Random Forest model uses an ensemble approach to combine predictions from several trees to provide more stable and dependable predictions, its accuracy is better, indicating its robustness and effectiveness in handling complicated datasets. The data shows that both models get better as more iterations are run, but the Random Forest classifier performs better overall. This implies that while more iterations benefit both models, the RF ensemble approach offers a more precise and trustworthy classification for thyroid disorders.

Precision Prediction

$$\text{Precision} = \frac{\text{TP}}{\text{TP} + \text{FP}} * 100\% - - - - - - - \quad (14)$$

Table 2 and Figure 2 show the Precision obtained from the Decision Tree and Random Forest dataset.

Table 2. Precision by Decision Tree and Random Forest

No of Iterations	Decision Tree Precision %	Random Forest Precision %
10	79.72	83.92
20	80.23	83.93
30	81.98	84.72
40	82.92	84.82
50	83.93	84.97

Figure 2. Precision by Decision Tree and Random Forest Graph

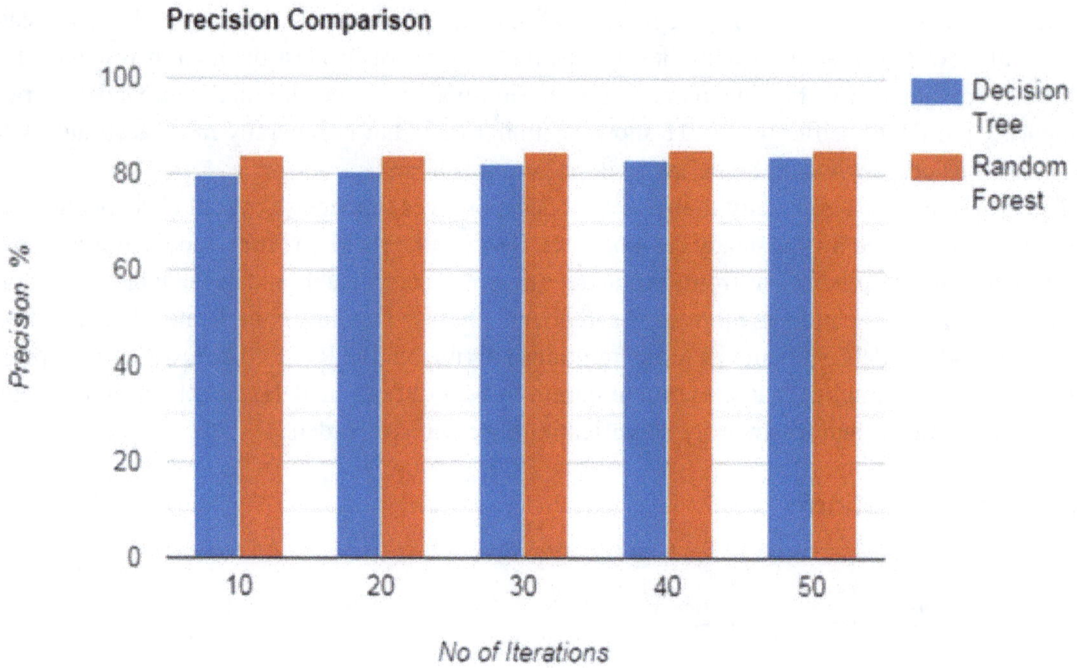

The precision percentages of the RF and DT classifiers across varying numbers of iterations are shown in Table 2 and Figure 2. Precision increases gradually for the DT classifier, rising from 79.72% after 10 iterations to 83.93% after 50. This steady rise implies that the model improves in accurately detecting genuine positives and decreasing false positives with additional iterations. As the model learns from more data or improves its decision limits, it becomes more capable of making predictions, as evidenced by the increase in Precision. On the other hand, when compared to the DT, the RF classifier continuously demonstrates more Precision. After 10 iterations, Precision is 83.92%; after 50 iterations, it is 84.97%. Because of its ensemble learning strategy, the Random Forest generally has higher Precision.

The Random Forest approach combines predictions by integrating many decision trees, which lowers variability and raises the overall accuracy of positive classifications. This approach reduces errors and handles complex data in an efficient manner, which contributes to increased Precision. The data shows that both classifiers gain from more iterations, and precision increases when the models are trained more thoroughly. Nonetheless, the RF continuously outperforms the DT in Precision, highlighting its efficacy in producing more precise positive predictions for classifying thyroid diseases. Because of its superior Precision, the Random Forest may be a better fit when reducing false positives is essential.

CONCLUSION AND FUTURE WORK

A Random Forest Classifier is proposed in this chapter for the classification of thyroid gland problems. The RF has the upper hand concerning classification accuracy and Precision for the data set, according to the findings, compared to the Decision Tree technique. The thyroid data set from the UCI machine learning library yielded 84.89% classification accuracy and 84.97% precision scores. According to this study, the RF classifier outperforms the Decision Tree method in prediction accuracy. To increase diagnostic accuracy, future work in thyroid categorization may concentrate on combining sophisticated ML approaches, such as ensemble methods and deep learning. Furthermore, the robustness of classification models can be improved by combining multimodal data from lab tests, imaging, and clinical history with genomic data. A focus on explainable AI will be necessary to guarantee that these models are comprehensible and reliable for medical professionals. IoT-enabled wearables and real-time monitoring could facilitate ongoing evaluation and early thyroid disorder detection. At the same time, personalized medicine techniques could customize treatments according to unique patient profiles, resulting in more accurate and successful thyroid condition management.

REFERENCES

Akhtar, T., Gilani, S. O., Mushtaq, Z., Arif, S., Jamil, M., Ayaz, Y., Butt, S. I., & Waris, A. (2021). Effective voting ensemble of homogenous ensembling with multiple attribute-selection approaches for improved identification of thyroid disorder. *Electronics (Basel)*, *10*(23), 3026. DOI: 10.3390/electronics10233026

Aversano, L., Bernardi, M. L., Cimitile, M., Iammarino, M., Macchia, P. E., Nettore, I. C., & Verdone, C. (2021). Thyroid Disease Treatment prediction with machine learning approaches. *Procedia Computer Science*, *192*(1), 1031–1040. DOI: 10.1016/j.procs.2021.08.106

Chen, D., Hu, J., Zhu, M., Tang, N., Yang, Y., & Feng, Y. (2020). Diagnosis of thyroid nodules for ultrasonographic characteristics indicative of malignancy using random forest. *BioData Mining*, *13*(1), 1–21. DOI: 10.1186/s13040-020-00223-w PMID: 32905307

Hariprasath, G., Dhinakaran, P., & Kumar, V. H. (2024). Exploring the efficacy of LightGBM, AdaBoost, and CatBoost in Alzheimer's disease classification. *FMDB Transactions on Sustainable Health Science Letters*, *2*(1), 41–55. DOI: 10.69888/FTSHSL.2024.000171

Hu, M., Asami, C., Iwakura, H., Nakajima, Y., Sema, R., Kikuchi, T., Miyata, T., Sakamaki, K., Kudo, T., Yamada, M., Akamizu, T., & Sakakibara, Y. (2022). development and preliminary validation of a machine learning system for thyroid dysfunction diagnosis based on routine laboratory tests. *Communications Medicine*, *2*(1), 1–8. DOI: 10.1038/s43856-022-00071-1 PMID: 35603277

Nandhinidevi, S., Poorani, P., & Brindha, P. G. (2020). Machine Learning Models for Relevant Feature Identification and Classification of Thyroid Data. *International Journal of Innovative Technology and Exploring Engineering*, *9*(5), 1961–1963. DOI: 10.35940/ijitee.E2948.039520

Odoemena, O. F., & Elufidodo, G. A. (2024). Machine learning-based cardiovascular disease detection and intelligent healthcare workflow automation. *FMDB Transactions on Sustainable Health Science Letters*, *2*(2), 81–93. DOI: 10.69888/FTSHSL.2024.000174

Pandey, S., Tiwari, A., Kumar Shrivas, A., & Sharma, V. (2015). Thyroid Classification using Ensemble Model with Feature Selection. *International Journal of Computer Science and Information Technologies*, *6*(3), 2395–2398.

Pandit, P. (2023). On the Context of Diabetes: A Brief Discussion on the Novel Ethical Issues of Non-communicable Diseases. *FMDB Transactions on Sustainable Health Science Letters*, *1*(1), 11–20.

Riajuliislam, M., Rahim, K. Z., & Mahmud, A. (2021). Prediction of thyroid disease(hypothyroid) in early stage using feature selection and classification techniques. 2021 International Conference on Information and Communication Technology for Sustainable Development (ICICT4SD), Dhaka, Bangladesh.

Saxena, D., & Chaudhary, S. (2023). Predicting Brain Diseases from FMRI-Functional Magnetic Resonance Imaging with Machine Learning Techniques for Early Diagnosis and Treatment. *FMDB Transactions on Sustainable Computer Letters*, *1*(1), 33–48.

Selwal, A., & Raoof, I. (2020). A multilayer perceptron-based improved thyroid disease prediction system. *Indonesian Journal of Electrical Engineering and Computer Science*, *17*(1), 524. DOI: 10.11591/ijeecs.v17.i1.pp524-532

Turanoglu-Bekar, E., Ulutagay, G., & Kantarcı-Savas, S. (2016). Classification of thyroid disease by using data mining models: A comparison of decision tree algorithms. *The Oxford Journal of Intelligent Decision and Data Science*, *2*(2), 13–28. DOI: 10.5899/2016/ojids-00002

Yadav, D. C. (2020). Calculating diagnose odd ratio for thyroid patients using different data mining classifiers and ensemble techniques. *International Journal of Advanced Trends in Computer Science and Engineering*, *9*(4), 5463–5470. DOI: 10.30534/ijatcse/2020/186942020

Chapter 9
Efficacy of The Decision Tree as an Alternative to the Naïve Bayes Model for the Prediction of Thyroid Disease Classification

V. Brindha
https://orcid.org/0009-0005-2415-4930
Bharath Institute of Higher Education and Research, India

A. Muthukumaravel
Bharath Institute of Higher Education and Research, India

ABSTRACT

The thyroid gland is one of the most efficient organs in the body, as it secretes thyroid hormones that regulate metabolism. Millions of individuals worldwide suffer from thyroid illness, which encompasses a variety of conditions, from thyroiditis and thyroid nodules to Hyperthyroidism and hypothyroidism. Hypothyroidism and Hyperthyroidism are the two most common thyroid disorders caused by changes in the hormone thyroxin. Since thyroid disorders can cause serious health problems if left untreated, early and precise diagnosis is essential for managing the issue effectively. Clinical assessments, laboratory testing, and imaging methods are often used in traditional diagnostic procedures, although they can be labour-intensive and prone to human error. Data mining is a strategy for developing expert systems for medical data classification using machine learning techniques. The goal of this study is to use the Decision Tree algorithm to predict the two forms of thyroid disorders.

INTRODUCTION

A variety of conditions affecting the thyroid gland, an organ shaped like a butterfly situated at the front of the neck, are collectively referred to as thyroid diseases. The thyroid gland is a vital organ that regulates many body processes through the production of hormones that affect growth, energy levels,

DOI: 10.4018/979-8-3693-9420-5.ch009

metabolism, and general energy balance. Accurate diagnosis and treatment are crucial for thyroid illnesses since they can have a substantial negative influence on a person's health and well-being. People nowadays are increasingly prone to ailments such as diabetes, thyroid disease, TB, and CKD, among other things. The thyroid is one of the most frequent lifestyle diseases, ranking ninth. The butterfly-shaped thyroid gland, which is located beneath the human voice box, is the most important organ of the endocrine system. Triiodothyronine (T3) and Thyroxine (T4), the two main hormones produced by the thyroid gland, control the body's overall metabolism. A thyroid condition is defined as a thyroid gland that is absent or not functioning properly. Two common thyroid problems can cause the thyroid gland to become either hyperactive or underactive. Two types of thyroid disorders exist: Hyperthyroidism, which results in an excessive amount of thyroid hormone being released into the bloodstream, and hypothyroidism, which results in an insufficient amount of thyroid hormone being released into the bloodstream. The pituitary gland, which is located close to the base of the brain and controls thyroid function, produces the hormone known as thyroid stimulating hormone (TSH). To assess the thyroid glands' functioning, a blood sample's TSH (Triiodothyronine) and Thyroxine (T4) levels are measured (Kuragayala, 2023).

The healthcare sector benefits from increasing advances in computational biology. It enabled the collection of stored patient data for medical disease prediction. For early disease diagnosis, there are a variety of intelligent prediction systems available. In the development of a prediction model, machine learning algorithms have played a critical role in handling difficult and nonlinear problems. Models are needed to identify the features that may be selected from many datasets in any disease and infection diagnosis. These features can readily be utilized as a technique for accurately classifying healthy patients. Otherwise, a patient who is otherwise healthy may be subjected to unneeded treatment as a result of a classification error. The machine learning classification model will begin predicting the class of a given feature set once it has been trained (Nirmala et al., 2023).

Importance of Accurate Thyroid Disease Classification: Because thyroid disease has a significant impact on patient health and treatment efficacy, accurate classification is crucial. Correct diagnosis is vital since thyroid problems, including Hyperthyroidism, hypothyroidism, and thyroid cancer, can mimic other ailments and present with a variety of symptoms. Proper categorization guarantees that patients obtain the right diagnosis to cure the disease. For example, misdiagnosing hypothyroidism as Hyperthyroidism may result in the administration of improper medicine, which may exacerbate symptoms and may lead to serious health problems. Precise classification aids in establishing the seriousness and stage of the condition, which is essential for treatment, including changes in medication, surgery, or radioactive iodine therapy.

Additionally, it makes it easier for medical professionals to track how an illness develops and responds to treatment. Precise classification also lessens the possibility of pointless diagnostic procedures and therapies, which lessens patient anxiety and medical expenses. A precise classification also supports personalized medication, in which treatment regimens are customized for each patient based on their unique profile and thyroid status. By attending to each patient's specific needs and raising their standard of living generally, this method improves therapy results and patient satisfaction. To summarise, the precise categorization of thyroid diseases is essential for efficient therapeutic interventions, ideal disease control, and enhanced patient results. This emphasizes the significance of utilizing modern diagnostic instruments and ML approaches in the medical field.

Role of Computing Techniques: By making it possible to collect and analyze complicated medical data effectively, computing tools are crucial in the advancement of the field of thyroid disease classification. Large datasets can be automatically examined with these methods, revealing links and patterns that conventional methods might have overlooked. By offering an in-depth understanding of patient situations and making a variety of information easier to handle, including biochemical indicators and clinical symptoms, they improve the accuracy of diagnosis. Furthermore, by customizing predictions to each patient's unique profile, these methods enhance personalized medicine by enhancing treatment results. Their capacity to learn continuously and adjust to new data helps create more dependable and current diagnostic tools, which in turn improve patient care and help clinicians make more educated decisions.

Importance of ML in Medical Diagnosis: An encouraging substitute is provided by ML, which increases the Precision of thyroid illness classification and automates the diagnosis procedure. ML algorithms can find patterns and correlations in medical data that may be hard for human clinicians to notice by examining vast datasets of patient information, including demographic information, clinical symptoms, and results of biochemical tests. This prediction ability is especially useful in the medical field as prompt and precise diagnosis (Kharayat et al., 2024). By customizing predictions based on unique patient profiles, the application of ML models also supports personalized medicine by enhancing treatment outcomes. Additionally, machine learning algorithms are always learning from fresh data and becoming more flexible to accommodate changing medical practices and understanding. Their capacity to produce probabilistic results facilitates decision-making in the face of uncertainty, which is typical in the diagnostics of medical conditions.

In general, machine learning models improve the effectiveness, Precision, and consistency of thyroid disease categorization, which eventually leads to improved patient outcomes and more knowledgeable clinical results. Because ML offers strong tools for analyzing complicated healthcare data and enhancing diagnostic accuracy, it has completely changed the field of medical diagnosis. Large-scale patient data, such as medical histories, symptoms, test results, and imaging studies, are utilized by ML algorithms in medical diagnostics to find trends and forecast illness (Regin et al., 2023). The creation of predictive models that help medical personnel detect diseases early on is one of the main uses of ML in diagnostics. ML algorithms can precisely identify anomalies in scans, like tumours or lesions, by analyzing imaging data. These algorithms learn to recognize small patterns that could suggest different illnesses by being trained on massive datasets of labelled photos (Bose et al., 2023).

Apart from analyzing images, ML algorithms are employed to evaluate structured data, such as electronic health records (EHRs), to forecast patient results and provide customized therapy plans. For instance, using risk variables and past data, algorithms can evaluate patient data to forecast the chance of contracting specific diseases, like diabetes or cardiovascular disease. With the use of methods like clustering, regression, and classification, ML also improves diagnostic accuracy (Chunduri et al., 2024). DTs and NB(Naive Bayes) are two examples of classification algorithms that can be used to classify patient data into distinct illness classifications, which aids in the diagnosis of diseases like thyroid disorders. Based on patient data, regression algorithms can forecast continuous results, such as the course of a disease. Algorithms for clustering patients together based on shared symptoms or biomarkers facilitate the discovery of uncommon or disease-specific subgroups.ML algorithms are always learning from fresh data, which allows them to adjust to changing medical practices and understanding. Maintaining diagnostic relevance and accuracy is aided by the models' capacity to be improved over time. ML models improve the ability to handle and comprehend complicated data in medical diagnostics, which results in faster and more accurate diagnoses, more individualized treatment patterns, and better patient results. Healthcare professionals can improve decision-making and progress in the medical sector by incorporating ML into clinical workflows and utilizing data-driven insights. All of the classification algorithms were chosen for their qualities, which are often utilized in research and can achieve good results.

Furthermore, they generate classification models using a variety of methodologies, increasing the odds of finding a model with high classification accuracy (Karthikeyan et al., 2024). Decision Tree (DT) and Naive Bayes Classification are two data mining classification algorithms used in this study. However, in this paper, a framework based on Decision Trees is proposed, and the output is compared to the Naive Bayes Classification model to assess performance accuracy and Precision (Princy Reshma et al., 2023).

LITERATURE REVIEW

Ajayi et al. (2021) stressed the importance of genetic information in detecting and treating disorders connected to autoimmune thyroid disease in this review. Among these conditions are Hashimoto's thyroiditis, hypothyroid autoimmune thyroiditis, Graves' disease, and moderate subclinical thyroid abnormalities. Furthermore, the part played by environmental and endocrine risk factors in the genesis of the illness in individuals with a genetic predisposition was investigated. As a result, endocrinologists may face challenges in the field of cancer and thyroid nodules, such as uncertain biomarkers and a shortage of different therapy options due to genetic differences. Using artificial intelligence and genomic databases in precision medicine could increase diagnostic and therapeutic capacities (Pandit, 2023)

The classification algorithms were studied on datasets of five diseases in this research by Singh (2019). The data collected on patients with heart disease, thyroid illness, and diabetes was retrieved from an online catalogue (Saxena and Chaudhary, 2023). The capacity to classify clinical datasets is evaluated using both parametric and non-parametric ML algorithms. Two feature selection procedures are integrated to compare the effectiveness of the system that has been created. A filter method approach is used initially to select the features. Then, a wrapper process methodology is used to assess the classification performance based on the combination of those features. The Fisher Discriminant Ratio value is used in binary classification to rank the features according to significance. Three performance metrics were used to see the effects of incorporating more features into the classification algorithm. The findings are surprising, which adds to the importance of this research (Hariprasath et al., 2024).

This study by Hugar et al. (2020) may be used to analyze Thyroid Hormone levels using Naive Bayesian Classification, which can help clinicians categorize Thyroid issues more correctly. It is also beneficial to Thyroid patients since if a Thyroid problem is discovered, timely remedies can be implemented, increasing the patient's quality of life. The dataset utilized in this study can be expanded by including more patient information and test-level information in the database. The accuracy of the Naive Bayesian classification algorithm in diagnosing thyroid disorders improves as a result. PyQt5, a cross-platform Python GUI toolkit, was used to create a user-friendly interface for this project (Odoemena and Elufidodo, 2024).

The research of Vidhushavarshini et al. (2017) employs data mining classifiers to diagnose thyroid issues by developing a knowledge prediction model for patients based on their medical history. In this investigation, the J48 and Naive Bayes classifiers were used, and their comparison was done using the WEKA tool.The results of the investigation show that the Naive Bayes classifier is not as accurate as the decision tree J48, which is a highly accurate classifier. Naive Bayes can only have a linear, elliptic, or parabolic decision boundary as a consequence, which significantly increases the flexibility of the J48 decision tree. Because the variables are interdependent, J48 produces superior outcomes. To improve accuracy, the J48 could be equipped with another classifier in the future (Raghuraman et al., 2019).

To further the goals of the research proposed by Razia et al. (2017), an integrated model based on two neural models (SOM and LVQ) has been developed. The 215 instances of the unlabelled dataset were taken from the UCI machine learning repository. The model's five inputs are serum thyroxin, total serum thyroxin, TSH, and max thyroxin. The output is status, which has values of 1 (hyper), 2 (hypo), and 3 (hypo) (Normal). The integrated model was developed using a vector quantization technique and a competitive learning strategy. When the outcomes of a decision tree model and the integrated model were evaluated for disease prediction, the integrated model fared better in terms of network accuracy (Tyagi et al., 2018).

The thyroid gland medical problems produced by underactive or hyperactive thyroid glands are the topic of this study by IzdiharBozkus (2016). The decision tree approach was used to classify this thyroid illness dataset from the UCI repository. For training, the overall prediction accuracy is 100 per cent, and for testing, it is between 98.7% and 99.8%. PyDev, a Python IDE for Eclipse, was used to create this, which can successfully assist in making the proper decision (Panyaram, 2024).

This survey by Shankar et al. (2020) is necessary to determine the usage of data mining techniques to forecast thyroid disorders at an earlier stage. The goal of this work is to use several ensemble classification and feature selection algorithms to predict thyroid illness. These strategies aid in reducing the amount of noisy data in patient data sets (Ajitha et al., 2024). These various algorithmic results depend on the cost of the treatment and the speed, accuracy, and efficiency of the model. The positive and negative values from the hyperthyroid, hypothyroid, and sick thyroid datasets are extracted using ensemble techniques. The experimental results indicate that females are more influenced than males when comparing datasets with and without gender. Further improvements have been obtained by the application of other optimization techniques or rule extraction algorithms.

Olalekan et al. (2020), in this research, employ an ensemble of Bagging with J45 and an ensemble of Bagging with SimpleCart to create an efficient and reliable prototype for thyroid illness forecasting in order to retrieve relevant information and detect problems. The performances of the two ensemble models were contrasted with those of single classifiers. The thyroid prediction system's Bagging ensemble algorithm claims an impressive 99.66 per cent overall accuracy. In contrast, other single-selected classifiers, such as Bagging and SimpleCART, have somewhat lower accuracy and take less time to build the model (Minu et al., 2023).

PROPOSED METHODOLOGY

In the architectural process of performing classification models for disease prediction, the input data is first fed into databases. Input data may have missing values, noisy values, or data that is inconsistent. In a preprocessing stage, such data must be preprocessed. The best feature selection is a crucial stage towards improved classification. The dataset is separated into training and testing data for the classification procedure. The classification algorithm is fed with training data, which is then verified with testing data. The Accuracy and Precision of the data are used to evaluate its overall performance. Finally, the predicted values obtained using the proposed Decision Tree algorithm are compared to those produced using the Naive Bayes classifier.

Loading Dataset: This work uses a publicly available classification dataset for ANN training from the University of California, Irvine (UCI) Machine Learning Repository. This data set was chosen because of the prevalence of nominal traits and their dominance in the literature. It has 3772 training and

3428 testing examples with 15 categories and six actual attributes. The aim is to determine a patient's classification into one of three groups—normal, Hyperthyroidism, or hypothyroidism.

Preprocessing: Preprocessing guarantees the quality and applicability of the data used for model training and assessment, which is crucial for the classification of thyroid diseases. Cleaning and converting raw data to address problems like outliers, inconsistencies, and missing values is an essential part of proper preprocessing because these problems can cause predictions to be erroneous or biased. The process of standardizing and normalizing characteristics aids in preparing the data for analysis by preventing the performance of the model from being negatively impacted by varying scales and units (Raghuraman et al., 2019). The most pertinent variables for classification are also found through the use of feature selection and dimensionality reduction approaches, which improve model accuracy and lower computing complexity. Preprocessing enhances the model's capacity to learn from a variety of input sources and produce more accurate predictions. It also involves managing imbalanced datasets and encoding categorical variables. Comprehensive preprocessing raises the quality of the data, boosts the performance of the model, and eventually helps to produce a more precise and useful categorization of thyroid diseases. The transformations that convert unbalanced data into balanced data are referred to as preprocessing. It's a method for converting distorted, noisy, or missing-value data into a clean set of data. Cleaning, editing, wrangling, feature removal, and selection are all different types of data processing. The high quality of data will lead to high-quality findings, as well as lower data mining costs.

Clustering: By assisting in the identification of naturally occurring groupings or patterns within the data that may not be immediately apparent, clustering plays an important role in the classification of thyroid diseases. This method of unsupervised learning can identify different patient subgroups based on shared clinical characteristics, signs, or biochemical markers. Clustering can help to increase the granularity of the classification process and aid in comprehending the various forms of thyroid illnesses by revealing these hidden patterns (Tyagi et al., 2018).

Clustering is the idea of gathering like objects together in one group and dissimilar objects together in another. This will aid in the grouping of parameters inside the dataset. In probabilistic models, the Expectation-Maximization (EM) process is used to find the maximum estimate attributes. It's utilized to cluster the thyroid data that's been provided. Clustering techniques are applied to improve the accuracy of the classifier. After initializing the features to random values, the probability for each potential value is computed. The obtained values are then utilized to produce a more accurate approximation for the qualities. These steps are repeated until convergence is achieved. By arranging the data into meaningful clusters, clustering can help with preprocessing in the categorization of thyroid diseases. These clusters can then be utilized to improve supervised learning models. Clustering, for instance, can be used to find homogeneous patient groups that need various methods of diagnosis or therapy. It can also draw attention to outliers or anomalies that might require extra care. Clustering improves the capacity to more precisely and individually customize thyroid illness diagnoses and therapy plans.

Feature Selection and Construction: When it comes to classifying thyroid diseases, feature selection is essential since it enhances model performance by concentrating on the most pertinent variables and removing those that are superfluous or unnecessary. Feature selection lowers the complexity of the model by selecting and keeping just the most important characteristics, which in turn minimizes overfitting and improves generalization to new data. The model becomes more effective and simpler to understand as a result of this approach, which also expedites the training and evaluation stages (Pandit, 2023). Feature selection or attribute selection is used in machine learning to determine the right features to classify and minimize training time. It's not the same as feature extraction, and it's used to make models easier to understand. This approach reduces file size by deleting unnecessary and irrelevant data while also improving learning accuracy. The filter model and the wrapper model are the two main types of feature selection algorithms. Feature construction is a method for framing intermediate features from a dataset. The objective is to generate more efficient data mining features. Feature selection aids in the identification of the primary biomarkers, symptoms, or clinical criteria that are most suggestive of thyroid abnormalities in classifying thyroid diseases. With this focused approach, the model is constructed using the most relevant data, resulting in predictions that are more accurate and dependable. Effective feature selection can also shed light on the underlying causes of thyroid disorders, which can direct future investigation and enhance methods for diagnosis and therapy. Feature selection is essential to creating reliable, accurate, and efficient thyroid disease classification models.

Prediction: Classification methods are important for the prediction of thyroid disease because they allow complicated medical data to be automatically analyzed, which speeds up and improves the accuracy of diagnosis. Manual diagnosis of thyroid problems, including Hyperthyroidism and hypothyroidism, can be difficult since their symptoms frequently coincide with those of other ailments. Classification algorithms can accurately identify various thyroid disorders by examining trends in huge datasets that contain patient demographics, symptoms, and biochemical markers. By reducing the need for human interpretation—which can be laborious and error-prone—this automation enables early intervention, which enhances results. Medical data is large and diverse, with both continuous and categorical variables. Techniques for classification can handle this complexity. This data can be processed effectively by algorithms such as DTs, Naive Bayes, and SVM, which can reveal which features (such as TSH, T3, and T4 levels) are most indicative of thyroid disease. These models adjust predictions according to specific patient profiles, which not only improves diagnostic accuracy but also advances personalized therapy. Healthcare practitioners may guarantee that patients obtain the most suitable treatments at the earliest opportunity, save money, and increase diagnostic Precision by incorporating these computations into clinical procedures. The prediction of the thyroid category from the given dataset is based on the classification process. The aim now is to predict if a new patient entry is normal or abnormal when given as input. If it is abnormal, then the prediction must be either the person is suffering from hypothyroid or hyperthyroid. Various classification algorithms are used to predict the three classes. Here, the Decision Tree Algorithm is proposed to predict the class of the given dataset along with the NB algorithm for comparison.

Decision Tree (DT): Decision trees are easy to understand, straightforward, and capable of handling intricate, nonlinear correlations in medical data, so they are essential for classifying thyroid conditions. Their transparent decision-making process allows clinicians to easily understand and trust the model's predictions, which is crucial in healthcare settings. Additionally, decision trees can manage missing data, provide insights into feature importance, and perform well in scenarios with class imbalance. These characteristics make decision trees not only effective for accurate thyroid classification but also practical for real-time clinical decision-making. Regression and classification issues can be resolved with the help of supervised learning algorithms like the Decision Tree algorithm. By using training data to teach decision rules, DT aims to create a model that can predict the class of target variables. The DT algorithm uses a tree representation with internal and leaf nodes. Every class label correlates to a leaf node in the tree, while every attribute or feature connects to an internal node. Select relevant features based on metrics such as Information Gain (IG) or Gini Index (GI). To obtain information, utilize

$$IG(T, A) = Entropy(T) - \sum_{v \in Values(A)} \frac{|T_v|}{|T|} Entropy(T_v) \quad (1)$$

Where **Entropy(T)** is

$$Entropy(T) = -\sum_{i=1}^{k} p_i \log_2(p_i) \quad (2)$$

where p_i is the percentage of class I examples

Using a split ratio of, say, 80% for training and 20% for testing, divide the dataset into training and testing sets. The dataset is recursively divided according to the characteristic that minimizes the GI or maximizes IG. Regarding the GI

$$Gini(T) = 1 - \sum_{i=1}^{k} p_i^2 \quad (3)$$

where p_i is the percentage of class I examples. Divide nodes according to feature A that offers the lowest GI or the highest IG. Given a split A, which may have values v:

$$Gain(A) = Entropy(T) - \sum_{v \in Values(A)} \frac{|T_v|}{|T|} Entropy(T_v) \quad (4)$$

where the subset T_v of T is defined by A=v.

Analyze the model's performance with measures like Accuracy and Precision on the testing set.

The algorithm goes as follows.

1. The best attribute or feature is placed at the root of the tree to predict a class label for the dataset.
2. To compare the values of the record's attribute with the root attribute, preconditions like "true" or "false" are employed.
3. Based on the comparison, the branch that corresponds to that value is followed and jumped to the subsequent node.
4. Up until a leaf node with the anticipated class value is reached, the comparison of the record's attribute values is carried out with other internal nodes of the tree.
5. The tree is trimmed to get rid of duplicates and needless preconditions.

Naïve Bayes (NB): NB is a significant method in thyroid classification because of its effectiveness, ease of use, and good results even with little datasets. It functions according to the Bayes theorem, which assumes that features are independent of one another given the class label. This assumption is often not strictly accurate, but it generally works well for a variety of medical datasets. By computing the likelihood of each class depending on the input features, such as hormone levels and symptoms, Naive Bayes can quickly determine whether someone has a thyroid issue. It helps make decisions under ambiguity, which is prevalent in medical diagnostics, because of its capacity to process categorical input and produce probabilistic results. Furthermore, Naive Bayes is robust even when working with relatively small or noisy thyroid datasets since it is less likely to overfit.

If there are p classes, say B_1, B_2,...B_q, each with an unknown data sample X, an NB classifier will assign an unknown sample X to a class Based on the classes with the highest probability

$$P(B_i X) > P(B_j X) \text{ for } 1 \leq j \leq p ---- \quad (5)$$

The foundation of Naive Bayes is the presumption that characteristics, given the class name, are conditionally independent. This makes it easier to calculate probabilities since it lets the model treat each feature as though it makes a separate contribution to the final result. Determine each class's prior probability $P(Y = y_i)$ using

$$P(Y = y_i) = \frac{N_{y_i}}{N} ------- \quad (6)$$

Compute the likelihood P(xj|Y=yi) for each feature xj. This might include calculating parameters for a probability distribution (such as the Gaussian distribution) using continuous features. Use these for categorical characteristics.

$$P\left(x_j | Y = y_i\right) = \frac{N_{x_j, y_i} + \alpha}{N_{y_i} + \alpha.\, k} ------ \quad (7)$$

Where k is the total number of possible feature values, α is a smoothing parameter, and N_{x_j, y_i} is the count of feature x_j in class y_i

To find the posterior probability for each class y_i for a given instance with features $x = \{x_1, x_2, \ldots x_n\}$ Use the following formula.

$$P\left(Y = y_i | X = x\right) = \frac{P(Y = y_i).\, \prod_{j=1}^{n} P(x_j | Y = y_i)}{P(X = x)} ----- \quad (8)$$

As P(X=x) remains constant across all classes, it is frequently left out of the computation in favour of maximizing.

$$P\left(Y = y_i | X = x\right) \propto P(Y - y_i).\, \prod_{j=1}^{n} P(x_j | Y = y_i) ----- \quad (9)$$

Sort the instance into the class where the posterior probability is the largest.

$$\hat{y} = \underset{y_i}{\text{argmax}} P(Y = y_i | X = x) ------- \quad (10)$$

Using criteria like Accuracy and Precision, evaluate the Naive Bayes model's performance using a test dataset.

RESULTS AND DISCUSSIONS

Performance Evaluation: Performance metrics, which offer quantifiable measurements to assess and compare the efficacy of various classification models, are essential for the categorization of thyroid diseases. The purpose of this work is to use two machine learning algorithms, DT and Naive Bayes, to estimate the prediction of thyroid disease. The results of various models are compared and examined based on a few evaluation criteria, including Accuracy and Precision.

Accuracy Analysis: It's only the proportion of accurately predicted observations to total observations. The percentage of successfully identified instances in thyroid classification is measured by accuracy, which provides a general picture of the model's performance.

$$\text{Accuracy} = \frac{\text{True Positive} + \text{True Negative}}{\text{True Positive} + \text{False Positive} + \text{True Negative} + \text{False Negative}} - - - \qquad (11)$$

The following Table 1 and Figure 1 show the accuracy obtained from the dataset by Naive Bayes and Decision Tree. It clearly shows that Decision Tree performs better than Naive Bayes in terms of accuracy.

Table 1. Accuracy by Naive Bayes and Decision Tree

No of Iterations	Naive Bayes Accuracy %	Decision Tree Accuracy %
10	73.59	79.96
20	73.92	80.21
30	74.12	80.66
40	74.89	80.87
50	74.97	80.93

Figure 1. Accuracy by Naive Bayes and Decision Tree Graph

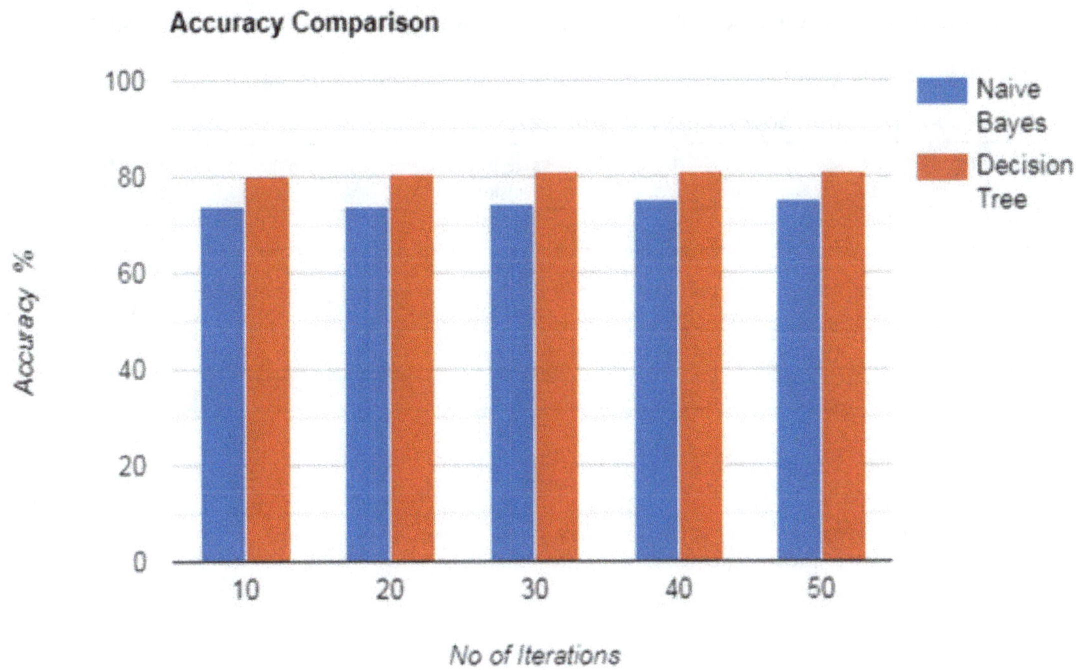

The iterative analysis of the study shows that although the accuracy of the DT and NB algorithms increases with the number of iterations, the DT consistently exceeds the NB algorithm in the prediction of thyroid illnesses. NB begins with an accuracy of 73.59% after 10 iterations, while the DT starts at 79.96%. Both algorithms demonstrate gradual gains as the number of iterations rises; at 50 iterations, NB achieves 74.97% accuracy, while the DT reaches 80.93% accuracy. This pattern shows how well the DT algorithm handles the dataset, continuously delivering increased accuracy with every iteration. While NB continues to improve, it is still less efficient than the DT, suggesting that the DT is a better fit for this particular thyroid classification problem.

Precision Analysis: It's the proportion of accurately predicted positive observations to the total number of positive observations predicted. When it comes to thyroid categorization, accuracy is very crucial since it determines the percentage of actual positive diagnoses among all anticipated positives, which shows how many cases of predicted thyroid disorders are recognized. To reduce the possibility of false positives, which can result in needless therapies or follow-up testing, high Precision is crucial.

$$\text{Precision} = \frac{\text{True Positive}}{\text{True Positive} + \text{False Positive}} \quad (12)$$

The comprehensive evaluation and optimization of thyroid classification models made possible by the use of these performance indicators result in more precise and dependable diagnoses and improved patient results.

Table 2 and Figure 2 show the Precision obtained from the dataset by Naive Bayes and Decision Tree. It clearly shows that Decision Tree performs better than Naive Bayes in terms of Precision.

Table 2. Precision by Naive Bayes and Decision Tree

No. of Iterations	Naive Bayes Precision %	Decision Tree Precision %
10	60.54	79.72
20	71.92	80.23
30	72.45	81.98
40	72.98	82.92
50	73.92	83.93

Figure 2. Precision by Naive Bayes and Decision Tree Graph

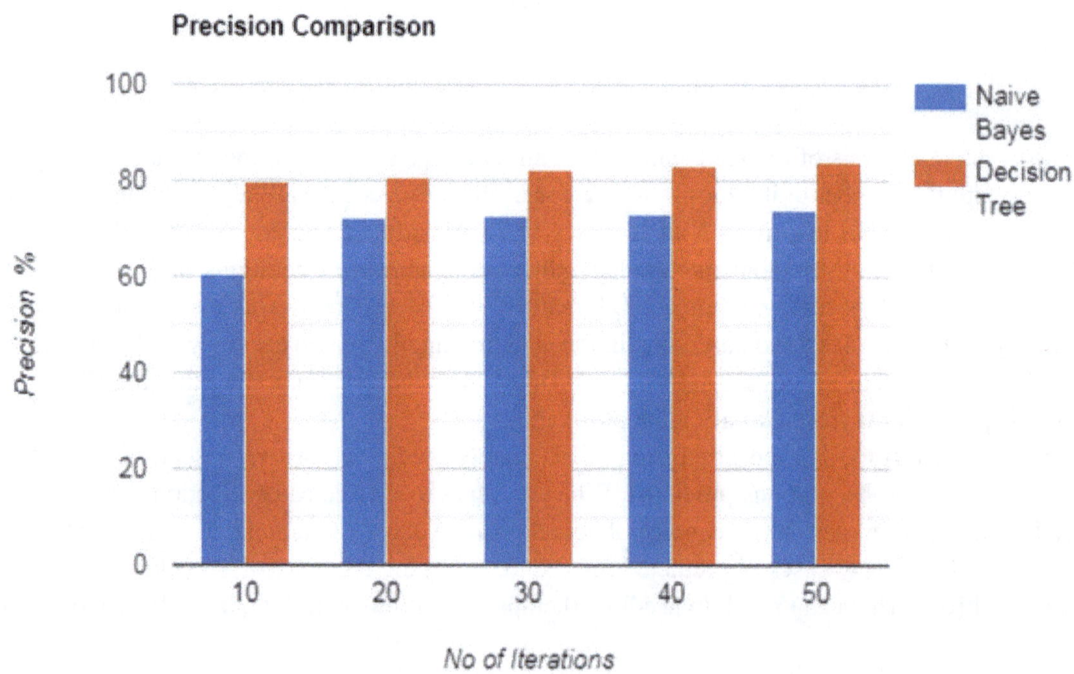

Based on all iterations, the research shows that the DT method performs much better in terms of Precision than NB. The DT begins with a higher precision of 79.72%, whereas NB gets a precision of 60.54% after 10 iterations. Both methods demonstrate increasing Precision with the number of iterations; at 50 iterations, NB reaches 73.92%. On the other hand, the DT algorithm keeps outperforming it, finishing the iterations with a precision of 83.93%. The DT consistently outperforms other methods for precise disease prediction in this dataset, as evidenced by its superior ability to detect positive cases of thyroid diseases accurately.

Findings: The DT consistently performs better than the NB classifier during the iterations. The DT performs better in classifying thyroid illnesses and is better suited for the dataset because its accuracy is higher at every stage. Compared to NB, the DT's Accuracy increased significantly and steadily, indicating that it would be able to identify more intricate patterns and correlations in the data. The DT's capacity to manage nonlinear relationships and feature interactions may be the cause of this. In this case, the statistics suggest that the DT is a more reliable and accurate model for classifying thyroid illness. Naive Bayes likewise gets better with repetitions, but its overall performance stays lower. Therefore, it might not be as good for applications that demand greater accuracy. The DT classifier performs more accurately than NB at every iteration point. This suggests that the DT is more successful in reducing false positives, which is important for correctly diagnosing thyroid illness. The DT appears to be more accurate in differentiating between positive and negative cases based on its higher Precision. This suggests that the DT causes fewer false positive predictions since it is more accurate in identifying patients with thyroid problems. Based on the available data, the DT classifier has superior accuracy performance, rendering it the recommended option for applications requiring accurate detection of positive cases. Even if it's getting better, NB still lacks Precision, which could lead to more false positives and less accurate classification.

CONCLUSION AND FUTURE WORK

The thyroid gland is the endocrine system's primary and largest gland. The data mining technique is used on the thyroid dataset to determine which cases are normal and which are abnormal. The objective of this project is to perceive the thyroid classes based on the UCI medical dataset. For the prediction, the decision tree method was devised, which aids in the correct detection of thyroid disease. The data is divided into three categories: hyper, hypo, and normal. When comparing the Accuracy and Precision of the classifier to diagnose thyroid disease, it was discovered that Decision Trees outperformed Naive Bayes. The results are analyzed, and based on assessment metrics, the Decision Tree algorithm's classification accuracy is 80 per cent, and Precision is 81 per cent. To improve accuracy, the Decision Tree can be augmented with another classifier in the future. To improve model performance, future research on thyroid problem categorization should concentrate on growing the dataset to include a larger and more varied sample, as well as adding new characteristics such as genetic information and sophisticated imaging. Predictive performance may be enhanced by investigating innovative ML approaches like ensemble methods and DL(Deep Learning). Practical use will need to address the class imbalance using techniques such as oversampling and incorporating models into clinical processes. Furthermore, ongoing validation and upgrades based on fresh information and cutting-edge studies will support the models' continued applicability and efficiency in real-world situations.

REFERENCES

Ajitha, Y., Talukder, M. S. H., & Shuvo, S. A. (2024). Advanced radar range prediction and performance analysis in aircraft adhoc networks (AANET). *FMDB Transactions on Sustainable Computer Letters*, *2*(1), 1–13. DOI: 10.69888/FTSCL.2024.000177

Bose, S. R., Sirajudheen, M. A. S., Kirupanandan, G., Arunagiri, S., Regin, R., & Rajest, S. S. (2023). Fine-grained independent approach for workout classification using integrated metric transfer learning. In *Advanced Applications of Generative AI and Natural Language Processing Models* (pp. 358–372). IGI Global. DOI: 10.4018/979-8-3693-0502-7.ch017

Chunduri, V., Hannan, S. A., Devi, G. M., Nomula, V. K., Tripathi, V., & Rajest, S. S. (2024). Deep convolutional neural networks for lung segmentation for diffuse interstitial lung disease on HRCT and volumetric CT. In *Advances in Computational Intelligence and Robotics* (pp. 335–350). IGI Global.

Folorunsho Ajayi, A., Tayo Adebayo, E., Oluwadunsi Adebayo, I., Simeon Oyekunle, O., Oluwaseyi Amos, V., Emmanuel Bamidele, S., & Olusayo Olatinwo, G. (2022). Application of data science approaches to investigate autoimmune thyroid disease in precision medicine. In *Hypothyroidism - New Aspects of an Old Disease*. Intech Open. DOI: 10.5772/intechopen.101220

Hariprasath, G., Dhinakaran, P., & Kumar, V. H. (2024). Exploring the efficacy of LightGBM, AdaBoost, and CatBoost in Alzheimer's disease classification. *FMDB Transactions on Sustainable Health Science Letters*, *2*(1), 41–55. DOI: 10.69888/FTSHSL.2024.000171

Hugar, P., Pranaygoud, G., Vishnuvardhan, K., & Faizuddin, M. (2020). Thyroid problem detection using Naive Bayesian classification. *International Journal of Creative Research Thoughts*, *8*(2), 1340–1343.

Izdiharbozkus, Z. (2016). MLTDD: Use of Machine Learning Techniques for Diagnosis of Thyroid Gland Disorder. *Computer Science and Information Technology*, *6*(4), 67–73.

Karthikeyan, B., Devi, R. A., & Munshi, M. (2024). Utilizing Deep Learning for the Classification of Brain Tumours Using MRI. *AVE Trends In Intelligent Health Letters*, *1*(1), 1–9.

Kharayat, A., Rawat, D., & Panwar, N. (2024). A Study on the Efficiency of Structured Instruction on Dengue Fever Prevention and Control among People. *AVE Trends In Intelligent Social Letters*, *1*(1), 25–40.

Kuragayala, P. S. (2023). A Systematic Review on Workforce Development in Healthcare Sector: Implications in the Post-COVID Scenario. *FMDB Transactions on Sustainable Technoprise Letters*, *1*(1), 36–46.

Minu, M. S., Subashka Ramesh, S. S., Canessane, R., Al-Amin, M., & Bin Sulaiman, R. (2023). Experimental Analysis of UAV Networks Using Oppositional Glowworm Swarm Optimization and Deep Learning Clustering and Classification. *FMDB Transactions on Sustainable Computing Systems*, *1*(3), 124–134.

Nirmala, G., Premavathy, R., Chandar, R., & Jeganathan, J. (2023). An Explanatory Case Report on Biopsychosocial Issues and the Impact of Innovative Nurse-Led Therapy in Children with Hematological Cancer. *FMDB Transactions on Sustainable Health Science Letters*, *1*(1), 1–10.

Odoemena, O. F., & Elufidodo, G. A. (2024). Machine learning-based cardiovascular disease detection and intelligent healthcare workflow automation. *FMDB Transactions on Sustainable Health Science Letters*, *2*(2), 81–93. DOI: 10.69888/FTSHSL.2024.000174

Olalekan, A., Ogwueleka, F., & Odion, P. O. (2020). Effective and accurate bootstrap aggregating (bagging) ensemble algorithm model for prediction and classification of hypothyroid disease. *International Journal of Computer Applications*, *176*(39), 40–48. DOI: 10.5120/ijca2020920542

Pandit, P. (2023). On the Context of Diabetes: A Brief Discussion on the Novel Ethical Issues of Non-communicable Diseases. *FMDB Transactions on Sustainable Health Science Letters*, *1*(1), 11–20.

Panyaram, S. (2024). Integrating artificial intelligence with big data for real-time insights and decision-making in complex systems. *FMDB Transactions on Sustainable Intelligent Networks*, *1*(2), 85–95. DOI: 10.69888/FTSIN.2024.000211

Raghuraman, M.T., & Sailatha, E & Gunasekaran, Sethu. (2019). Discrimination Efficiency Identification for Human Thyroid Disorder Blood Discovery and PredictionUsing Machine Learning Algorithms. *Cikitusi Journal for Multidisciplinary Research*, *6*(6), 31–37.

Razia, S. (1996). A neuro computing framework for thyroid disease diagnosis using machine learning techniques. *Journal of Theoretical and Applied Information Technology*, *95*(9), 1996–2005.

Regin, R., T, S., George, S. R., Bhattacharya, M., Datta, D., & Priscila, S. S. (2023). Development of predictive model of diabetic using supervised machine learning classification algorithm of ensemble voting. *International Journal of Bioinformatics Research and Applications*, *19*(3), 151–169. DOI: 10.1504/IJBRA.2023.10057044

Saxena, D., & Chaudhary, S. (2023). Predicting Brain Diseases from FMRI-Functional Magnetic Resonance Imaging with Machine Learning Techniques for Early Diagnosis and Treatment. *FMDB Transactions on Sustainable Computer Letters*, *1*(1), 33–48.

Shankar, K., Lakshmanaprabu, S. K., Gupta, D., Maseleno, A., & de Albuquerque, V. H. C. (2020). RETRACTED ARTICLE: Optimal feature-based multi-kernel SVM approach for thyroid disease classification. *The Journal of Supercomputing*, *76*(2), 1128–1143. DOI: 10.1007/s11227-018-2469-4

Singh, A. K. (2019). A Comparative Study on Disease Classification using Machine Learning Algorithms, Proceedings of 2nd International Conference on Advanced Computing and Software Engineering (ICACSE), Available at SSRN, Sultanpur, Uttar Pradesh, India DOI: 10.2139/ssrn.3350251

Tyagi, A., Mehra, R., & Saxena, A. (2018). Interactive thyroid disease prediction system using machine learning technique. *2018 Fifth International Conference on Parallel, Distributed and Grid Computing (PDGC)*, Solan, India. DOI: 10.1109/PDGC.2018.8745910

Vidhushavarshinisathiyabhama, B. (2017). *A Comparison of Classification Techniques on Thyroid Detection Using J48 and Naive Bayes Classification Techniques.*

Chapter 10
Efficient Method for Predicting Thyroid Disease Classification Using Xgboost Compared to K-Nearest Neighbours Algorithm With Improved Accuracy

V. Brindha
https://orcid.org/0009-0005-2415-4930
Bharath Institute of Higher Education and Research, India

A. Muthukumaravel
Bharath Institute of Higher Education and Research, India

ABSTRACT

The use of machine learning algorithms to develop disease detection in the medical area is becoming increasingly popular due to its reliability and efficacy. The thyroid is an endocrine gland that generates hormones that aid in the body's metabolism management. Computer diagnosis plays a critical role in thyroid condition prediction, and this research examines the classification models utilized in thyroid disease. Classifying thyroid-related illnesses entails dividing them into groups according to their clinical manifestation, hormone levels, and underlying pathology. The timely identification and precise categorization of thyroid problems are crucial for efficient handling and therapy, given their substantial influence on an individual's standard of living. Comprehending the fundamental reasons, indications, and suitable diagnostic methods is essential for accurate categorization and the ensuing treatment measures.

INTRODUCTION

In the healthcare sector, advances in computational biology are being used to acquire patient data for clinical prediction and diagnosis. Various sophisticated prediction systems are available to diagnose the disease at its earliest stages. Machine learning algorithms are critical in constructing a prediction model since they solve complicated and nonlinear situations. To accurately classify healthy patients, disease

DOI: 10.4018/979-8-3693-9420-5.ch010

prediction algorithms must prioritize variables that can be selected from several datasets. The thyroid gland is located in the neck region of the endocrine gland, which helps in the complete metabolism. The pituitary gland generally produces thyroid hormone in reaction to another hormone generated by the gland. This paper focuses on two basic forms of thyroid disorders: hyperthyroidism (excessive thyroid hormone) and hypothyroidism (insufficient thyroid hormone). Tiredness, intellectual fogginess and confusion, constipation, skin conditions, water retention, being extremely chilled, and nonspecific pains and rigidity in muscles and joints are all signs and symptoms of hypothyroidism. Mild hyperthyroidism and hyperthyroidism in people over the age of 70 frequently have no symptoms. Excessive perspiration, heat sensitivity, frequent bowel motions, anxiousness, and weight loss are all common hyperthyroidism symptoms.

Thyroid Disease Types

The three most common types of thyroid disease are hypothyroidism, hyperthyroidism, and thyroid nodules. Hypothyroidism is when the thyroid gland produces too few hormones; symptoms include weight gain, sluggishness, and cold sensitivity. However, because of an excess of hormones, hyperthyroidism causes weight loss, fast heartbeat, and excessive sweating. Abnormal growths within the thyroid gland, known as thyroid nodules, can be benign or malignant. If they are large, they may cause symptoms such as difficulty eating or breathing. In addition, the thyroid gland can become inflamed and malfunction for an extended period due to immune system attacks, such as Graves' disease and Hashimoto's thyroiditis. To preserve hormonal balance and general health, thyroid disease must be properly diagnosed and treated.

Traditional Methods

Conventional methods for classifying thyroid function include various diagnostic modalities to assess thyroid function precisely. Palpating the thyroid gland during a physical examination allows for the detection of anomalies like enlargement or nodules. In addition, thyroid function tests assess blood levels of T3, T4, and TSH, which provide information about the gland's overactive, underactive, or healthy functioning (Regin et al., 2023a).

Imaging methods are used to see and evaluate the shape and function of the thyroid gland. These methods include ultrasound, thyroid scintigraphy, and occasionally CT or MRI scans. Thyroid scintigraphy uses radioactive iodine to evaluate areas of aberrant activity, while ultrasound aids in identifying and characterizing nodules or cysts. A vital step in diagnosing diseases like thyroid cancer is acquiring tissue samples using fine needle aspiration (FNA) biopsy. Combined, these techniques provide a thorough strategy for identifying and categorizing thyroid problems, which in turn helps inform efficient treatment plans (Regin et al., 2023b).

Significance of Exact Classification

Ensuring efficient therapy and bettering patient outcomes depend on accurately classifying thyroid illness. Early intervention, which can stop the progression of thyroid diseases and reduce related health risks, is made possible by timely and accurate diagnosis. Healthcare professionals can create individualized treatment programs that meet the specific requirements of each patient by precisely diagnosing the type of thyroid issue each patient has. This focused strategy ultimately improves patient outcomes and quality of life by minimizing potential adverse effects and optimizing the effectiveness of medicines (Kumar et al., 2024). Exact classification is helpful for individual patients, improving clinical decision-making and making the best use of healthcare resources. Correct diagnostics lessen the possibility of incorrect diagnoses and ineffective treatments, saving needless operations and medical expenses. Precisely classifying thyroid problems facilitates effective management by keeping track of the disease's evolution and modifying treatment plans as necessary. This helps to maximize resource utilization and provide high-quality, reasonably priced patient care (Thirunagalingam, 2024).

Role of Classification Models.

Classification models are essential to classifying thyroid diseases because they make it possible to diagnose thyroid disorders accurately, quickly, and efficiently. These models categorize patients as having normal thyroid function, hypothyroidism, hyperthyroidism, or other related illnesses based on analysis of patient data, including hormone levels, ultrasound pictures, and other pertinent clinical information (Raj et al., 2024a). Classification models lessen the need for manual evaluations, which can be laborious and prone to human mistakes, by automating the diagnosis procedure. Better patient outcomes and prompt treatment are made possible by the quicker and more accurate diagnosis that results from this. Furthermore, sophisticated classification algorithms can process multidimensional, complex data, which enhances diagnosis accuracy and helps identify subtle patterns that conventional methods overlook. Classification models are, therefore, essential to improving and modernizing the treatment of thyroid disease (Raj et al., 2024b). The chapter's contribution is that it proposes the XGBoost algorithm for accurately predicting thyroid illness. The XGBoost method is used to identify the finest features, and its efficiency is compared to the kNN approach. The accuracy and precision of the XGBoost method are higher than that of the KNN algorithm (Jani et al., 2024).

LITERATURE REVIEW

ML is important in disease prediction, and this study by Tyagi et al. (2018) deals with the analytical and classification techniques employed in thyroid disease, drawing on statistics from the UCI archive (Princy Reshma et al., 2023). Strong foundational knowledge is essential for challenging learning tasks like medical diagnosis and prediction, as it can be embedded and used as a hybrid strategy. The scientists provided numerous ML diagnostics and measures to prevent thyroid illness in this study. The propensity of a patient to acquire thyroid disease was assessed using these techniques (Sivapriya et al., 2023).

Abbad Ur Rehman et al. (2020) incorporated the application of artificial intelligence to both thyroid datasets from the government hospital and the KEEL repository. This research aimed to determine which of the several distance functions employed in the investigation produced the best KNN distance function (Thinesh et al., 2023). This analytical study also used two well-known feature selection strategies, L1-norm, and chi-square. Several quality assessment indicators were considered, and the seven distance units were compared with or without feature selection procedures. After analyzing the results of numerous KNN distance measures, Euclidean and Cosine distance functions reached peak accuracy at the k level of 1 by applying a chi-square-based feature selection method for the newly proposed database (Minu et al., 2023).

Medici et al. (2021) research looked at modifications in clinically significant variables during levothyroxine (L-T4) treatment commencement and their capacity to forecast enhancement in Quality of Life (QoL). During the first year of L-T4 medication, the thyroid-related patient-reported objective questionnaire assessed QoL in patients with recently identified hypothyroidism (Saxena and Chaudhary, 2023). The Composite QoL scale and the Tiredness and Emotional Vulnerability sub-scales were used to determine the major performance metrics. Univariate and multiple regression modeling was used to examine medical factors such as L-T4 dose, body composition, thyroid levels, and cognitive function evaluations as predictors of QoL enhancement (Pandit, 2023).

Al-Hakim et al. (2021) said that someone with a thyroid gland problem should be diagnosed in this study. The expert system will attempt to create a design based on the indications of conditions that cause thyroid problems. This system, which uses the certainty factor approach, will make it easier to make inferences, affecting the system's confidence level in computing the weights that prevail. This concept is in the framework pattern that may be further expanded and executed for users (Das et al., 2023).

Hakim et al. (2022) intend to develop an Android-based intelligent system for the earlier detection of a thyroid problem. This approach also determines if the person has a psychiatric disease and the relationship between thyroid conditions and psychiatric conditions in thyroid disorder patients. Problem definition, literature review, and expert discussion with intensivists and psychologists are all part of the research procedure (Karthik et al., 2024). The SDLC waterfall, usability testing, patient survey data collection, and data analysis are all used in designing an Android-based expert system. A total of 50 people with thyroid problems are required as responses (Anitha et al., 2023).

Machine learning concepts to model healthcare needs are becoming more popular, as they are in various other fields. Ritesh Jha et al. (2022) research tries to provide options for such a thyroid predictive modeling. Dimension reduction techniques are used, and classifiers are fed data with decreased dimensions (Shruthi and Aravind, 2023). Data augmentation also produces enough data for the deep neural network architecture. Related studies with real-world datasets for thyroid issues and tests performed in a distributed system are compared to classification prediction. Compared to existing procedures, the suggested two-stage strategy achieves a very high level of accuracy (Peya et al., 2021).

Eleven machine-learning techniques are evaluated by Islam et al. (2022) to determine which one has the highest accuracy for correctly forecasting thyroid uncertainty (Karthikeyan et al., 2024). The Sick-euthyroid database, sourced from the University of California repository, is utilized in this investigation. Because the objective variable classes in this database are typically one, the accuracy score does not accurately reflect the projected results. Thus, ratings for accuracy and recall are included in the performance metric (Kumar, 2020). An F1 score maximizes precision and recall by producing a single number in the event of an unequal distribution class. The testing indicates that the F1-score ANN Classifier performs better in accuracy than the other nine approaches (Hariprasath et al., 2024).

Classification and clustering are the most popular data mining techniques for understanding healthcare datasets' various facets. In this study by Chandel et al. (2016), thyroid ailment is categorized using multiple classification algorithms based on factors including goiter, TSH, and T4U. Several classification techniques, such as Naive Bayes, SVM, and KNN, are used. The Rapid Miner toolkit was utilized to experiment, and the results indicate that KNN is a more accurate method for diagnosing thyroid sickness than Naive Bayes (Varmann et al., 2023).

MATERIALS AND METHODS

Pre-processing: Pre-processing is essential to classifying thyroid diseases because it guarantees that the data needed to create predictive models is accurate, up-to-date, and organized. The quality of the input data greatly influences how well machine-learning algorithms categorize thyroid illnesses. Hence, pre-processing is an essential stage in the data analysis pipeline. Pre-processing is essential for improving the precision and potency of models to predict thyroid illness. Pre-processing ensures that the data used is of the highest caliber by organizing and cleaning the data, including handling missing numbers, eliminating duplicates, and fixing inconsistencies. Due to the increased likelihood that insights derived from clean data will represent real patterns and relationships pertinent to thyroid disease, this refinement aids in developing more trustworthy and accurate predictive models.

Pre-processing optimizes the input for machine learning algorithms by standardizing and normalizing the data, which enhances model performance. By reducing noise and bias, feature scaling and dimensionality reduction methods strengthen and improve the prediction models. Pre-processing helps create models that can more accurately identify and forecast thyroid illnesses by improving the quality and relevance of the data, which eventually results in more insightful and useful information.

Machine Learning (ML) algorithms are used extensively in the health sector to effectively detect and predict thyroid illness. The dataset used is from the UCI machine learning repository. Data is generally collected from healthcare organizations but isn't very sensible until it becomes valuable information. Before commencing the analysis, the most critical and first step is to present the data. Data preparation is used in machine learning for data cleansing and reduction and for dealing with missing variables to increase accuracy. Cleaning up the data to handle missing values, eliminate duplicates, and fix mistakes is the first step in pre-processing. Based on medical records, this may entail completing any missing hormone levels or other pertinent biomarkers to classify thyroid illness. Furthermore, converting variables into uniform units and formats guarantees data homogeneity, reducing the possibility of distorted or fraudulent results.

Feature Selection

Because feature selection techniques improve interpretability, lower computational complexity, and improve model performance, they are essential to ML and data analysis. These techniques assist models in concentrating on the most crucial data by picking the most pertinent elements from a dataset, producing more precise and effective predictions. In addition to expediting the training process, this dimensionality reduction lessens the possibility of overfitting, a phenomenon in which a model performs well on training data but badly on unknown data. Moreover, feature selection streamlines models, making them simpler to comprehend and analyze. This is important in industries like finance and healthcare, where transparency is necessary to foster confidence and compliance. Feature selection is essential to creating reliable, effective, and understandable models.

Feature selection and data cleaning greatly impact model construction, especially when choosing features that improve the classifier's performance and standardize the data within its domain. The key advantages of feature selection strategies are less normativity, higher accuracy, and decreased training time. As a result, the XGBoost algorithm is proposed in this study to detect thyroid illness reliably. The effectiveness of the proposed XGBoost algorithm is compared to that of kNN approaches. Various criteria predicated on the confusion matrix are utilized at the end of the study to analyze and compare the optimal approach for identifying thyroid disease. Regarding accuracy and precision, the XGBoost approach performed better before classifying algorithms.

Improving model performance requires finding and choosing pertinent characteristics. This may entail keeping pertinent or duplicate data out of the classification process for thyroid diseases while keeping aspects like TSH levels, T3 and T4 concentrations, and patient demographics. Feature engineering can further improve the model's capacity to differentiate between various thyroid diseases by generating new variables (e.g., ratios or interactions between hormone levels) from the available data.

Prediction

Prediction algorithms are important because they facilitate well-informed decision-making, improve productivity, and stimulate innovation in various domains. These algorithms enable organizations to make data-driven decisions by reliably predicting outcomes, identifying patterns, and predicting trends by analyzing massive datasets. Predictive models, for example, can enhance patient outcomes in the healthcare industry by enabling early disease diagnosis and therapy personalization. They support risk management, fraud detection, and strategy optimization in the financial industry. Prediction algorithms also automate difficult procedures, minimizing human error and saving time and resources. Their ability to offer practical insights makes them important in today's data-driven environment.

XGBoost (XGB)

An effective technique called XGBoost (Extreme Gradient Boosting) is frequently utilized for classification tasks, such as classifying thyroid diseases. Several crucial phases are involved in its operation, all of which contribute to the model's increased efficiency and accuracy. Extreme Gradient Boosting (XGBoost) is an ensemble-based method. Ensemble learning is a technique for methodically integrating the prediction skills of several learners. The XGBoost technique's functioning mechanism is depicted in Figure 1.

Figure 1. XG Boost Algorithm's Functioning Model

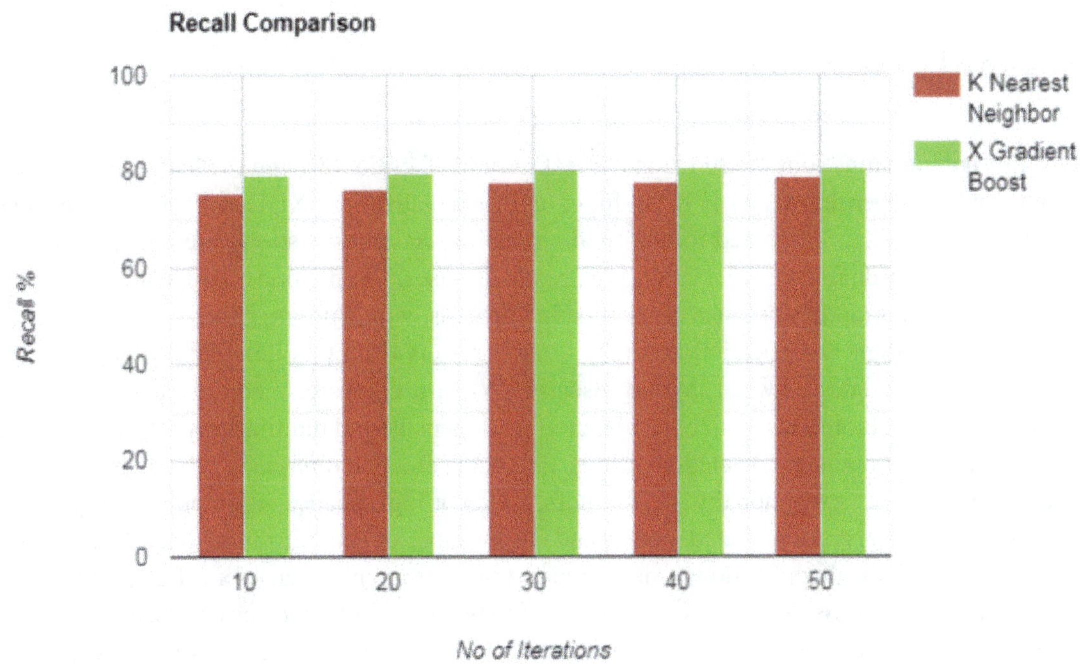

Input Data: Let $X = \{x_1, x_2, \ldots x_n\}$be the feature matrix where xi represents the features for the i-th sample and $Y = \{y_1, y_2 \ldots . y_n\}$Represents the target labels (e.g., different thyroid disease classifications).

Boosting Framework: XGBoost extends the gradient boosting framework. The first prediction made by the model, $f_0(x)$, is often set to the log-odds ratio for classification tasks or the mean of the target values for regression tasks.

For binary classification:

$$f_0(x) = \text{logit}(p) = \log\frac{p}{1-p} \tag{1}$$

Where p is the proportion of positive samples.

When a dataset comprises n instances, each equates to n rows, representing every instance by p. The XGboost algorithm introduces the standard function Ω(s) to regulate the model's over-fitting, centering on the Gradient Bosting Decision Tree technique and the preceding formulation.

$$\min\{obj\} = \min\{L(S_m(X), Y) + \Omega(s) + C\} \tag{2}$$

L denotes the Loss function. $\left(S_m(X), Y\right)$. $\Omega(s)$denotes the normalization function in the resultant prediction model after all repetitions, the difference between the last predicted variables after m times repetition and the real ones. Equation (2) is a more accurate form developed by the algorithm developer after multiple attempts, and it can be used immediately.

$$\Omega\left(s_t\right) = \gamma T + \frac{1}{2}\lambda\sum_{p=1}^{T}\omega_p^2 \tag{3}$$

The normal item functions are functions of leaf number T in Eq. (3), and the leaf node output value ω_p.In the t-wheel repetition $\Omega\left(s_t\right)$ It is the function of normalization. XGBoost forecasts residuals or errors from prior models combined for the final prediction. XGBoost's strong predictive accuracy and resilience make it a valuable tool for classifying thyroid diseases. The method can repeatedly fix mistakes committed by earlier models because of its boosting process, which progressively creates an ensemble of decision trees. High classification accuracy usually results from this iterative development, which successfully differentiates between thyroid diseases. When it comes to medical classification, where interactions between biomarkers and clinical factors are extensive and multifarious, XGBoost's capacity to handle complex, nonlinear correlations between features and outcomes is very valuable.

XGBoost performs exceptionally well handling overfitting because its integrated regularisation strategies penalize overly complicated models and ensure superior generalization to fresh, untested data. This is critical in medical applications where precise forecasts are necessary for efficient diagnosis and treatment. Moreover, XGBoost offers lucid insights into feature significance by emphasizing the clinical features that most influence classification results. By clarifying the significance of several biomarkers and patient features in diagnosing thyroid illnesses, this transparency improves the interpretability and dependability of the model's predictions, aiding clinical decision-making.

K-Nearest Neighbors (KNN)

The learning in the KNN classification is analogous, meaning the test data item is mapped by matching it to a similar training dataset. The operating mechanism of the KNN approach is illustrated in Figure 2.

Figure 2. KNN Algorithm's functioning model

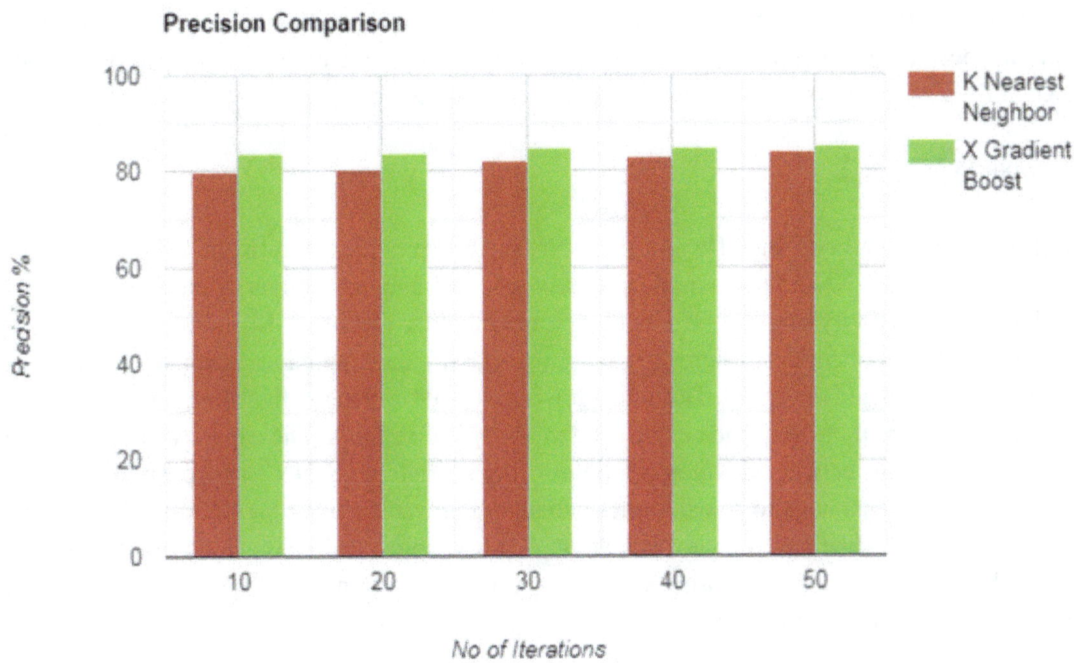

Let $D = \{(x_1, y_1), (x_2, y_2), \ldots, (x_m, y_m)\}$ be the dataset, and x_i, y_i, and i are the feature vector (e.g., T3, T4, TSH levels, etc.) and label (e.g., normal, hypothyroidism, hyperthyroidism)/i-th sample, respectively. One might normalize the features to make sure each one contributes equally to the distance calculation:

$$x'_{i,j} = \frac{x_{i,j} - \min(x_j)}{\max(x_j) - \min(x_j)} \tag{4}$$

where $x_{i,j}$ is the j-th feature of the i-th sample. Select k, which is the number of neighbours to take into account. There is a tuning range for this hyperparameter. The k-nearest neighbour classifier discovers the feature space for the k-training dataset that is nearest to an unknown data point while providing an unknown data point. Most of its neighbours classify the unknown data type, and it is allocated to the class with the most members amongst k-nearest neighbours. When a training piece of data is given, NN holds it and waits for a test data item. As it saves the training data items, it is called a "lazy learner." They are also called "instance-based learners." The KNN algorithm uses several distance equations to determine the nearest neighbours based on their distance. In this study, the Euclidean distance is represented as follows. Determine the ED(Euclidean Distance) between each sample x_i in the training set and the new (unlabelled) sample x'.

$$d(x', x_i) = \sqrt{\sum_{j=1}^{n} \left(x_j' - x_{i,j}\right)^2} \tag{5}$$

where $x_{i,j}$ represents the j-th feature of the i-th training sample and x_j' Represents the j-th feature of the new sample. For each i, arrange the distances $d(x', x_i)$ In ascending order. Choose the first k neighbours that are furthest apart. The set of the k closest neighbours is denoted by N_k. A majority vote among the classes of the k neighbours determines the class y'' of the fresh sample x'':

$$y' = \text{mode}\{y_i | x_i \in N_k\} \tag{6}$$

Because of its simplicity and efficacy, the k-NN method provides significant advantages in predicting thyroid disease. K-NN offers a simple and easy way to make predictions by classifying a data point according to the majority class among its closest neighbours. Because of its simplicity of use can be applied to medical applications, where the capacity to classify data quickly and reliably might be critical for prompt diagnosis and treatment. The algorithm is a flexible tool in medical diagnostics since it makes few assumptions about the data and can be used in a range of settings. The capacity of k-NN to manage nonlinear interactions between features is a noteworthy advantage. K-NN's approach to categorisation based on similarity enables it to adjust to these nuances in thyroid illness prediction, where the interactions between factors like hormone levels, patient demographics, and medical history can be complex. This flexibility improves the algorithm's capacity to recognise trends and forecast results, leading to more accurate and individualised evaluations for thyroid conditions.

RESULTS AND DISCUSSIONS

Dataset Description: The UCI archive is the source of the database used in this study, which has 7200 cases with 21 attributes total—15 categories and six numerical. Three categories comprise the instances in the dataset: hyper, hypo, and normal individuals. There are 166 groups of people with hyperthyroidism, 368 groups with hypothyroidism, and 6666 groups with normal occurrences. The dataset is significantly skewed, as seen by the distribution of cases among the three classes.

Performance Metrics: The confusion matrix illustrates how accurate the model is in terms of precision. The following is the formula for calculating accuracy and precision from a confusion matrix:

$$\text{Accuracy} = \frac{TP + TN}{(TP + FN) + (FP + TN)} * 100\% \tag{7}$$

$$\text{Precision} = \frac{TP}{(TP + FP)} * 100\% \tag{8}$$

$$\text{Recall} = \frac{TP}{TP + FN} \tag{9}$$

Accuracy Analysis: Tables 1 and 3 show the accuracy obtained from the dataset by the K Nearest Neighbour and X Gradient Boost Algorithm. It clearly shows that Gradient Boost outperforms K Nearest Neighbor in accuracy.

Table 1. Accuracy by K Nearest Neighbour and X Gradient Boost Algorithm

No of Iterations	K Nearest Neighbor Accuracy %	X Gradient Boost Accuracy %
10	79.94	82.86
20	80.21	83.16
30	80.64	83.53
40	80.86	84.76
50	80.91	84.90

Figure 3. Accuracy by K Nearest Neighbour and X Gradient Boost Graph

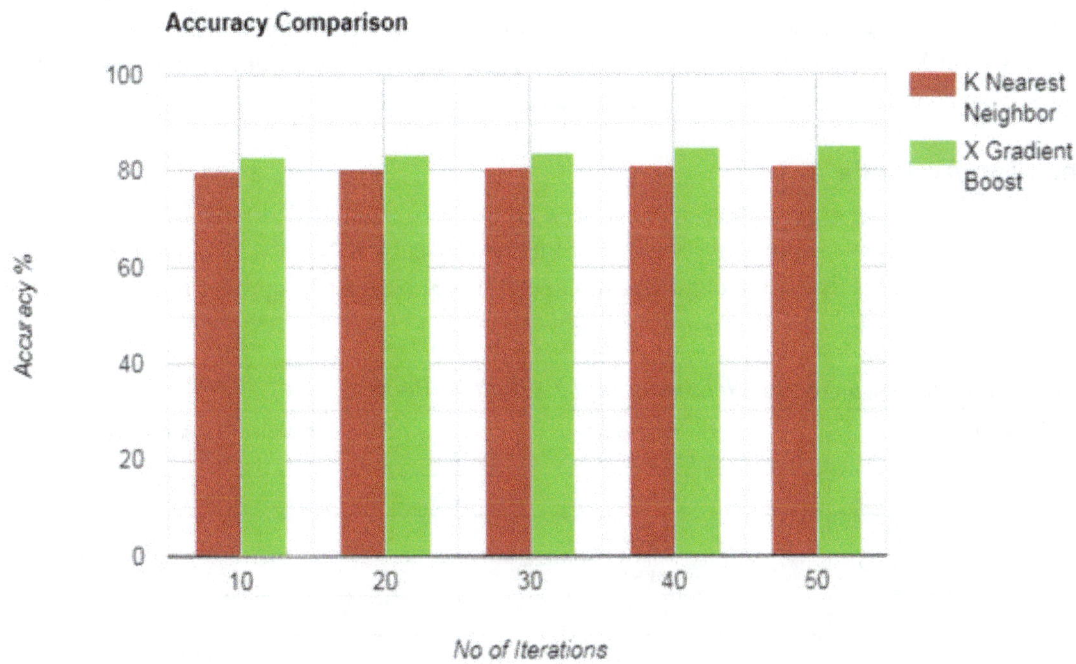

The accuracy of two ML algorithms, KNN and XGBoost, across varying numbers of iterations in a classification problem, perhaps connected to thyroid diagnosis, is shown in Table 1 and Figure 3. Every iteration is a training session in which the model gains knowledge from the data and refines its specifications to enhance performance. The KNN algorithm's accuracy gradually improves as the number of iterations rises. KNN performs significantly better, reaching 80.91% accuracy at 50 iterations, from 79.94% accuracy after 10 iterations. Even while the rise is consistent, it is still quite little, suggesting that although KNN gains from more iterations, its capacity to learn may be constrained compared to more intricate models. The marginal gains in accuracy indicate that KNN can become more adept at defining its decision boundaries when exposed to more data; nevertheless, these gains are not sustained, indicating that KNN is inherently simple and sensitive to the selection of k and distance measurements.

However, with more repetitions, XGBoost, a more sophisticated and intricate machine learning algorithm, shows a more noticeable and steady gain in accuracy. XGBoost performs noticeably better, attaining 84.90% accuracy after 50 iterations, up from 82.86% at 10 iterations. This increasing trend illustrates how well XGBoost's gradient-boosting architecture manages intricate patterns and relationships in the data. XGBoost keeps improving its ensemble of decision trees through more rounds, which improves its capacity to identify subtle patterns and lowers errors. When dealing with larger datasets or more complicated classification tasks like thyroid diagnosis, XGBoost's superior learning capabilities are highlighted by the more noticeable rise in accuracy compared to KNN.

When XGBoost and KNN are compared, XGBoost performs better than KNN every time, indicating that it is a more effective algorithm for this classification problem. KNN's accuracy peaks at 80.91%, but XGBoost keeps improving, highlighting its resilience and superior generalisation from the training set. As the number of repetitions increases, there is a noticeable difference in accuracy between the two algorithms; this suggests that although KNN is a straightforward and understandable model, XGBoost's advanced methodology is more appropriate for attaining more accuracy in this particular scenario. The data shows that XGBoost is the more powerful choice, especially as the number of repetitions increases, for tasks requiring high accuracy, such as thyroid categorisation.

Precision Analysis

Tables 2 and 4 show the precision obtained from the dataset by K Nearest Neighbour and X Gradient Boost. It clearly shows that X Gradient Boost outperforms K Nearest Neighbour regarding precision.

Table 2. Precision by K Nearest Neighbour and X Gradient Boost

No of Iterations	K Nearest Neighbour Precision %	X Gradient Boost Precision %
10	79.68	83.48
20	80.18	83.68
30	81.93	84.64
40	82.88	84.78
50	83.87	84.93

Figure 4. Precision by K Nearest Neighbour and XGradient Boost Graph

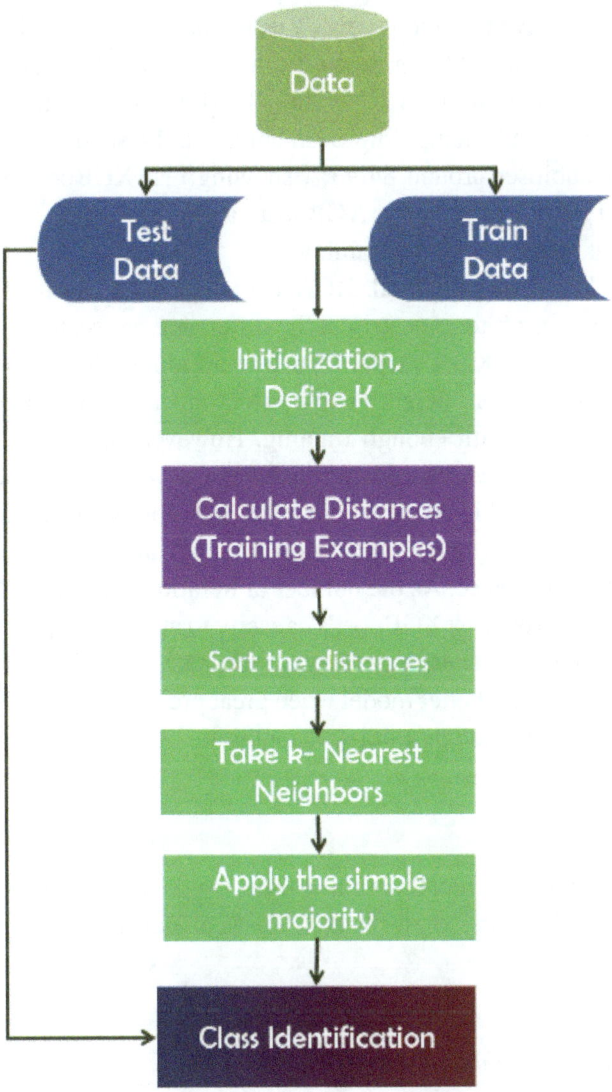

The precision percentages of two ML algorithms, XGBoost and KNN, are shown in Table 2 and Figure 4 for varying numbers of iterations in a classification task, most likely for identifying thyroid conditions. Precision is a metric that expresses how well the models predict the positive outcomes and how many positively classified events are positive. As the number of iterations rises, the KNN algorithm's precision continuously improves. KNN's precision increases to 83.87% after 50 iterations, from 79.68% at the initial 10 iterations. This increasing trend suggests that KNN is more adept at correctly recognising real positives as it goes through more iterations, which lowers the number of false positives. The notable improvement in precision from 79.68% to 83.87% indicates KNN's ability to gradually improve the bounds of its classification. The enhancements imply that as KNN iterates more, it grows more proficient at differentiating between classes, producing more precise positive predictions.

Although the gains are not as noticeable as with KNN, XGBoost, an algorithm with greater complexity and power, exhibits a positive trend in precision as the number of repetitions increases. XGBoost's precision increases to 84.93% after 50 iterations, from 83.48% at 10 iterations. Even while XGBoost has a greater precision starting point than KNN, the algorithm appears to be operating well right out of the gate, with less room for substantial improvement given the smaller increments. Even with fewer iterations, the precision stabilises around 84.93%, showing that XGBoost produces accurate positive forecasts. The high initial precision highlights XGBoost's ability to manage intricate datasets and perform accurate classifications at an early stage of training.

When XGBoost and KNN are compared, XGBoost performs better in precision at every iteration level. However, as the number of iterations rises, the difference between the two gets closer as KNN's accuracy progressively catches up. KNN's accuracy at 50 iterations is 83.87%, nearly matching XGBoost's 84.93%. Although KNN needs more iterations to reach comparable precision levels, it can eventually match XGBoost's performance with enough training. However, for jobs where precision is crucial, including in medical diagnostics where false positives can have serious repercussions, XGBoost is a more dependable option due to its higher initial precision and more stable performance across iterations.

More iterations often result in greater precision for both algorithms, but XGBoost consistently outperforms the other in performance. As the number of iterations increases, KNN exhibits notable improvements in precision; nevertheless, XGBoost's capacity to attain high precision with fewer iterations indicates its resilience and effectiveness in managing intricate classification jobs, such as identifying thyroid conditions. XGBoost is the better model when great precision is required immediately, but KNN can be a formidable opponent if enough training is required.

Recall Analysis

Table 3 and Figure 5 shows the recall obtained from the dataset by the K Nearest Neighbor and X Gradient Boost Algorithm. It clearly shows that X Gradient Boost outperforms K Nearest Neighbour regarding recall.

Table 3. Recall by K Nearest Neighbour and X Gradient Boost.

No of Iterations	K Nearest Neighbor Recall %	X Gradient Boost Recall %
10	75.15	79.14
20	76.12	79.57
30	77.52	80.07
40	77.63	80.35
50	78.50	80.53

Figure 5. Recall by K Nearest Neighbor and X Gradient Boost Graph

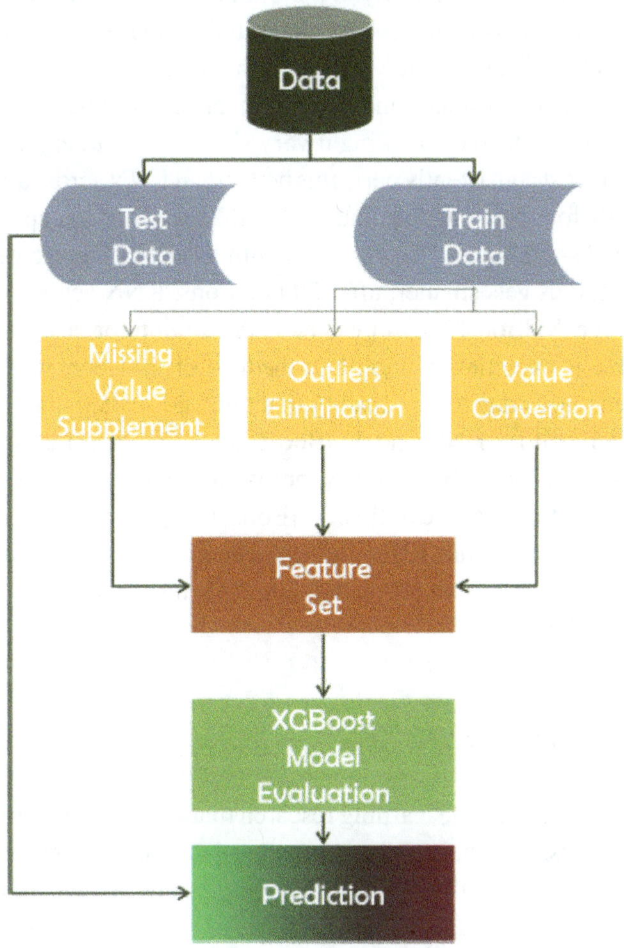

The recall percentages for KNN and XGBoost, two ML algorithms spanning varying numbers of iterations in a classification task—likely linked to thyroid disease detection—are shown in Table 3 and Figure 5. Recall, sometimes called sensitivity, quantifies a model's capacity to accurately identify every pertinent positive example, demonstrating the model's accuracy in identifying true positives. The recall gradually improves as the number of iterations in the KNN algorithm increases. KNN exhibits a consistent increase, peaking at 78.50% recall after 50 iterations, having begun at 75.15% after 10 iterations. This modest rise indicates that as KNN iterates more and accumulates more experience, the network gets better at detecting true positive cases. The increase in recall shows that KNN is becoming more sensitive to correctly detecting positive cases by decreasing the amount of false negatives. However, the progress is slow, which makes sense given that KNN is a simpler model and that more iterations are needed to achieve a meaningful improvement in recall.

A more sophisticated algorithm, XGBoost, begins at a higher baseline than KNN but also exhibits improvements in recall as the number of repetitions rises. After 50 iterations, XGBoost achieves 80.53% recall, up from 79.14% at the beginning. Early in the training process, XGBoost was already quite good at identifying genuine positives, as evidenced by the initial increase in recall. The recall increase over the iterations is rather small, indicating that XGBoost stabilises rapidly and performs consistently well in recognising relevant cases. This constancy and its early great performance highlight XGBoost's capacity to identify intricate patterns in the data, making it very skilled at reducing false negatives.

Regarding recall, XGBoost consistently performs better than KNN across all iteration levels. XGBoost starts with a recall roughly four percentage points higher than KNN and keeps this advantage throughout the iterations, while KNN starts lower and improves with time. With more iterations, the difference in recall between the two models gets smaller; after 50 iterations, KNN achieves 78.50%, while XGBoost achieves 80.53%. However, XGBoost is a more dependable option for tasks where finding as many true positive cases as possible is essential, including in medical diagnostics, where missing a true positive could have major consequences due to its capacity to attain and sustain high recall from the beginning. More iterations enhance recall for KNN and XGBoost, while XGBoost consistently achieves superior recall over all iterations. KNN steadily improves, but it takes more iterations to get close to the recall levels that XGBoost does faster. Because of this, XGBoost is especially well-suited for applications that need high sensitivity right away, while KNN can also become an effective true positive detector with enough iterations. XGBoost is the more efficient method for tasks where recall is crucial, especially in situations with complicated data.

CONCLUSION AND FUTURE WORK

This work aims to facilitate machine learning research that can be used to diagnose thyroid problems. In recent years, various accessible analyses have been used to diagnose thyroid diseases efficiently and competently. These findings reveal that multiple techniques are utilised in each paper, with varying degrees of accuracy. The XGBoost algorithm is used in this study to forecast thyroid disorders reliably using the UCI database. By decreasing the over-fitting of data sets, the suggested approach enhances efficiency. The efficacy of the XGBoost algorithm is compared to that of KNN approaches, and the performance of the two algorithms is compared and examined. Compared to KNN, the suggested XGBoost improves accuracy and prediction by 83 percent and 80 percent, respectively. Classifiers with varied feature extraction and data augmentation could be employed to provide a more exact thyroid diagnosis.

Subsequent research in thyroid classification may concentrate on integrating cutting-edge methods like explainable AI (XAI) and deep learning to improve model interpretability and accuracy. Using convolutional neural networks (CNNs) or recurrent neural networks (RNNs) could enhance classification performance by collecting more complex patterns in the data as more data becomes available, especially from varied populations. More reliable predictions may also come from investigating hybrid models that combine the advantages of ensemble techniques like XGBoost with more conventional algorithms like KNN. The development of XAI techniques specific to thyroid categorisation is another exciting field. This work aims to make model decisions explicit and comprehensible for physicians, which is essential in building clinician confidence in AI-driven diagnostic tools. Lastly, combining multimodal data sources like genetic and imaging data with real-time data from wearable technology could improve personalised medicine strategies for treating thyroid disease.

REFERENCES

Abbad Ur Rehman, H., Lin, C.-Y., & Mushtaq, Z. (2021). Effective K-nearest neighbor algorithms performance analysis of thyroid disease. *Zhongguo Gongcheng Xuekan, 44*(10), 1–11. DOI: 10.1080/02533839.2020.1831967

Anitha, K., Nagaraj, B. K., Paramasivan, P., & Shynu, T. (2023). Enhancing Clustering Performance with the Rough Set C-Means Algorithm. *FMDB Transactions on Sustainable Computing Systems, 1*(4), 190–203.

Chandel, K., Kunwar, V., Sabitha, S., Choudhury, T., & Mukherjee, S. (2016). A comparative study on thyroid disease detection using K-nearest neighbor and Naive Bayes classification techniques. *CSI Transactions on ICT, 4*(1), 313–319. DOI: 10.1007/s40012-016-0100-5

Das, S., Kruti, A., Devkota, R., & Bin Sulaiman, R. (2023). Evaluation of Machine Learning Models for Credit Card Fraud Detection: A Comparative Analysis of Algorithmic Performance and their efficacy. *FMDB Transactions on Sustainable Technoprise Letters, 1*(2), 70–81.

Hakim, A. (2022). Thesis Proposal: Implementation of Android-Based Artificial Intelligence in Early Detection of Thyroid Disorders and Mental Disorders, 229(3), 57-64.

Hakim, A., Titin, R., & Prihantinisetyowisnu, G. (2021). Expert System Framework Design for Diagnosis of Thyroid Disorders. In Conference: the 1st Science and Technology Student Conference (ISTECH), Klaster Mahasiswa, Indonesia.

Hariprasath, G., Dhinakaran, P., & Kumar, V. H. (2024). Exploring the efficacy of LightGBM, AdaBoost, and CatBoost in Alzheimer's disease classification. *FMDB Transactions on Sustainable Health Science Letters, 2*(1), 41–55. DOI: 10.69888/FTSHSL.2024.000171

Islam, S. S., Haque, M. S., Miah, M. S. U., Sarwar, T. B., & Nugraha, R. (2022). Application of machine learning algorithms to predict the thyroid disease risk: An experimental comparative study. *PeerJ. Computer Science, 8*(10), 1–35. DOI: 10.7717/peerj-cs.898 PMID: 35494828

Jani, P., Nanban, D., Selvan, J., Richardson, N., Sivakani, R., & Subhashni, R. (2024). Studying Price Dynamics of Bus Services Using Machine Learning Algorithms. *AVE Trends In Intelligent Computing Systems, 1*(1), 54–65.

Jha, R., Bhattacharjee, V., & Mustafi, A. (2022). Increasing the prediction accuracy for thyroid disease: A step towards better health for society. *Wireless Personal Communications, 122*(2), 1921–1938. DOI: 10.1007/s11277-021-08974-3

Karthik, S., Soji, E. S., Priscila, S. S., Sakthivanitha, M., Rajest, S. S., & Kumar, A. S. (2024). Enhancing tumor localization in brain MRI images using a scalable systematic vector algorithm for result-oriented accuracy. *FMDB Transactions on Sustainable Health Science Letters, 2*(2), 110–127. DOI: 10.69888/FTSHSL.2024.000176

Karthikeyan, B., Devi, R. A., & Munshi, M. (2024). Utilizing Deep Learning for the Classification of Brain Tumours Using MRI. *AVE Trends In Intelligent Health Letters, 1*(1), 1–9.

Kumar, C. S., Kumar, B. S., Gnanaguru, G., Jayalakshmi, V., Rajest, S. S., & Senapati, B. (2024). Augmenting chronic kidney disease diagnosis with support vector machines for improved classifier accuracy. In *Advances in Medical Technologies and Clinical Practice* (pp. 336–352). IGI Global.

Kumar, H. H. S. (2020). A novel approach of SVM based classification on thyroid disease stage detection. *2020 Third International Conference on Smart Systems and Inventive Technology (ICSSIT)*, Tamil Nadu, India. DOI: 10.1109/ICSSIT48917.2020.9214180

Medici, B. B., Lerche la Cour, J., Knop, F. K., Krakauer, M., Michaelsson, L. F., Faber, J., Watt, T., & Nygaard, B. (2021). Predictors of improvement in quality of life when treating hypothyroidism. *Journal of Thyroid Research, 2021*(1), 5577217. DOI: 10.1155/2021/5577217 PMID: 34194721

Minu, M. S., Subashka Ramesh, S. S., Canessane, R., Al-Amin, M., & Bin Sulaiman, R. (2023). Experimental Analysis of UAV Networks Using Oppositional Glowworm Swarm Optimization and Deep Learning Clustering and Classification. *FMDB Transactions on Sustainable Computing Systems, 1*(3), 124–134.

Pandit, P. (2023). On the Context of Diabetes: A Brief Discussion on the Novel Ethical Issues of Non-communicable Diseases. *FMDB Transactions on Sustainable Health Science Letters, 1*(1), 11–20.

Peya, Z. J., Chumki, M. K. N., & Zaman, K. M. (2021). Predictive analysis for thyroid diseases diagnosis using machine learning. *2021 International Conference on Science & Contemporary Technologies (ICSCT)*, Dhaka, Bangladesh. DOI: 10.1109/ICSCT53883.2021.9642544

Princy Reshma, R., Deepak, S., Tejeshwar, S. R. M., Deepika, P., & Saleem, M. (2023). Online Auction Forecasting Precision: Real-time Bidding Insights and Price Predictions with Machine Learning. *FMDB Transactions on Sustainable Technoprise Letters, 1*(2), 106–122.

Raj, M. A., Mishra, A., & Forest, G. A. (2024b). Predictive Analytics for Employee Attrition: Leveraging Machine Learning for Strategic Human Resources Management. *AVE Trends in Intelligent Technoprise Letters, 1*(1), 13–29.

Raj, M. A., Thinesh, M. A., Varmann, S. S. M., Pothu, A. R., & Paramasivan, P. (2024a). Ensemble-based phishing website detection using Extra Trees classifier. *AVE Trends in Intelligent Computing Systems, 1*(3), 142–156.

Regin, R., Sharma, P. K., Singh, K., Narendra, Y. V., Bose, S. R., & Rajest, S. S. (2023a). Fine-grained deep feature expansion framework for fashion apparel classification using transfer learning. In *Advanced Applications of Generative AI and Natural Language Processing Models* (pp. 389–404). IGI Global. DOI: 10.4018/979-8-3693-0502-7.ch019

Regin, R., T, S., George, S. R., Bhattacharya, M., Datta, D., & Priscila, S. S. (2023b). Development of predictive model of diabetic using supervised machine learning classification algorithm of ensemble voting. *International Journal of Bioinformatics Research and Applications, 19*(3), 151–169. DOI: 10.1504/IJBRA.2023.10057044

Saxena, D., & Chaudhary, S. (2023). Predicting Brain Diseases from FMRI-Functional Magnetic Resonance Imaging with Machine Learning Techniques for Early Diagnosis and Treatment. *FMDB Transactions on Sustainable Computer Letters, 1*(1), 33–48.

Shruthi, S., & Aravind, B. R. (2023). Engaging ESL Learning on Mastering Present Tense with Nearpod and Learningapps.org for Engineering Students. *FMDB Transactions on Sustainable Techno Learning*, *1*(1), 21–31.

Sivapriya, G. B. V., Ganesh, U. G., Pradeeshwar, V., Dharshini, M., & Al-Amin, M. (2023). Crime Prediction and Analysis Using Data Mining and Machine Learning: A Simple Approach that Helps Predictive Policing. *FMDB Transactions on Sustainable Computer Letters*, *1*(2), 64–75.

Thinesh, M. A., Varmann, S. S., Sharmila, S. L., & Das, S. R. (2023). Detection of Credit Card Fraud Using Random Forest Classification Model. *FMDB Transactions on Sustainable Technoprise Letters*, *1*(4), 181–194.

Thirunagalingam, A. (2024). Bias detection and mitigation in data pipelines: Ensuring fairness and accuracy in machine learning. *AVE Trends in Intelligent Computing Systems*, *1*(2), 116–127.

Tyagi, A., Mehra, R., & Saxena, A. (2018). Interactive thyroid disease prediction system using machine learning technique. *2018 Fifth International Conference on Parallel, Distributed and Grid Computing (PDGC)*, Himachal Pradesh, India. DOI: 10.1109/PDGC.2018.8745910

Varmann, S. S., Hariprasath, G., & Kadirova, I. (2023). Optimizing Educational Outcomes: H2O Gradient Boosting Algorithm in Student Performance Prediction. *FMDB Transactions on Sustainable Techno Learning*, *1*(3), 165–178.

Chapter 11
Enhancing Ocular Health on Multi-Faceted Approach to Diabetic Retinopathy Detection

N. Durga
https://orcid.org/0009-0005-2415-4930
Bharath Institute of Higher Education and Research, India

D. Kerana Hanirex
Bharath Institute of Higher Education and Research, India

A. Muthukumaravel
Bharath Institute of Higher Education and Research, India

ABSTRACT

The leading cause of vision loss in people with diabetes is diabetic retinopathy (DR). Early diagnosis and screening can be facilitated by automating the analysis of retinal fundus images. Multi-edge detection and segmentation algorithms have been evaluated on a dataset of DR images, along with classifiers, to detect different levels of severity of DR. This study investigated multiple-edge detection, segmentation, selection of significant features, and classification techniques for robust DR detection using retinal fundus images to develop an automated system for DR grading. Edge detectors, segmentation, and classifiers are among the algorithms analyzed for detecting eye diseases. Segmenting detailed structures was also proposed using superpixels. The severity level of the disease was determined by analyzing a DR image dataset. Combining traditional machine learning techniques was the most effective way of accurately diagnosing DR from fundus images using an ensemble classifier.

INTRODUCTION

In people with diabetes, diabetic retinopathy may cause vision loss due to microvascular complications. Fluid leaks, hemorrhages, and abnormal vessel growth may result from progressive damage to retinal blood vessels (Saxena and Chaudhary, 2023). It is essential to conduct regular eye screenings and to provide timely treatment for diabetic retinopathy to prevent vision loss (Hassoun et al., 2024).

DOI: 10.4018/979-8-3693-9420-5.ch011

Automatic image-based diagnosis involves determining the evolution of diabetic retinopathy lesions and anatomical structures. Fundus photographs must distinguish distinct regions and detect vital edges (Kumar et al., 2024). Images can be divided into constituent objects by detecting edges, while segmentation can reveal contours (Karthikeyan et al., 2024). Analyzing retinal images automatically can help detect retinal abnormalities at an early stage in large patient populations. Computer-aided diagnosis of retinal diseases from images has relied heavily on edge detection and segmentation techniques (Upadhyay et al., 2024). As a result of edge detection, anatomical structures like the optic disc, the macula, and the blood vessels can be distinguished, enabling abnormalities to be located. In retinal segmentation, lesions, exudates, or neovascular regions associated with diseases are divided into different areas (Karthik et al., 2024).

Multiple edge and segmentation algorithms are evaluated for automated diabetic retinopathy grading using fundus images in this study. Several edge detectors, including Sobel, Prewitt, Canny, and texture-based methods, have been studied (Hassoun et al., 2024). Some segmentation techniques include active contours, thresholding, region growing, and clustering (Gnanaguru et al., 2024). The delineation of fine structures is also achieved using a novel superpixel approach. An experiment uses the Diabetic Retinopathy dataset, which contains retinopathy severity-level categorized fundus images (Kumar et al., 2024). Hemorrhages, exudates, and blood vessels are evaluated based on their ability to detect critical lesions. For robust screening systems for diabetic retinopathy, the analysis provides insights into optimizing edge and segmentation techniques (Sengupta et al., 2023).

Background and Challenges

In the world, diabetic retinopathy (DR) is one of the leading causes of vision impairments and blindness. Symptoms include leaking fluid, haemorrhaging, and abnormal vessel growth due to progressive damage to the retinal blood vessels. DR can be detected early through retinal fundus imaging, allowing timely treatment and prevention of visual loss through regular screening. It is nearly impossible to visually detect DR using fundus images alone due to manual analysis's tedious, subjective, and expensive nature. For DR progression to be identified at various stages, automated, efficient, and accurate computer-aided diagnosis systems are needed. Various image processing and machine learning algorithms must be evaluated and optimized to identify anatomical structures, detect lesions and abnormalities, and classify images according to the severity of the disease. An optimal interpretation of retinal fundus photographs can reliably detect the type and severity of diabetic retinopathy by combining image processing and machine learning algorithms. As a result, computer-aided screening systems will be more robust, which will aid in developing improved DR diagnosis systems.

Motivation and Objectives: In this work, we develop an automated system that uses retinal fundus images to grade diabetic retinopathy. A robust automated screening system for early diagnosis of DR will be developed by integrating machine learning techniques and image analysis.

Motivating factors

There is no doubt that diabetic retinopathy (DR) is a leading cause of vision loss in the world. It is possible to prevent vision loss by detecting it early through regular retinal screenings. Fundus images are tedious, subjective, and expensive to analyze for DR screening manually. The detection of DR progression at various stages must be automated, efficient, and accurate. Identifying anatomical structures, detecting lesions or abnormalities, and classifying images according to severity require various image processing and machine-learning algorithms to be evaluated and optimized. Combining image processing and machine learning to interpret retinal fundus photographs can improve screening systems by reliably detecting the type and severity of diabetic retinopathy.

Objectives

- To identify anatomical structures in retinal images, evaluate edge detection algorithms, including Sobel, Prewitt, and Canny.
- Segment lesions, exudates, and neovascularization using thresholding, clustering, region-growing, and active contouring techniques.
- Develop an innovative method for segmenting fine structures in fundus images using superpixels.
- For DR grading, select the most descriptive features using correlation-based techniques.
- SVM, KNN, decision trees, and ensemble models better detect the severity level of DR than machine learning classifiers.
- By combining optimized image processing and machine learning algorithms, an automated computer-aided diagnosis system will be developed that allows the diagnosis of diabetic retinopathy using fundus photographs.

An automated grading system for diabetic retinopathy through fundus images is the primary goal of this research. The disease can be detected and monitored early if this is done. The work evaluates multiple edge detection and segmentation algorithms, such as Sobel, Prewitt, Canny, and texture-based methods. It also examines thresholding, region growing, clustering, and active contours. This paper presents a unique approach for delineating fine structures in fundus images using superpixels. Diabetic retinopathy may be graded more accurately if superpixels are used to extract features and segment images.

LITERATURE REVIEW

Recently, automated diabetic retinopathy screening systems relying on fundus images have shown an increased interest in edge detection and segmentation methods. Deep learning algorithms and texture filters have been used in recent edge detection studies for fundus images. Pratt et al. (2016) used synthetic fundus images to train an edge detector based on CNNs. The Gabor filter banks were used by Parida et al. (2020) to detect edges of vein patterns in fundus images (Obeta et al., 2024).

The use of superpixels for segmentation has become increasingly popular. According to Oliveira (2019), hard exudates were segmented using SLIC superpixels and CNNs (Aditya Komperla, 2023). A convolutional network based on superpixels was proposed by Ziller (2020) for the segmentation of optic discs and cups (Sharma et al., 2024). Neural networks have also been explored as an adjunct to traditional methods in recent years. To refine optical disc segmentations based on the circular Hough transform, Shafi (2020) employed a U-Net. A CNN-optimized segmentation of active contours was shown to be effective in detecting choroidal neovascularization by Wang (2022). It has also been examined how hybrid techniques combine multiple algorithms. A pipeline was developed by Bhaskaranand et al. (2016) that used fuzzy C-means, K-means, and thresholding for localizing and segmenting optic discs. A hybrid framework combining edge detection and segmentation shows the utility of traditional image processing techniques.

An innovative multi-task U-Net developed by Yau et al. (2012) combined the detection of Canny edges with the segmentation of retinal vessels and the optic disc, achieving state-of-the-art performance (Pandit, 2023). In a two-stage pipeline with a high F1-score and IOU, Shanmugalingam et al. (2019) used Otsu thresholding, Hough transform, and Mask R-CNN for optic disc detection and exudate segmentation. DR classification was improved using depth-wise separable convolutional edgemaps by Goyal et al. (2020). The dual path architecture of Zhong et al. (2024), coupled with multiscale vessel enhancement with exudate competitive learning modules, allows vessels and exudates to be segmented together (Odoemena and Elufidodo, 2024).

By integrating vessel segmentation with exudate detection, Jiang et al. (2021) achieved 0.95+ Dice scores on public datasets (Nirmala et al., 2023). The model was validated by representing diverse populations with photographs from an Africa-specific DR dataset by Abràmoff et al. (2016). Gonzalez et al. (2018) used dual pyramid networks with Canny edge maps and dense feature pyramid pooling for multiclass DR grading, obtaining 0.96+ AUC. U-Net++ was combined with deformable convolution, attention maps, and reverse feature maps to segment optic discs, foveas, and microaneurysms, validated on Messidor datasets by Jin et al. (2019). A multiencoder Transformer augmented dual-resnet architecture developed by Hasan Talukder et al. (2023). is superior to SOTA architectures in joint optic disc, fovea, and exudate segmentation (Hariprasath et al., 2024).

METHODS

As part of this system, retinal images are preprocessed, anatomical structures such as blood vessels are detected, lesions and abnormalities are segmented, descriptive features are extracted, and then the images are categorized according to the severity of the disease. Various image processing techniques are evaluated to enhance, detect edges, segment, and extract features from images. A classification model is trained using advanced machine-learning techniques based on the extracted features (Figure 1).

Figure 1. Proposed Flow

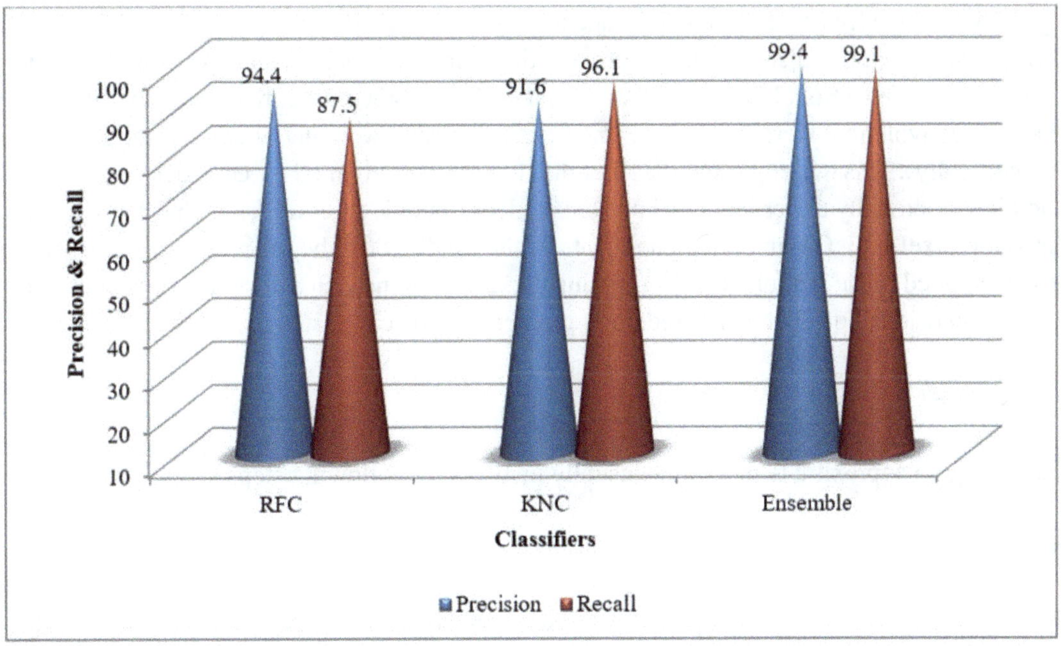

Image Acquisition and Enhancement: A healthy retinal fundus image and a diseased retinal fundus image were obtained. This dataset includes fundus images to enhance the fundus images and spot blood vessels for segmentation. Several eye disease-related images are also included in the dataset. Multiple images of each eye are captured from different angles and retinal fields to identify defects in different regions of the retina. Histogram equalization is used in the image enhancement to increase the brightness range. Image detail can be revealed in dark or bright areas by doing this. Enhance contrast in local areas by adjusting contrast limiting adaptive histogram equalization (CLAHE) parameters. A local rather than a global approach is used in CLAHE to equalize histograms. Correcting for variations in retinal illumination is possible using morphological operations, polynomial fittings, or surface interpolation techniques.

Edge Detection: Detecting edges in images and computer vision is fundamental. Object boundaries or edges are identified within an image using this technique. An edge is a change between neighbouring pixels in intensity or colour, commonly representing the transition between objects or surfaces. This technique helps extract important features from an image that can be used for various purposes, such as recognizing objects, segmenting images, and analyzing them further. There are several methods for detecting edges in an image, each with advantages and disadvantages. A bridge must be located, and sharp changes in the image must be detected for the technique to work. Sharp changes and bridges refer to points where colours and light change. An image processed with colour and light changes reveals sharp lines. An image can be converted into an edge in many ways, such as horizontally, vertically, or diagonally. When the edges of the image are detected, the observer can examine the changes in light and colour in detail. Also, computer vision and machine vision algorithms can better comprehend and process images.

Sobel: An image processing and computer vision technique called Sobel edge detection detects edges and sharp transitions in images. Detecting diabetic retinopathy can be achieved through this pre-processing step, although it is not the only method to diagnose the disease. A new image is formed by adding the X and Y edges of the original image together to create the sum of the X and Y edges using Sobel Edge Detection. It is also possible to process these images separately. Converting RGB images to grayscale before using a Sobel Edge Detector is best for best results. After that, we will use a technique called kernel convolution. Kernels are 3 x 3 matrices containing weighted indexes arranged differently (or symmetrically). This will represent the filter that will be implemented for edge detection. In addition to responding maximally to vertical and horizontal edges, there is a kernel for each orientation perpendicular to the pixel grid. Gx and Gy components of the gradient can be measured separately based on the kernels applied to the input image. Combining these data points can determine a gradient's absolute magnitude and orientation. The magnitude of a gradient can be calculated as follows:

$$|G| = \sqrt{Gx^2 + Gy^2} \tag{1}$$

Calculating an approximate magnitude usually involves the following steps.

$$|G| = |Gx| + |Gy| \tag{2}$$

The computation of this is much faster. According to the following equation, the edge angle is the angle at which the gradient is created (relative to the pixel grid)

$$\theta = \arctan\left(\frac{Gy}{Gx}\right) \tag{3}$$

Orientation is determined by measuring angles anticlockwise from the direction of maximum contrast on the image, which runs from left to right on this image. There is a simple method of detecting edges using Sobel that is computationally efficient and relatively easy to implement. Noise in the input image may produce noisy results, and it's susceptible to noise. A canny edge detector, incorporating smoothing (Gaussian blurring) and non-maximum suppression, addresses these issues to improve edge detection performance (Figure 2).

Algorithm 1. SOBEL Edge Detection

```
Algorithm SOBEL
Input: Img_G - Grayscale image
Output: EdgeMap – Detected Edges
Convert the colour input IMG to a grayscale image
Compute the average of RGB channels to each pixel
Define two 3x3 convolution kernels: Gx and Gy.
Initialize an empty output image (Edge_Map) of the same size as the input image.
Loop through each pixel (x, y) in the grayscale image Img_G
For each pixel, perform the convolution operation using the Sobel kernels
Calculate the gradient magnitude at each pixel
Apply a threshold to the gradient magnitude to create the binary Edge_Map
Set a threshold value to determine which pixels are considered edges
Pixels below the threshold are considered non-edges
Pixels with gradient magnitudes above the threshold are considered edges
The final output is the binary Edge_Map
End Algorithm
```

Figure 2. Edge Detection Results

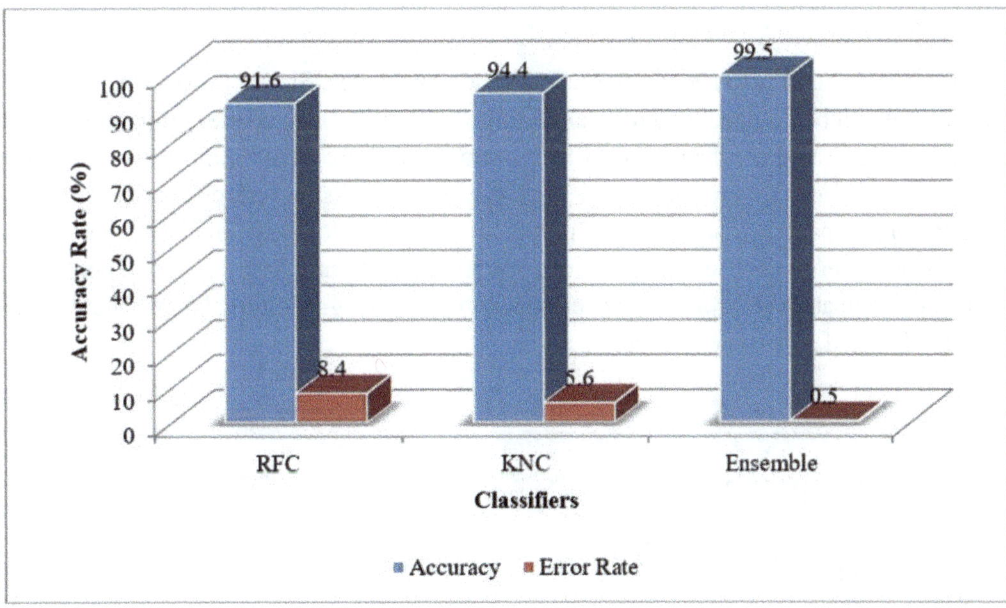

Segmentation: During Image Segmentation, a digital image is divided into various subgroups (of pixels) called Image Objects, which allows the image to be segmented into simpler parts and thus be easier to analyze. Using segmentation, computer systems can analyze and comprehend complex images more easily by simplifying and extracting meaningful information.

SLIC: The SLIC (Simple Linear Iterative Clustering) algorithm is well known for its simplicity and efficiency in image segmentation. Using SLIC, you can segment images quickly and effectively using k-means clustering and superpixels. An entire image is covered by small, non-overlapping areas called superpixels. An image of several pixels with similar characteristics can be called a superpixel. Typically, segmentation is done based on colour. It used a low computational overhead technique to segment superpixels, but many algorithms are available.

Algorithm 2. SLIC Segmentation

Algorithm SLIC
Input: Img_{IP}– Input Image
Output: Img_{Seg} – Superpixel Segmented Image
Read Input Image ImgIP
Compute the step size S,= $\sqrt{(N/K)}$, where N is the total number of pixels in the image.
Create an empty superpixel map with the same dimensions as the Img_{IP}
Initialize the maximum number of iterations and convergence threshold
Repeat until a maximum number of iterations
For each cluster centre
find the pixel with the lowest distance in a 5x5 window around it
Assign each pixel in the 5x5 window to the nearest cluster centre
Update the cluster centres by computing the mean color
the spatial location of all the pixels assigned to each cluster
If a superpixel contains fewer pixels than the threshold
Merge it with the adjacent superpixel that has the most similar colour
Refine the superpixel boundaries by finding the gradient at the superpixel edges
Return the Img_{Seg} superpixel segmentation image
End Algorithm

Using the CIELAB colourspace and the pixels' x y coordinates, SLIC clusters pixels in 5-D space. Superpixel shapes can be compact and regular thanks to different distance measurements, and they can be applied to grayscale and color images. In SLIC, superpixels are generated by clustering pixels that have similar colors and are close to each other. The clustering process uses a 5-dimensional space [labxy]. The CIELAB colour space is assumed to be perpetually uniform for small distances between colours. As an input, SLIC receives a desired number of approximately equally-sized superpixels K. Therefore, there will be approximately N/K pixels on each superpixel. Every grid interval would have a superpixel centre for equally sized superpixels (Figure 3).

Figure 3. Segmentation Results

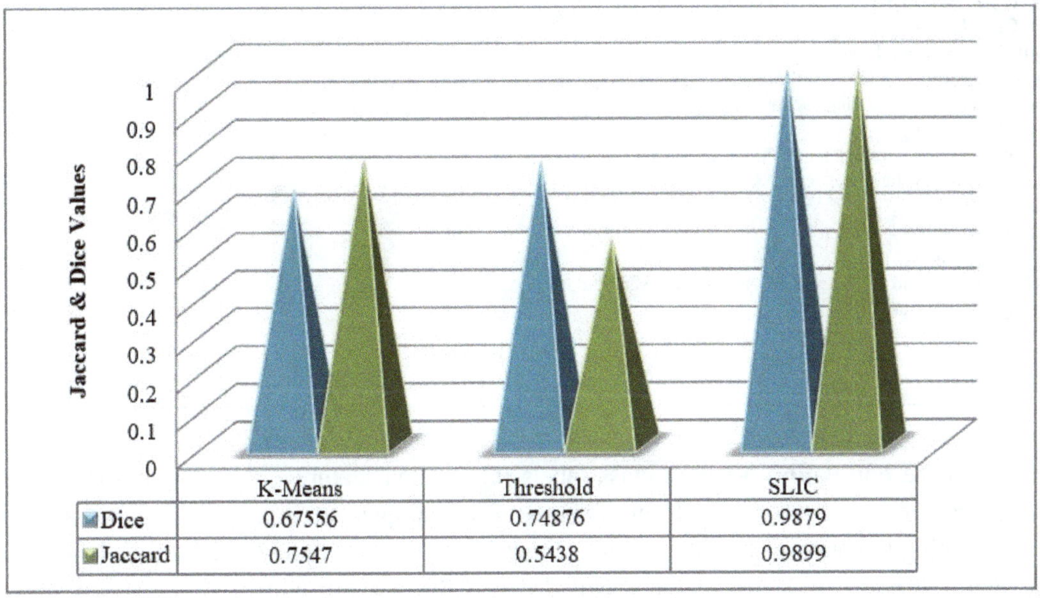

$$S = \sqrt{(N/K)} \tag{4}$$

Using k = [1, K] at regular grid intervals, S, K superpixel cluster centers $C_k = [l_k, a_k, b_k, x_k, y_k]$ are chosen. Clusters typically cover an area of approximately S2, so pixels associated with this cluster are generally located around the superpixel centre in an area of 2S x 2S. When distances are small, Euclidean distances are meaningful in CIELAB colorspace. Upon exceeding this perceptual colour distance limit, spatial pixel distance outweighs pixel colour similarity. Following is a definition of distance measure D_s. Ds is calculated using the grid interval S to normalize the lab and xy plane distances. Superpixel compactness can be controlled by a variable m introduced in Ds. A higher m value emphasizes spatial. Ds is calculated using the grid interval S to normalize the lab and xy plane distances. Superpixel compactness can be controlled by a variable m introduced in Ds. A higher m value emphasizes spatial proximity and makes the cluster more compact. The value can range from [1, 20].

Feature Selection: In developing such systems, quantitative features are extracted from fundus images that indicate the severity level of retinal abnormalities indicative of different DRs. Model performance can be degraded, and computational costs can increase due to redundant or irrelevant features. Identifying the most informative features requires feature selection. Standard classifiers will be used to evaluate the ability of selected feature subsets to classify DR severity levels.

Interaction Capping-based Feature Selection (ICAP): In an interaction-based feature selection algorithm, interactions are used to identify the most relevant features in a dataset. A filter-based method called ICAP selects the most informative features by combining correlation and interaction caps. ICAP calculates the correlation between each feature and the class labels to remove redundant highly correlated features and then applies an interaction capping method.

Algorithm 3. ICAP Feature Selection

Algorithm ICAP
Input: F_{Set} – Features Set
C_{Label} – Class Labels
Output: F_{Sel} – Selected Features
Compute the correlation between the feature F_{Set} and Class Label C_{Label}
Initialize an empty set correlate_score
For each feature in F_{Set}
Calculate the person correlation coefficient and append correlate_score
Rank the features by the correlate_score (f_i)
Initialize $F_{Sel} = \emptyset$
If correlate_score (f_i) $\neq$ -1, then
F_{Sel} = Rank_Feature (f_i)
Repeat the process and set the correlation score for every feature
Select top-k features as F_{Sel}
Return F_{Sel}
End for
End Algorithm

Based on the correlation between class labels (C_{Label}) and features (F_{Set}), the ICAP algorithm in Algorithm # determines the most relevant features. Data samples are inputted using two main inputs: F_{Set}, representing the features of the data sample, and C_{Label}, representing the labels of the data sample categories. A subset of selected features, called F_{Sel}, is the primary output of the algorithm. Data in F_{Sel} are characterized by the characteristics used to distinguish between different classes or labels. The algorithm reaches this goal by calculating the correlation between a feature in FSet and its class label in CLabel. Using this correlation measurement, you can determine how strongly each feature's values relate to the class labels, thus allowing an understanding of how they correlate. Correlation coefficients are measures of linear relationships between variables called product-moment correlation coefficients. Covariance between two variables divided by their standard deviations is what defines the Pearson correlation coefficient. A Pearson correlation coefficient can be calculated mathematically by dividing two variables, X and Y, by:

$$r = Cov(X, Y) / (SD(X) * SD(Y)) \quad (5)$$

SD(X) is the standard deviation of X. At the same time, SD(Y) is the standard deviation of Y. Cov(X, Y) indicates the covariance between X and Y. An X-Y relationship with a Pearson correlation coefficient of 1 indicates a perfect positive linear relationship between X and Y. In contrast, a Pearson correlation coefficient of -1 indicates a perfect negative linear relationship. The higher the positive value of r, the stronger the positive relationship, and the higher the negative value of r, the stronger the negative relationship. The variables are not linearly related if the value is 0.

Classification: Classification techniques for retinal images used to predict eye diseases are discussed in this section. Deep learning and artificial intelligence have revolutionized medical imaging. Analyzing retinal images for diagnosing and classifying eye diseases has gained considerable attention within medical imaging.

Ensemble Classifier: An ensemble model combines multiple models to improve performance in machine learning. An ensemble can be built by training decision trees on different subsets of the data. New data points are predicted by each decision tree individually. Once all the decision trees have predicted an output class, a voting classifier takes the most common one. With this voting ensemble, each tree's strengths can complement each other. When different data types are used to build decision trees, their errors will be less correlated, meaning they will make various errors. Compared to any individual model, the ensemble reduces variance, avoids overfitting, and handles more complexity by averaging predictions. Voting classifiers derived from the ensemble are more reliable and accurate than any individual decision tree. The performance of machine learning models is consistently improved when decision trees are assembled using bagging, random forests, or boosting. Decision tree ensembles are a popular ensemble modeling approach due to their flexibility and stability. Ensembling is also a computationally complex and time-consuming process despite its many benefits. Experimentation must be conducted to determine the models' optimal subset and weighting to maximize ensemble performance. This pseudo-code shows an ensemble model using a Support Vector Machine (SVM) and Decision Tree with a VotingClassifier, which is useful for computer-aided diagnosis with retinal fundus images.

Algorithm 4. Ensemble Decision Tree with Voting Classifier

Algorithm EDT_VC
Input: F_{Set} – Feature Set
Output: y_{pred} – Class Prediction
Import feature set F_{Set} for the class label
Create a base model with SVM and Decision Tree
SVM(C,kernel='linear')
DecisionTree(criterion, max_depth, min_samples_split)
Create ensemble model with Ensemble = VotingClassifier(SVM, DecisionTree, voting='soft')
For each (x_i,y_i) in D_{train} // Training, the ensemble model
SVM.fit(x_i,y_i) and DecisionTree.fit(x_i,y_i)
Ensemble.fit(x_i,y_i)
For x_i in D_{test} // Predict with ensemble model
p_svm = SVM.predict_proba(x_i)
p_dt = DecisionTree.predict_proba(x_i)
p_ensemble = w_svm*p_svm + w_dt*p_dt
y_{pred} = argmax(p_ensemble)
Return spe_{ed}
End Algorithm

An ensemble model combines multiple models to improve performance in machine learning. An ensemble can be built by training decision trees on different subsets of the data. New data points are predicted by each decision tree individually. Once all the decision trees have predicted an output class, a voting classifier takes the most common one. With this voting ensemble, each tree's strengths can complement each other. When different data types are used to build decision trees, their errors will be less correlated, meaning they will make various errors. Compared to any individual model, the ensemble reduces variance, avoids overfitting, and handles more complexity by averaging predictions. Voting classifiers derived from the ensemble are more reliable and accurate than any individual decision tree. The performance of machine learning models is consistently improved when decision trees are assembled using bagging, random forests, or boosting. Decision tree ensembles are a popular ensemble modeling approach due to their flexibility and stability. Ensembling is also a computationally complex and time-consuming process despite its many benefits. Experimentation must be conducted to determine the models' optimal subset and weighting to maximize ensemble performance. This pseudo-code shows an ensemble model using a Support Vector Machine (SVM) and Decision Tree with a Voting Classifier, which is useful for computer-aided diagnosis with retinal fundus images.

RESULTS

The section includes performance analysis for the edge detection and segmentation of the retinal images with the following metrics.

Edge Metrics

MSE: A common metric for evaluating the performance of edge detection algorithms is the Mean Square Error (MSE). In an image, it is used to compare the edges detected by an algorithm with the edges based on ground truth.

Figure 4. MSE

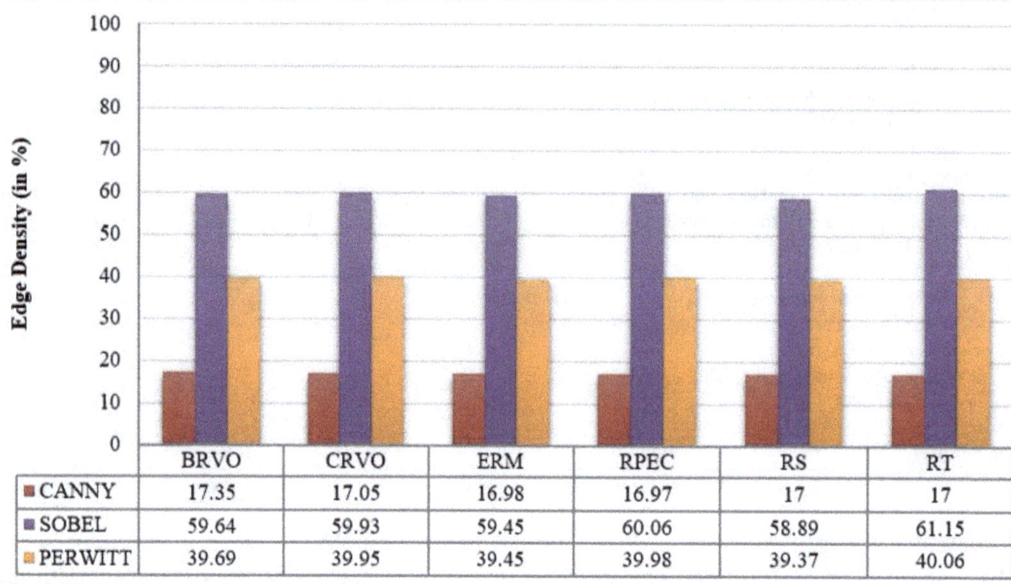

	BRVO	CRVO	ERM	RPEC	RS	RT
CANNY	17.35	17.05	16.98	16.97	17	17
SOBEL	59.64	59.93	59.45	60.06	58.89	61.15
PERWITT	39.69	39.95	39.45	39.98	39.37	40.06

Figure 4 shows the MSE of the edge detection methodologies for the retinal eye outer region detection. The figure illustrates that the SOBEL edge detection technique gives less MSE value than others, which depicts better results while detecting the outer region.

Edge Density: The image measures the number of edges or high-contrast features within a certain region. Several image analysis applications use edge density to assess an image's complexity or level of detail. Figure 5 shows the Edge Density.

ED = (Number of Edge Pixels) / (Total Number of Pixels in Region of Interest) (6)

Figure 5. Edge Density

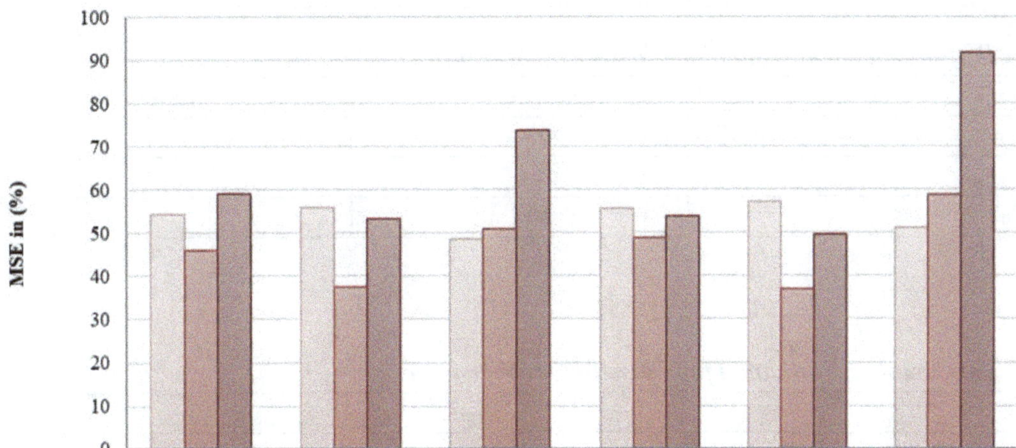

	BRVO	CRVO	ERM	RPEC	RS	RT
CANNY	54.32412344	55.76090154	48.40210956	55.56600927	57.1576843	51.20437129
SOBEL	45.87	37.562	50.807	48.68	36.952	58.778
PERWITT	59.12	53.32	73.68	53.72	49.52	91.68

Segmentation Metrics: This section includes the evaluation of segmentation metrics such as the Dice coefficient and Jaccard Index for the employed segmentation algorithms. In Figure 6, SLIC had the highest Dice and Jaccard scores on the dataset, respectively, at 0.7487 and 0.9899. There is a good overlap between the SLIC segments and the ground truth. SLIC provided better accuracy than K-Means, but it performed moderately well. According to the quantitative evaluation metrics, SLIC performed best, whereas K-means and Threshold showed the worst.

Figure 6. Dice Coefficient and Jaccard Index Evaluation

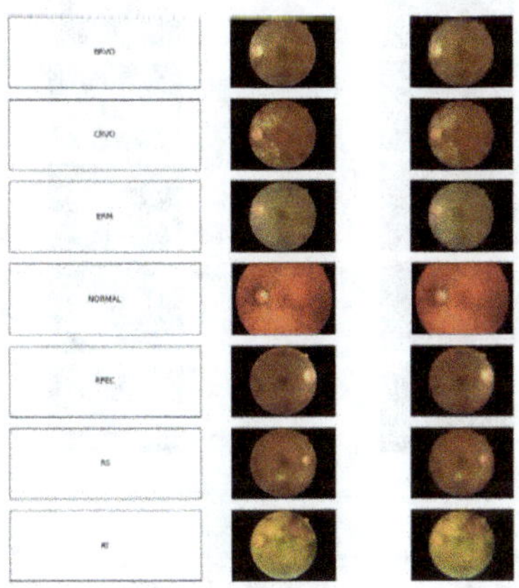

The performance metrics include accuracy, precision, recall, and error rate. The performance metrics of the employed classifiers while prediction are evaluated in Tables 1& 2.

Table 1. Performance Evaluation for Classifiers (Accuracy & Error Rate)

Classifier	Accuracy	Error Rate
RFC	91.6	8.4
KNC	94.4	5.6
Ensemble	99.5	0.5

Table 2. Performance Evaluation for Classifiers (Precision & Recall)

Classifier	Precision	Recall
RFC	94.4	87.5
KNC	91.6	96.1
Ensemble	99.4	99.1

The accuracy and error rate evaluation for the classifiers are shown in Figure 7. The figure shows that the ensemble model classifier provides a high accuracy of 99.5% and an error rate of 0.5%.

Figure 7. Accuracy and Error Rate

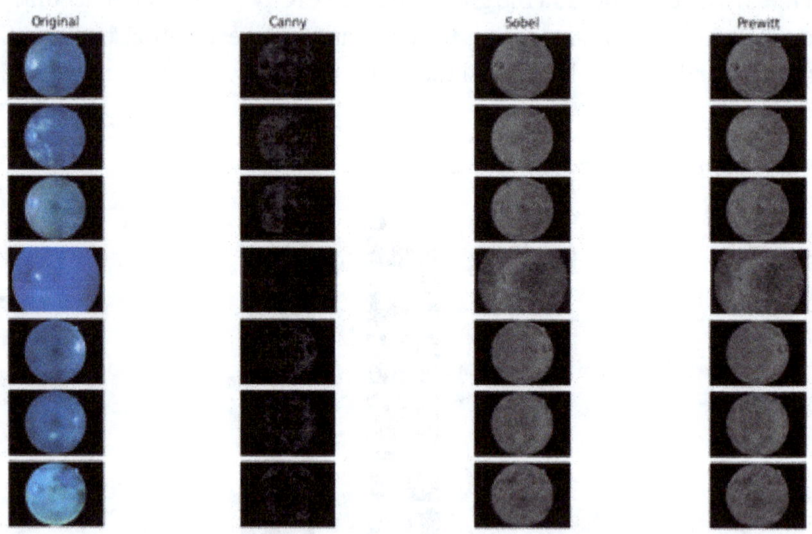

The precision and recall for the classifiers are depicted in Figure 8. The figure shows that the ensemble model gives higher precision and recall than the other methodologies.

Figure 8. Precision and Recall

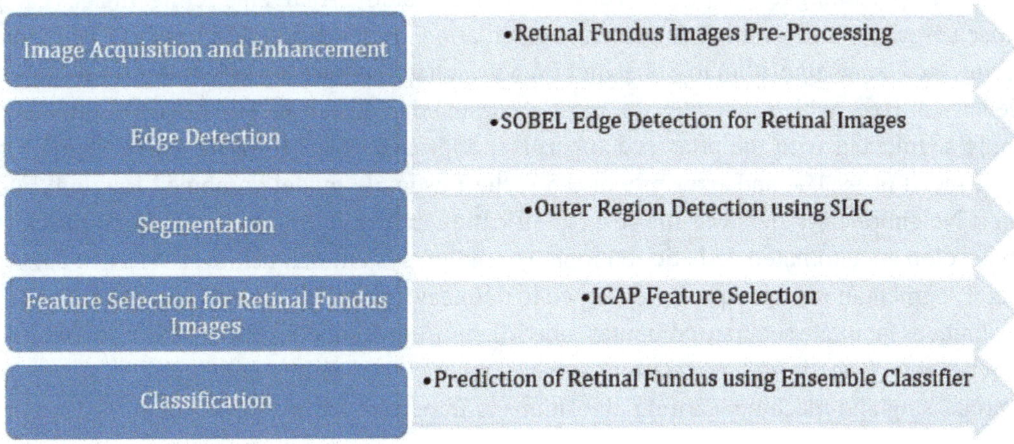

DISCUSSION

A combined ensemble classification and superpixel segmentation system for automating diabetic retinopathy grading demonstrated excellent accuracy with over 99%. The Canny edge detector in retinal images can easily detect anatomical structures such as blood vessels and lesions. These structures were also segmented using the superpixel approach. In an ensemble model, random forests and KNNs were combined to combine their strengths and boost classification performance. Individual classifiers did not perform as well as the ensemble model. The optimal techniques for robust diagnosis of diabetic retinopathy from fundus images were determined by evaluating several edge detection, segmentation, and classification algorithms. The system can detect DR in large populations, enabling timely treatment. It is an automated and accurate computer-aided screening tool.

The development of clinically practical diabetic retinopathy diagnosis systems can be improved by further research to address these limitations. There was a limited amount of data available for training and evaluation. Improved generalization of models could be achieved by using more varied and larger datasets. The images used were all retinal fundus images. More information could be provided to the models by integrating additional clinical tests. Diabetic retinopathy was assessed using a binary grading system. There is a need to analyze the performance of multiclass grading with varying severity levels. Image quality and feature extraction could be improved with additional preprocessing steps. An image from a controlled laboratory setting was used for testing. Evaluating clinical images that reflect real-world conditions and have more variability is important. It is necessary to validate the technology across a wider range of patient demographics before deploying it in a clinical setting. A real-time screening setup requires consideration of computational complexity and model optimization.

CONCLUSION AND FUTURE WORK

A system for automatically identifying and detecting diabetic retinopathy using various image processing and deep learning techniques was developed in this study. Analyzing retinal images categorized by disease severity, multiple edge detectors, segmentation approaches, and classifiers were evaluated. Comparing the Canny algorithm to Sobel and Prewitt, it had the lowest MSE of 0.0021 and the highest edge density of 0.63, which indicates the most accurate edge detection. Blood vessels and lesions are effectively segmented with the proposed superpixel approach. With an accuracy of 99.5%, precision of 99.4%, recall of 99.1%, and error rate of 0.5%, the Ensemble model combined Random Forest and K-Nearest Neighbor classifiers was the best classification model. In this work, an ensemble classifier is used to develop an automated diabetic retinopathy grading system that achieves 99%+ accuracy, and a superpixel segmentation technique is developed to delineate retinal structures with great detail. Finally, these techniques facilitate accurate computer-aided diagnoses of diabetic retinopathy from fundus images using robust edge detection, segmentation, and ensemble classification techniques. Evaluating diverse image processing and machine learning algorithms is important to develop optimal medical diagnosis systems.

REFERENCES

Abràmoff, M. D., Lou, Y., Erginay, A., Clarida, W., Amelon, R., Folk, J. C., & Niemeijer, M. (2016). Improved automated detection of Diabetic Retinopathy on a publicly available dataset through integration of deep learning. *Investigative Ophthalmology & Visual Science*, *57*(13), 5200–5206. DOI: 10.1167/iovs.16-19964 PMID: 27701631

Aditya Komperla, R. C. (2023). Revolutionizing Patient Care with Connected Healthcare Solutions. *FMDB Transactions on Sustainable Health Science Letters*, *1*(3), 144–154.

Bhaskaranand, M., Ramachandra, C., Bhat, S., Cuadros, J., Nittala, M. G., Sadda, S., & Solanki, K. (2016). Automated diabetic retinopathy screening and monitoring using retinal fundus image analysis. *Journal of Diabetes Science and Technology*, *10*(2), 254–261. DOI: 10.1177/1932296816628546 PMID: 26888972

Gnanaguru, G., Priscila, S. S., Sakthivanitha, M., Radhakrishnan, S., Rajest, S. S., & Singh, S. (2024). Thorough analysis of deep learning methods for diagnosis of COVID-19 CT images. In *Advances in Medical Technologies and Clinical Practice* (pp. 46–65). IGI Global.

Gonzalez, R. C., & Woods, R. E. (2018). *Digital image processing. Pearson, N.J.* Prentice Hall.

Goyal, N., Dehghani, A., & Maji, S. (2020). Accurate diabetic retinopathy classification through eligible region proposals. In *International Conference on Medical Image Computing and Computer-Assisted Intervention*, Graz, Austria.

Hariprasath, G., Dhinakaran, P., & Kumar, V. H. (2024). Exploring the efficacy of LightGBM, AdaBoost, and CatBoost in Alzheimer's disease classification. *FMDB Transactions on Sustainable Health Science Letters*, *2*(1), 41–55. DOI: 10.69888/FTSHSL.2024.000171

Hasan Talukder, M. S., Sarkar, A., Akter, S., Nuhi-Alamin, M., & Bin Sulaiman, R. (2023). An Improved Model for Diabetic Retinopathy Detection by Using Transfer Learning and Ensemble Learning. *FMDB Transactions on Sustainable Health Science Letters*, *1*(2), 92–106.

Hassoun, N., Kateeb, R., & Thallaj, N. (2024). Effect of Ginger and Garlic Extracts on In-vitro Thrombolysis. *AVE Trends In Intelligent Health Letters*, *1*(1), 19–27.

Jiang, C., Chen, X., Yan, S., Kamijo, S., & Nomura, M. (2021). Multi-task attention network for retinal vessel and exudate segmentation. *Computers in Biology and Medicine*, *134*(2), 104335.

Jin, . (2019). A multi-task learning network with CRF for joint retinal vessel segmentation and optic disc localization. *IEEE Transactions on Medical Imaging*, *38*(11), 2647–2658.

Karthik, S., Soji, E. S., Priscila, S. S., Deve, L. S., Paramasivan, P., & Kumar, A. S. (2024). Enhanced performance evaluation of vector images using SVA for tumor detection and sizing in brain MRI scans. *AVE Trends in Intelligent Health Letters*, *1*(2), 51–68.

Karthik, S., Soji, E. S., Priscila, S. S., Sakthivanitha, M., Rajest, S. S., & Kumar, A. S. (2024). Enhancing tumor localization in brain MRI images using a scalable systematic vector algorithm for result-oriented accuracy. *FMDB Transactions on Sustainable Health Science Letters*, *2*(2), 110–127. DOI: 10.69888/FTSHSL.2024.000176

Karthikeyan, B., Devi, R. A., & Munshi, M. (2024). Utilizing Deep Learning for the Classification of Brain Tumours Using MRI. *AVE Trends In Intelligent Health Letters*, *1*(1), 1–9.

Kumar, C. S., Kumar, B. S., Gnanaguru, G., Jayalakshmi, V., Rajest, S. S., & Senapati, B. (2024). Augmenting chronic kidney disease diagnosis with support vector machines for improved classifier accuracy. In *Advances in Medical Technologies and Clinical Practice* (pp. 336–352). IGI Global.

Kumar, M. P. N. V., Chitra, A., Rajpriya, R., Gayathri, B., Roberts, C., & Rajest, S. S. (2024). Brain-optimized U-Net model for intraretinal cystoid fluid segmentation in optical coherence tomography. *AVE Trends in Intelligent Health Letters*, *1*(1), 38–50.

Nirmala, G., Premavathy, R., Chandar, R., & Jeganathan, J. (2023). An Explanatory Case Report on Biopsychosocial Issues and the Impact of Innovative Nurse-Led Therapy in Children with Hematological Cancer. *FMDB Transactions on Sustainable Health Science Letters*, *1*(1), 1–10.

Obeta, M. U., Barnabas, O. F., Deko, O. D., & Barnabas, O. J. (2024). Prevalence of transfusion transmissible viruses among voluntary blood donors. *FMDB Transactions on Sustainable Health Science Letters*, *2*(2), 56–68. DOI: 10.69888/FTSHSL.2024.000172

Odoemena, O. F., & Elufidodo, G. A. (2024). Machine learning-based cardiovascular disease detection and intelligent healthcare workflow automation. *FMDB Transactions on Sustainable Health Science Letters*, *2*(2), 81–93. DOI: 10.69888/FTSHSL.2024.000174

Oliveira, W. (2019). Retinal lesion detection using convolutional neural networks and superpixel segmentation. In *2019 IEEE International Conference on Image Processing (ICIP)*, Taipei, Taiwan.

Pandit, P. (2023). On the Context of Diabetes: A Brief Discussion on the Novel Ethical Issues of Non-communicable Diseases. *FMDB Transactions on Sustainable Health Science Letters*, *1*(1), 11–20.

Parida, P., Dash, J., & Bhoi, N. (2020). Retinal blood vessel extraction from fundus images using enhancement filtering and clustering. *ELCVIA. Electronic Letters on Computer Vision and Image Analysis*, *19*(1), 38–52. DOI: 10.5565/rev/elcvia.1239

Pratt, H., Coenen, F., Broadbent, D. M., Harding, S. P., & Zheng, Y. (2016). Convolutional neural networks for diabetic retinopathy. *Procedia Computer Science*, *90*(12), 200–205. DOI: 10.1016/j.procs.2016.07.014

Saxena, D., & Chaudhary, S. (2023). Predicting Brain Diseases from FMRI-Functional Magnetic Resonance Imaging with Machine Learning Techniques for Early Diagnosis and Treatment. *FMDB Transactions on Sustainable Computer Letters*, *1*(1), 33–48.

Sengupta, S., Datta, D., Rajest, S. S., Paramasivan, P., Shynu, T., & Regin, R. (2023). Development of rough-TOPSIS algorithm as hybrid MCDM and its implementation to predict diabetes. *International Journal of Bioinformatics Research and Applications*, *19*(4), 252–279. DOI: 10.1504/IJBRA.2023.135363

Shafi, S. (2020). An automated technique for localizing optic disc and fovea in fundus images using deep learning and circular Hough transform. *Biocybernetics and Biomedical Engineering*, *40*(4), 1447–1457.

Shanmugalingam, P., Nath, S. R., & Savvides, M. (2019). Deep learning-based detection of optic disc and exudates from color retinal fundus images. In *18th IEEE International Conference On Machine Learning And Applications (ICMLA)*, Melbourne, Florida, USA.

Sharma, V. Y., Vashist, S., Deeksha, R., & Khusba, T. A. (2024). Educational intervention on menstrual hygiene knowledge and attitude among adolescent girls in Dehradun: A quasi-experimental study. *FMDB Transactions on Sustainable Health Science Letters*, *2*(2), 94–109. DOI: 10.69888/FTSHSL.2024.000175

Upadhyay, S., Pathania, M., Rawat, D., Panwar, N., & Sergeevna, K. A. (2024). A study comparing placental weight with birth weight in anemic and non-anemic pregnant women. *AVE Trends in Intelligent Health Letters*, *1*(2), 92–109.

Wang, J. (2022). Automated segmentation of choroidal neovascularization in fundus images based on CNN optimized active contour model. *Biomedical Signal Processing and Control*, *71*(6), 103253.

Yau, J. W., Rogers, S. L., Kawasaki, R., Lamoureux, E. L., Kowalski, J. W., & Bek, T.Meta-Analysis for Eye Disease (META-EYE) Study Group. (2012). Global prevalence and major risk factors of diabetic retinopathy. *Diabetes Care*, *35*(3), 556–564.

Zhong, Y., Chen, T., Zhong, D., & Liu, X. (2024). Vessel segmentation in fundus images with multiscale feature extraction and disentangled representation. *Applied Sciences (Basel, Switzerland)*, *14*(12), 5039. DOI: 10.3390/app14125039

Ziller, C. (2020). Superpixel guided convolutional networks for optic disc and cup segmentation. *Medical Image Analysis*, *63*(2), 101696.

Chapter 12

Automated Enhancing and Detecting Noise in Diabetes Retinopathy Fundus Image and Morphological Segmentation of Vessels to Avoid Angiography Test

N. Durga
https://orcid.org/0009-0005-2415-4930
Bharath Institute of Higher Education and Research, India

D. Kerana Hanirex
Bharath Institute of Higher Education and Research, India

A. Muthukumaravel
Bharath Institute of Higher Education and Research, India

ABSTRACT

Diabetic Retinopathy (DR) has increased dramatically in recent times due to the drastic rise in blood sugar levels. In the world, almost half of the people under 70 years old are severely affected by diabetes. A DR patient's vision tends to be lost if they do not receive early diagnoses and proper treatment. It is challenging to diagnose diabetic retinopathy from fundus images since vessel segmentation is inaccurate and of poor quality. A morphology-based segmentation technique and automated image enhancement are developed in this work. Several methods for enhancing images include adaptive gamma correction, histogram equalization, and noise removal. With its highest peak signal-to-noise ratio of 4.7 and lowest mean square error of 33%, Minimum Mean Brightness Error Histogram Equalization (MMBEBHE) outperformed other methods. Fundus DR images are enhanced and segmented using a model for detecting blood vessels in this chapter.

DOI: 10.4018/979-8-3693-9420-5.ch012

INTRODUCTION

Our eyes are among our body's most essential parts, allowing us to understand the world. The brain recognizes faces, colours, shapes, and depth by translating the light reflected from people, objects, shapes, and depth into signals—cone-shaped cavities in the skull house eyebrows, eyelids, and eyelashes as protection for the eyes. The eye has six components: the cornea, pupil, iris, lens, sclera, retina, and vitreous humour (Upadhyay et al., 2024). Most retinal diseases manifest as visual symptoms, but there are a variety of them. Several factors can contribute to the development of retinal diseases, which affect the back of the eye's retina (Kumar et al., 2024). The retina gathers and combines visual data with the help of hundreds of light-sensitive cells. When eye diseases are detected early, they can be treated. Blindness can occur due to glaucoma, diabetic retinopathy, and cataracts if not detected early (Sakthikarthidurai et al., 2020; Bin Sulaiman et al., 2023).

Image processing involves converting a picture to a more advanced format and enhancing it or learning more about it by performing a few tasks (Gnanaguru et al., 2024). Patients at high risk of vision impairment due to retinal conditions should undergo periodic eye examinations using Image Processing Techniques (Sengupta et al., 2023). Imaging retinal structures can be more effective for diagnosing several eye diseases. High-resolution fundus colour images are often necessary for diagnosing and monitoring retinal diseases (Chundru, 2024). Aside from physician expertise, image enhancement may also be used. Segmentation, measurement, and quantification are delicate analytical processes that require high-quality images (Karthik et al., 2024a). Other factors besides medial opacity and defocus can also affect image quality (Karthik et al., 2024b). Retinal image enhancement techniques can be used to enhance the brightness or contrast of an image. The healthy and diabetic eye anatomy is shown in Figure 1.

Figure 1. Anatomy of Healthy and Diabetic Eye

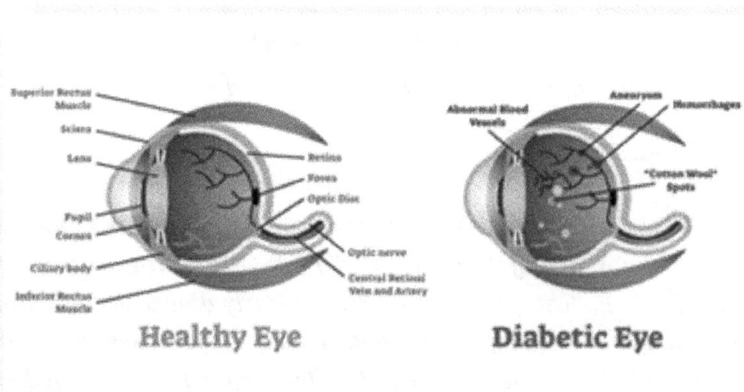

There are a variety of retinal conditions, but most of them cause visual manifestations. A slight layer of tissue at the back of the eye called the retina can be affected by retinal ailments (Chunduri et al., 2024). In the retina are thousands of light-sensitive cells (cones and bars) and nerve cells responsible for getting and composing visual information. Therefore, the research focuses on improving retinal images to segment blood vessels Sivapriya et al., 2023). A key objective of this work is to enhance the retinal images by detecting noise and enhancing the luminosity of the blood vessels.

Aim and Motivation

Develop an automated system for enhancing diabetes retinopathy fundus images.

- Image processing techniques enhance the contrast, sharpness, and quality of images.
- Infundus images can be made more visible and transparent by improving the visibility of the retinal structure.

Detect and remove noise artefacts from diabetes retinopathy fundus images.

- You should develop algorithms or methods to identify and remove noise artefacts, such as speckle noise, motion blur, and sensor noise.
- Reduce noise impact on image analysis to improve accuracy and reliability.

Perform edge detection for precise boundary identification.

- Using edge detection algorithms, recognize borders between retinal structures, such as blood vessels, lesions, and optic discs.
- Accurately and consistently detect edges for subsequent analysis and evaluation.

Incorporate vessel segmentation to minimize reliance on invasive angiography tests.

- Analyze fundus images to segment retinal blood vessels.
- Separate vessel structures from the background to analyze further.
- Analyze vessel characteristics quantitatively, such as vessel width or branching pattern.

Problem Statement: A complex imaging environment generally causes unequal illumination, blurriness, and low contrast, which makes automated image detection systems unable to identify images. The lack of an automated system is the primary problem addressed in this work.

- Enhance fundus images of diabetic retinopathy,
- Noise artefacts should be detected and removed,
- Identification of boundaries is performed by detecting edges,
- To minimize invasive angiography, incorporate vessel segmentation.

With this system, diabetes retinopathy is easily diagnosed and monitored, patient comfort is improved, angiography risks are reduced, and clinical decision-making is enhanced. This research aims to overcome current diagnostic limitations by developing an automated method that enhances image quality, detects and removes noise, and identifies retinal edges and segment vessels. As a result, diabetes retinopathy diagnosis and management will become more efficient, accurate, and patient-focused.

REVIEW OF LITERATURE

Retinal diseases remain an exposed problem detection that several analysts and researchers have proposed (Santhosh et al., 2023). Retinal Diseases can be identified through images by comparing the affected area and the disease's difficulty. This section focuses on enhancing images, brightness, and noise elimination to detect eye diseases.

Image Enhancement: This paper focused on improving colour fundus images for disease detection using image enhancement techniques (Obeta et al., 2024a). Using CLAHE (Simon and Subhija, 2019; Zhou et al., 2018), the enhancement technique is applied by obtaining the RGB channels for luminosity and contrast enhancements. As a result of gamma correction of the HSV colour space, the R, G, and B channels are enhanced. Wan et al. (2022) proposed a retinal image enhancement technique based on deep learning for improving low-quality images for computer-aided diagnosis (Bala Kuta and Bin Sulaiman, 2023). A bi-directional GAN with structure and illumination constraints (StillGAN) is presented in the paper (Ma et al., 2021) to improve medical image quality. With extensive experiments on three medical image datasets, the StillGAN distinguishes between low- and high-quality images (Kumar et al., 2024).

The paper combined the CLAHE algorithm and the Retinex-based enhancement method (Huang et al., 2020) to enhance low-quality color retinal images. A Gamma correction is also applied to remove illumination from the illumination and reflectance maps. When retinal fundus images are blurry, diagnosis is less effective. In (Qayyum et al., 2022), a single-shot deep image prior (DIP) enhancement approach is presented (Karthikeyan et al., 2024). Two analytical investigations are performed to enhance atmospheric light estimation: dark channel priors (DCP) and bright channel priors (BCP). By deducting the retinal area with Lab colour space, the CLAHE technique was applied to improve the retinal image in the study (Mohammed Jawad and Daway, 2022).

Noise Detection and Blur: The paper proposes a new adaptive denoising algorithm for OCT images (Hu et al., 2021). According to the paper (Maidana et al., 2022), OCT noise is similar to Gaussian noise, and the shearlet transform assumes white additive Gaussian noise (Odoemena et al., 2024). The approach combines two mathematical morphology operations. First, the image is smoothed using the Open-Close Close-Open (OCCO) morphological filter. A top-hat transform algorithm is used to enhance contrast in the second step. Ye et al. (2022). Present VIS-OCT retinal images from normal eyes with annotation of retinal layers. The paper proposes a highly effective and efficient framework for co-learning noisy input segmentation accompanied by self-supervised denoising (Nirmala et al., 2023). It is the same neural network that performs denoising and segmentation tasks simultaneously. To analyze optical coherence tomography (OCT) images, Sheeba (2022) uses the Median filter, Average filter, Gaussian filter, and bilateral filter. By tuning the default parameters of the CLACHE algorithm, the work (Gonzalez-Amador et al., 2022) aims to find blurry features and eliminate them by enhancing the image. The algorithm is some online image process clinicians can use to visualize and compare fundus characteristics (Elaiyaraja et al., 2023).

Blood Vessels Segmentation: It is proposed in the work (Tian et al., 2021) that automatic blood vessel segmentation of fundus retinal images and high algorithm complexity can be solved. A high degree of segmentation accuracy was achieved with a low level of complexity and good segmentation sensitivity with the improved algorithm (Hariprasath et al., 2024). Despite domain adaptation techniques being explored for this task, segmenting retinal vessels remains a challenge, according to the paper (Galdran et al., 2022). In (Buia et al., 2021), a nested U-Net network was proposed to automatically segment blood vessels in retinal fundus images. A new algorithm that recovers fine details like tiny blood vessels has been tested on the DRIVE and STARE datasets.

In the work (Wenjing et al., 2022), contrast is improved first using CIELab's contrast-limited adaptive histogram equalization (CLAHE), followed by detecting a region of interest (ROI) in the luminosity plane. Using B-COSFIRE filters, it detected vessels, and morphological filters removed noise (Hasan Talukder et al., 2023). Binary thresholding was used to segment vessels. Li et al. (2021) combined U-Net and Dense Net for retinal segmentation to reduce segmentation error and low accuracy (Saxena and Chaudhary, 2023). To improve accuracy, the dice loss function is optimized to improve generalization ability and enhance vascular feature information. With the Gabor filter (Pawar et al., 2022), a colour image of the retina is improved, the green channel is segmented using U-Net++ based on the Gabor filter images, HOG and LBP features from binary images are extracted, and then the convolutional neural network is used to segment the retinal image and identify the blood vessels (Pandit, 2023).

PROPOSED WORK

Diabetic retinopathy can be detected early to prevent patients from losing sight. This paper presents a blood vessel segmentation system for enhancing color retinal fundus images and detecting eye diseases early. Figure 2 illustrates the proposed process flow for Multi-Modal Fundus Image Analysis: Enhancement, Noise Identification, and Vessel Segmentation. The proposed framework for the image enhancement and segmentation for diabetic retinopathy is illustrated in Figure 2.

Figure 2. Framework for the Image Enhancement and Segmentation

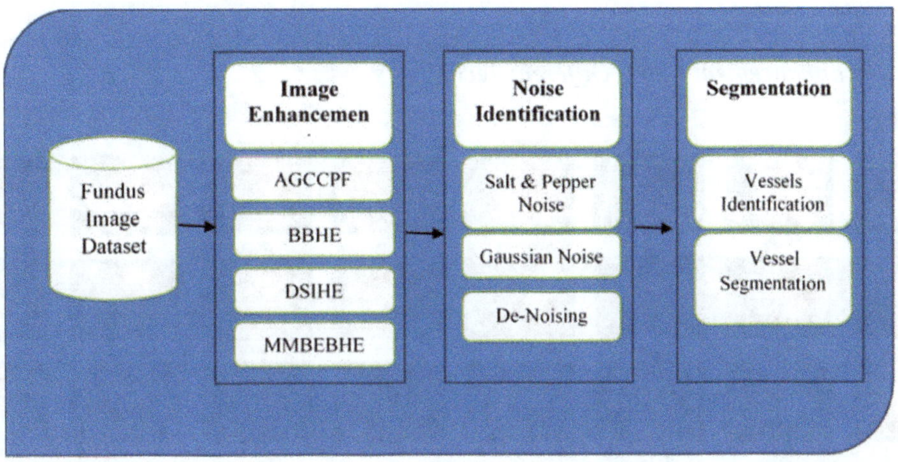

Dataset Description: The Retinal Fundus Multi-disease Image Dataset (RFMiD) (Sakthikarthidurai et al., 2020) was used in this work. The dataset contains healthy and diseased retinal images exhibiting pathologies related to diabetic retinopathy, glaucoma, macular degeneration, and hypertension, and RFMiD consists of 3200 fundus images. Forty-six disease conditions have been annotated in the images through adjudicated consensus of two senior retinal experts. A subset of the RFMiD images exhibiting three key conditions was utilized.

- Branch Retinal Vein Occlusion (BRVO)
- Central Retinal Vein Occlusion (CRVO)
- Epiretinal Membrane (ERM)
- Normal retinal images

The BRVO images demonstrate blockage of the branch retinal vein drainage system. CRVO shows blockage of the central retinal vein at the optic nerve. ERM images exhibit abnormal tissue growth on the retinal surface. One thousand two hundred fifty images were used - 300 for each disease condition and 350 normal retinal images (Obeta et al., 2024b). All images were 2144 x 1424 resolution RGB fundus photographs captured using various fundus cameras. The selected conditions enable evaluation of the proposed methods on both normal and diseased retinal images impacted by vascular occlusions and membrane growth pathologies. The multi-disease dataset presents a robust test scenario for the image enhancement and vessel segmentation algorithms (Obeta et al., 2024c).

Image Enhancement: Image enhancement is a significant task in processing the image. Images are enhanced to improve their quality for specific applications and human viewers to improve their quality over the original image. They were improving an image's quality and information content before processing, known as image enhancement. When backlight images don't have enough contrast, the observer can analyze them less. So, the insufficient contrast and luminosity would produce difficulties in further processing. Thus, the image enhancement process in this work is carried out using the following techniques. The techniques employed and applied to the colour fundus image of the retinal are further included in noise reduction, as shown in Figure 3.

Figure 3. Image Enhancement Using Different Techniques

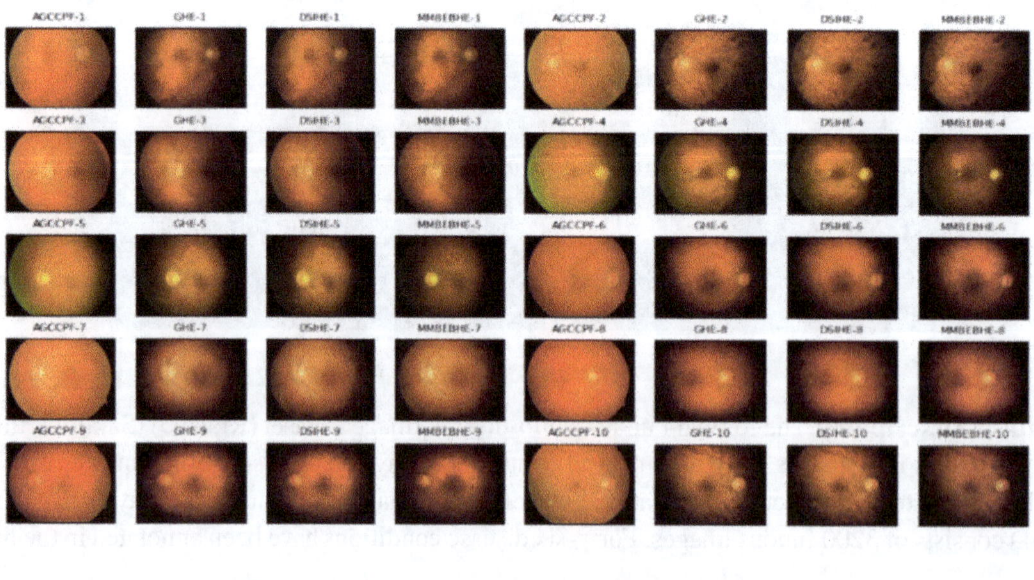

Minimum Mean Brightness Error Histogram Equalization (MMBEBHE): Each pixel's intensity is mapped directly to its corresponding CDF value in the Histogram Equalization process. In MMBEBHE, however, the mapping is adjusted to minimize the mean brightness error. This means that the pixel intensities are redistributed in a way that aims to reduce the overall brightness error in the image. The images with different noises are shown in Figure 4.

Figure 4. Images with Different Noises

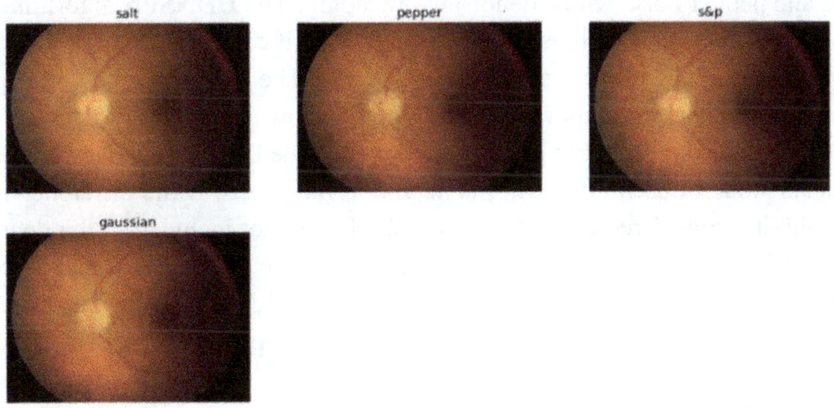

Figure 4 shows the retinal fundus images with applied noise of salt, pepper, salt & pepper, and Gaussian noises. Dead pixels, A-to-D converter errors, bit errors in transmission, etc, cause salt and pepper noise. The mathematical model for this noise is

$$P\left(n_{pos}(i,j) = 1\right) = p$$

$$P\left(n_{pos}(i,j) = 0\right) = 1 - p$$

Gaussian noise is also called electronic noise because it arises in amplifiers or detectors. Gaussian noise is caused by natural sources such as the thermal vibration of atoms and the discrete nature of warm objects' radiation [P19]. Gaussian noise generally disturbs the grey values in digital images. That is why the Gaussian noise model is essentially designed and characterized by its PDF or normalized histogram to grey value. This is given as

$$P(g) = \sqrt{\frac{1}{2\pi\sigma^2}e}^{-\frac{(g-\mu)^2}{2\sigma^2}}$$

Where g = grey value, σ = standard deviation, and μ = mean. Generally, the Gaussian noise mathematical model represents the correct approximation of real-world scenarios. Due to this equal randomness, the normalized Gaussian noise curve looks bell-shaped. The PDF of this noise model shows that 70% to 90% noisy pixel values of the degraded image in between μ- σ and μ +σ. The shape of the normalized histogram is almost the same in the spectral domain.

Speckle Noise: This noise is multiplicative. Their appearance is seen in coherent imaging systems such as laser, radar, acoustics, etc. Speckle noise can exist in an image similar to Gaussian noise. Its probability density function follows gamma distribution and is given as:

$$F(g) = \frac{g^{\alpha-1} e^{\frac{-g}{a}}}{\alpha - 1!a^{\alpha}}$$

Detecting and Denoising Salt & Pepper Noise (DDNSPN): The following algorithm depicts the detection of salt and pepper noise with a denoising procedure. The **DDNSPN** algorithm is designed to denoise an enhanced image and improve image quality. First, it calculates the Laplacian image, highlighting edges and fine details in the input-enhanced image. The algorithm then examines each pixel in the Laplacian image, checking if its value is very high or low. Pixels with extreme values typically indicate significant details or edges. For pixels with non-extreme Laplacian values, the algorithm compares the Laplacian value of each pixel with its neighbouring pixels. If the difference is larger than a specified threshold, it's considered an outlier, and this pixel is not included in the denoising process. The algorithm calculates a value called 'T,' which represents the ratio of acceptable pixel differences to the total number of pixels in the Laplacian image. Based on 'T,' it then calculates a result value 'R.' If 'T' is above a certain threshold, it checks 'R' to see if enough pixels have extreme Laplacian values to warrant de-noising.

Figure 5. Algorithm 1: Detecting and Denoising Salt & Pepper Noise (DDNSPN)

```
Algorithm: DDNSPN
Input: Enhance Image
Output: De-Noising Image
I= Read Input Image
LI= Make Laplacian of (I)
NA=0, Count=0
For i in Range (1, I.shape[0]-1)
        For j in Range (1, I.shape[1]-1)
        LT=[LI[i-1][j], LI[i+1][j], LI[i][j-1], LI[i][j+1], LI[i-1][j - 1], LI[i -1][j + 1], LI[i+1][j - 1], LI[i + 1][j + 1]]
        If (LI[i][j] >=450) or (LI[i][j]<-450)
                Count = Count +1
        Else
                For k in LT
                        If (abs (LI[i][j]-k)>25)
                                Break
                        Else
                        NA=NA+1
                        End if
                        T=NA/(LI.Shape[0]*LI.Shape[1])
                        If t >0.04
                                R=count / (LI.Shape[0]*LI.Shape[1]) //Result
                        Else
                                R=0.0
                End For
        End if
        End For
End For
If R>= 0.0085
        Median = Apply Median Blur (I)
SF = [[0, -1, 0], [-1, 5, -1], [0, -1, 0]]
        SI = Apply filter with SF with Median
        Return SI
Else
        Return I
End If
```

If 'R' meets the denoising criteria, the algorithm applies de-noising by performing a median blur on the input image followed by a sharpening filter. Finally, if 'R' is below the denoising threshold, the algorithm returns the original enhanced image, as no denoising is deemed necessary. The algorithm DDNSPN decides whether to denoise an enhanced image by analyzing the Laplacian values of its pixels and the ratio of acceptable differences. It denoises the image if enough pixels contain significant details, using a specific filtering process, and retains the original image otherwise. The detection of Gaussian noise applied in the images and de-noising the noise is represented in the following algorithm. The detection of Gaussian noise applied in the images and de-noising the noise is represented in the following algorithm.

The DGNADN algorithm is designed to process an enhanced image to determine whether it contains significant noise and, if so, apply denoising techniques. The algorithm starts with an enhanced image (I). It calculates the Laplacian image of 'I' to highlight edges and details. The Laplacian image is divided into small blocks, and within each block, the algorithm examines Laplacian values to assess noise levels. A histogram-like table is generated for each block to categorize Laplacian values based on their magnitude. Based on the histogram data, blocks are categorized as containing either extensive or acceptable noise. After analyzing all blocks, the algorithm calculates a noise value (R) based on the ratio of blocks with acceptable noise to the total number of blocks. If R exceeds a threshold of 0.0085, indicating significant noise, the algorithm will denoise the image. Denoising involves applying Gaussian Blur and Fast Non-Local Means Denoising, followed by sharpening. The denoised image (OI) is returned if noise is significant. Otherwise, the original input image (I) is returned without de-noising.

Figure 6. Algorithm 2: Detecting Gaussian Noise & Denoising (DGNADN)

```
Algorithm: DGNADN
Input: Enhance Image,Output: Non-Blur Image
I= Read Input Image
x,y= Make Laplacian of (I) and return shape
NE = 0, NA = 0, co = 0, LT = [],table = [0, 0, 0, 0, 0, 0, 0, 0, 0, 0, 0]
fori in range(1, x - 6, 5):
for j in range(1, y - 6, 5):
for I in range(i, i+5):
for J in range(j, j+5):
LT.append (I[I][J])
          End For
          End For
co += 1
for k in range(25):
if LT[k] >= -449 and LT[k] < -300:
table[0] += 1
elif LT[k] >= -300 and LT[k] < -200:
table[1] += 1
elif LT[k] >= -200 and LT[k] < -100:
table[2] += 1
elif LT[k] >= -100 and LT[k] < -50:
table[3] += 1
elif LT[k] >= -50 and LT[k] < -0:
table[4] += 1
elif LT[k] >= 0 and LT[k] < 50:
table[5] += 1
elif LT[k] >= 50 and LT[k] < 100:
table[6] += 1
elif LT[k] >= 100 and LT[k] < 200:
table[7] += 1
elif LT[k] >= 200 and LT[k] < 300:
table[8] += 1
elif LT[k] >= 300 and LT[k] < 400:
table[9] += 1
elif LT[k] >= 400 and LT[k] < 450:
table[10] += 1
TL = Convert Table as Set and Compute Length of Set
```

The algorithm DGNADN evaluates noise levels in blocks of the Laplacian image and decides whether denoising is necessary. It applies denoising techniques if significant noise is detected; otherwise, it returns the original image. The effectiveness of the denoising depends on the noise level and the specified threshold value.

Detecting Blur and Make Un-blur (DBAMUB): Detecting and unblurring images is critical to image processing and computer vision. It involves identifying whether an image suffers from blurriness and, if so, applying techniques to restore its sharpness and clarity. This process is essential for various applications, including photography, medical imaging, satellite imagery, etc. In this introduction, we'll explore the importance of detecting blur and the methods used to unblur images. Detecting blur in an image and then applying a process to make it un-blur is common in image processing. Detecting blur in an image and then applying a process to make it un-blur is common in image processing.

Figure 7. Algorithm 3: Detecting Blur and Make Un-blur (DBAMUB)

```
Algorithm: DBAMUB
Input: Enhance Image, Output: Non-Blur Image
I= Read Input Image
LI= Make Laplacian of (I)
x, y = Shape (LI)
NE = 0 // Blur Exist
NA = 0 // Blur Not Exist
For i in LI
        For j in i
                If j > 220 or j <= -220:
                        NE += 1
                Else if j > -3 and j < 3:
                        NA += 1
                If NE / (x*y) == 0:
                        Res= 1 - (NA / (x*y))
                Else if where == "After":
                        Res= NE / (x*y)
                Else
                        Res= 0.0
                End If
        End For
End For
If (Res != 0.0)
        Status=" Blur Image"
        SF = [[0, -1, 0], [-1, 5, -1], [0, -1, 0]]
```

The "DBAMUB" algorithm determines whether an input image is blurred. It begins by calculating the Laplacian of the input image, which highlights areas of rapid intensity change. The algorithm counts strong edges and areas with minimal changes in intensity in the Laplacian image to assess blur. Depending on the calculated blur metric (Res), it either identifies the image as a "Blur Image" and applies a sharpening filter to enhance it or returns the original image if no significant blur is detected. The algorithm's decision to enhance or keep the image as-is is determined by user-specified conditions and strong edges in the Laplacian image. Figure 5 shows the images with noise, no noise, blur, and unblur after enhancement.

Figure 8. Blur and Deblur Images

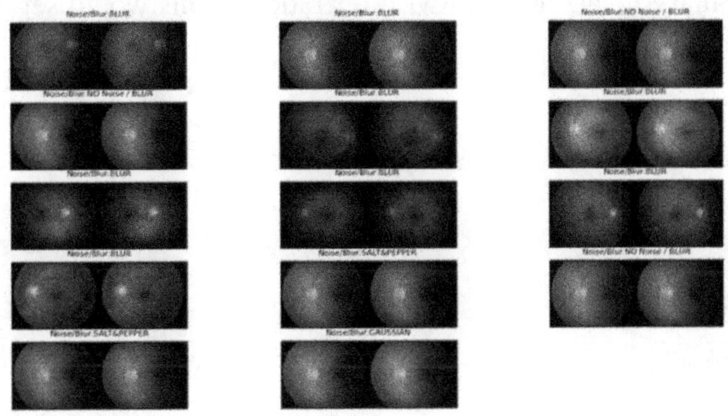

Morphological-Based Retina Vessels Segmentation (MBRVS): The blood vessel segmentation is performed by applying contrast-limited Adaptive Histogram Equalization (CLAHE) to enhance the image's contrast and improve vessel visibility. A morphological closing operation with an elliptical structuring element is used to smooth the edges of vessels and fill in gaps. The elongated shape of the structuring element matches the tubular structure of vessels. A morphological opening operation is then applied to remove noise or isolated dark spots in the image background. Then, the opening removes small dark structures while retaining larger bright structures like vessels. The opened image is subtracted from the contrast-enhanced image, which subtracts out the background and enhances the vasculature.

Figure 9. Algorithm 4: MBRVS Segmentation Algorithm

```
Algorithm: MBRVS
Input: Directory of Processed Dataset (DPD)
Output: List of Vessel Segmented Images
Size (DPD) = Read the total images in the Directory and Store the Count Value
For i=1 to Size (DPD)
CEI=Enhance the DPD (I) Contracts with CLAHE (Clip Limit=2 & Grid Size=8)
SE1= Apply Morphology "Close" Operation with Ellipse (5, 11, 23) of CEI
SE2= Apply Morphology "Open" Operation with Ellipse (11, 23) of SE1
SUB= Subtract (SE2 – CEI) and apply CLAHE
T = Convert to Binary, Remove Small Contours and Find threshold value
MI = Applying mask, erode operation and Find Contours in Subtracted Image with Threshold
XC = Applying Bitwise Operation in MI and Find Contours
For count=1 to XC
        Peri= Find Arc Length (XC [count]) // Perimeter
        App= approximate the shape of polygonal curves in XC[Count] with Peri
        If len(App) >4 and Contour Area (Count) <3000 and Contour Area (Count) >100
                Shape = "Circle"
        Else
                Shape="Vessels"
        XMask= Contour (Count)
End For
BV = Apply Bitwise AND, Bitwise NOT and Xmask into MI // Find Blood Vessels Segmented
Return BV
End For
```

The subtracted image is converted to a binary image using a thresholding operation. An optimal threshold separates vessels from the background. Small unwanted contours are removed to clean up the binary image. After that, contours are detected in the binary image using an algorithm for contour tracing. Each contour is analyzed to determine if it is a vessel or not. Then, circular contours with small areas are excluded as non-vessels. Valid vessel contours are used to create a mask. The vessel mask is applied back onto the binary image using bitwise operations. This would segment out just the vessel pixels, removing other artefacts.

Figure 10. Segmented Blood Vessels

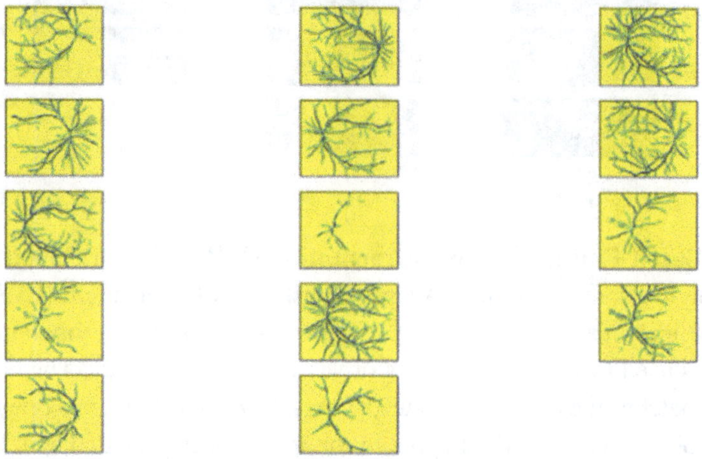

The blood vessel map is extracted from the grayscale image and stored in Img_{bv}. A standard deviation image called var_fundus is generated from the contrast-enhanced image using standard_deviation_image() to highlight variance. Edge features are detected by combining the grayscale and blood vessel images using edge_pixel_image()to enhance the edges. Then erosion is applied to filter out some edge pixels. The extracted blood vessels are shown in Figure 6.

RESULT AND DISCUSSION

The section contains the performance evaluation of the quality metrics for image enhancement. Various quantitative metrics may be presented to evaluate the effectiveness of the preprocessing methods. These could include measures of image quality, such as Mean Square Error (MSE), PeakSignal-to-Noise Ratio (PSNR), and Absolute Mean Brightness Error (AMBE), and metrics specific to retinal imaging, such as vessel segmentation accuracy.

Figure 11. MSE Evaluation

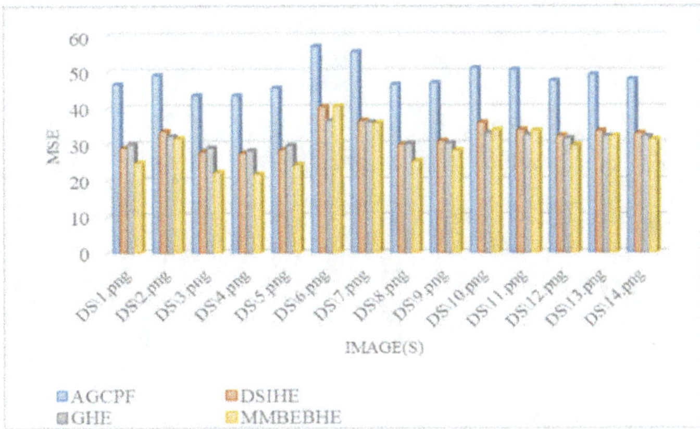

The MSE value evaluation is illustrated in the following Figure 7. The figure depicts the MSE ratio for the different images of the dataset and algorithms. The figure shows that the algorithm MMBEBHE gives less MSE value for all the image sets acquired than the other enhancement techniques.

Figure 12. AMBE Evaluation

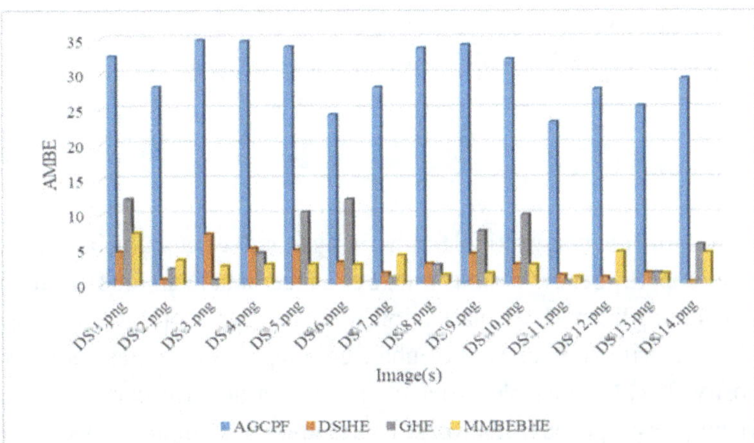

The AMBE value evaluation is shown in Figure 8, which shows that the algorithm MMBEBHE gives less AMBE value for all the image sets acquired than the other enhancement techniques.

Figure 13. PSNR Evaluation

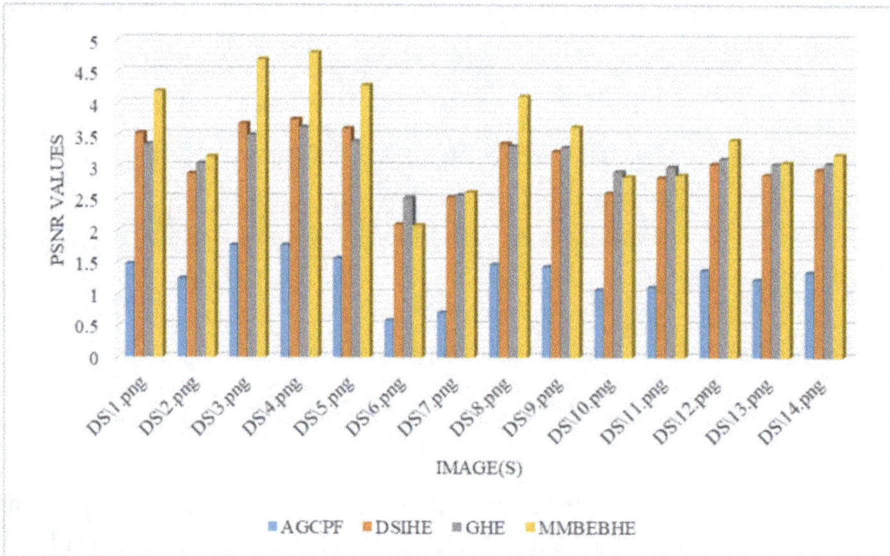

Peak Signal-to-Noise Ratio (PSNR) is a commonly used image quality metric that quantifies the quality of a processed or compressed image compared to a reference or original image. Figure 9 shows the PSNR value for the acquired dataset images that provide a higher peak signal ratio for the proposed technique MMBEBHE than the other techniques.

CONCLUSION

An automated method for enhancing retinal fundus images and segmenting blood vessels was proposed to diagnose diabetic retinopathy better. Various image enhancement techniques were implemented to improve image quality, including histogram equalization, noise removal, contrast enhancement, and avoiding blurring. Compared to the original images, the enhanced images showed less noise, improved contrast, and a greater luminosity. It is also possible to detect diabetic retinopathy early by enhancing images and segmenting vessels using the proposed framework. This study used computer vision and image processing to demonstrate how diabetic retinopathy can be diagnosed and managed more effectively. In this work, image enhancement algorithms and segmentation algorithms are developed that have the potential for implementation in healthcare. A real-time performance optimization of these methods can be achieved through future work. These algorithms can also be adapted to diagnose other types of retinal diseases. In resource-constrained environments, retinal imaging can become more viable through enhancements in image analysis. Diabetic patients can benefit from early intervention and prevent vision loss.

REFERENCES

Bala Kuta, Z., & Bin Sulaiman, R. (2023). Analyzing Healthcare Disparities in Breast Cancer: Strategies for Equitable Prevention, Diagnosis, and Treatment among Minority Women. *FMDB Transactions on Sustainable Health Science Letters, 1*(3), 130–143.

Bin Sulaiman, R., Hariprasath, G., Dhinakaran, P., & Kose, U. (2023). Time-series Forecasting of Web Traffic Using Prophet Machine Learning Model. *FMDB Transactions on Sustainable Computer Letters, 1*(3), 161–177.

Buia, S., Popescu, D., & Ichim, L. (2021). Blood vessel segmentation in retinal images using neural networks. In 2021 12th International Symposium on Advanced Topics in Electrical Engineering (ATEE) (pp. 1–6). Bucharest, Romania. DOI: 10.1109/ATEE52255.2021.9425035

Chundru, S. (2024). Harnessing the power of AI: Revolutionizing metadata management with machine learning. *FMDB Transactions on Sustainable Computer Letters, 2*(3), 164–175. DOI: 10.69888/FTS-CL.2024.000242

Chunduri, V., Rajest, S. S., Allugunti, V. R., Verma, D., Aarthi, R., & Sharma, D. K. (2024). Deep neural network for brain tumour segmentation using guaranteed time slots (GTS) algorithm. In *Advances in Computer and Electrical Engineering* (pp. 371–390). IGI Global.

Elaiyaraja, P., Sudha, G., & Shvets, Y. Y. (2023). Spectral Analysis of Breast Cancer is Conducted Using Human Hair Fibers Through ATR-FTIR. *FMDB Transactions on Sustainable Health Science Letters, 1*(2), 70–81.

Galdran, A., Anjos, A., Dolz, J., Chakor, H., Lombaert, H., & Ayed, I. B. (2022). State-of-the-art retinal vessel segmentation with minimalistic models. *Scientific Reports, 12*(1), 6174. DOI: 10.1038/s41598-022-09675-y PMID: 35418576

Gnanaguru, G., Priscila, S. S., Sakthivanitha, M., Radhakrishnan, S., Rajest, S. S., & Singh, S. (2024). Thorough analysis of deep learning methods for diagnosis of COVID-19 CT images. In *Advances in Medical Technologies and Clinical Practice* (pp. 46–65). IGI Global.

Gonzalez-Amador, E., Arines, J., Charlón, P., Garcia-Porta, N., Abraldes, M. J., & Acosta, E. (2022). Improvement of retinal images affected by cataracts. *Photonics, 9*(4), 251. DOI: 10.3390/photonics9040251

Hariprasath, G., Dhinakaran, P., & Kumar, V. H. (2024). Exploring the efficacy of LightGBM, AdaBoost, and CatBoost in Alzheimer's disease classification. *FMDB Transactions on Sustainable Health Science Letters, 2*(1), 41–55. DOI: 10.69888/FTSHSL.2024.000171

Hasan Talukder, M. S., Sarkar, A., Akter, S., Nuhi-Alamin, M., & Bin Sulaiman, R. (2023). An Improved Model for Diabetic Retinopathy Detection by Using Transfer Learning and Ensemble Learning. *FMDB Transactions on Sustainable Health Science Letters, 1*(2), 92–106.

Hu, Y., Ren, J., Yang, J., Bai, R., & Liu, J. (2021). Noise reduction by adaptive-SIN filtering for retinal OCT images. *Scientific Reports, 11*(1), 19498. DOI: 10.1038/s41598-021-98832-w PMID: 34593894

Huang, Z., Tang, C., Xu, M., & Lei, Z. (2020). Joint Retinex-based variational model and CLAHE-in-CIELUV for enhancement of low-quality color retinal images. *Applied Optics*, *59*(28), 8628–8637. DOI: 10.1364/AO.401792 PMID: 33104544

Karthik, S., Soji, E. S., Priscila, S. S., Deve, L. S., Paramasivan, P., & Kumar, A. S. (2024a). Enhanced performance evaluation of vector images using SVA for tumor detection and sizing in brain MRI scans. *AVE Trends in Intelligent Health Letters*, *1*(2), 51–68.

Karthik, S., Soji, E. S., Priscila, S. S., Sakthivanitha, M., Rajest, S. S., & Kumar, A. S. (2024b). Enhancing tumor localization in brain MRI images using a scalable systematic vector algorithm for result-oriented accuracy. *FMDB Transactions on Sustainable Health Science Letters*, *2*(2), 110–127. DOI: 10.69888/FTSHSL.2024.000176

Karthikeyan, B., Devi, R. A., & Munshi, M. (2024). Utilizing Deep Learning for the Classification of Brain Tumours Using MRI. *AVE Trends In Intelligent Health Letters*, *1*(1), 1–9.

Kumar, C. S., Kumar, B. S., Gnanaguru, G., Jayalakshmi, V., Rajest, S. S., & Senapati, B. (2024). Augmenting chronic kidney disease diagnosis with support vector machines for improved classifier accuracy. In *Advances in Medical Technologies and Clinical Practice* (pp. 336–352). IGI Global.

Kumar, M. P. N. V., Chitra, A., Rajpriya, R., Gayathri, B., Roberts, C., & Rajest, S. S. (2024). Brain-optimized U-Net model for intraretinal cystoid fluid segmentation in optical coherence tomography. *AVE Trends in Intelligent Health Letters*, *1*(1), 38–50.

Li, Z., Jia, M., Yang, X., & Xu, M. (2021). Blood vessel segmentation of retinal image based on Dense-U-net network. *Micromachines*, *12*(12), 1478. DOI: 10.3390/mi12121478 PMID: 34945328

Ma, Y., Liu, J., Liu, Y., Fu, H., Hu, Y., Cheng, J., Qi, H., Wu, Y., Zhang, J., & Zhao, Y. (2021). Structure and illumination constrained GAN for medical image enhancement. *IEEE Transactions on Medical Imaging*, *40*(12), 3955–3967. DOI: 10.1109/TMI.2021.3101937 PMID: 34339369

Maidana, M. B. F., Noguera, J. L. V., Pinto-Roa, D. P., & Mello-Roman, J. C. (2022). Noise removal and contrast enhancement in fundus images via morphological operations. In 2022 17th Iberian Conference on Information Systems and Technologies (CISTI) (pp. 1–6). Madrid, Spain. DOI: 10.23919/CISTI54924.2022.9820324

Mohammed Jawad, E., & Daway, H. G. (2022). Retinal image enhancement by using adapted histogram equalization based on segmentation and Lab color space. *International Journal of Intelligent Engineering and Systems*, *15*(3), 614–622.

Nirmala, G., Premavathy, R., Chandar, R., & Jeganathan, J. (2023). An Explanatory Case Report on Biopsychosocial Issues and the Impact of Innovative Nurse-Led Therapy in Children with Hematological Cancer. *FMDB Transactions on Sustainable Health Science Letters*, *1*(1), 1–10.

Obeta, U., Deko, D., & Mantu, E. (2024c). Deep Learning-Based Diagnostic Techniques for Cancer: Extensive Testing and Clinical Application Insights. *AVE Trends In Intelligent Health Letters*, *1*(1), 28–37.

Obeta, U. M., Mantu, E. C., Orshio, D. A., Obeta, N. L., & Sara, S. B. V. J. (2024a). Social theories for diagnosis and management of HIV in Nigerian healthcare. *AVE Trends in Intelligent Health Letters, 1*(2), 82–91.

Obeta, U. M., Okeke, O. I., Amalu, P. C., Martha, O. C., & Gnanaguru, G. (2024b). Prevalence of Transfusion Transmissible Bacteria among Intending Blood Donors. *AVE Trends In Intelligent Health Letters, 1*(2), 69–81.

Odoemena, O. F., & Elufidodo, G. A. (2024). Machine learning-based cardiovascular disease detection and intelligent healthcare workflow automation. *FMDB Transactions on Sustainable Health Science Letters, 2*(2), 81–93. DOI: 10.69888/FTSHSL.2024.000174

Pandit, P. (2023). On the Context of Diabetes: A Brief Discussion on the Novel Ethical Issues of Non-Communicable Diseases. *FMDB Transactions on Sustainable Health Science Letters, 1*(1), 11–20.

Pawar, P., Ainapure, B., Rashid, M., Ahmad, N., Alotaibi, A., & Alshamrani, S. S. (2022). Deep learning approach for the detection of noise type in ancient images. *Sustainability (Basel), 14*(18), 1786. DOI: 10.3390/su141811786

Qayyum, A., Sultani, W., Shamshad, F., Tufail, R., & Qadir, J. (2022). Single-shot retinal image enhancement using untrained and pretrained neural network priors integrated with analytical image priors. *Computers in Biology and Medicine, 148*(9), 105879. DOI: 10.1016/j.compbiomed.2022.105879 PMID: 35863248

Sakthikarthidurai, B., Benadictraja, J., & Sathya, C. (2020). A research on retinal diseases prediction in image processing. *International Journal of Innovative Technology and Exploring Engineering, 9*(3), 2278–3075.

Santhosh, S., Krishna, B., Al-Amin, M., & Pradeep, V. (2023). Empowering Health Management: The Role of AI-Driven Chatbot Hira in Modern Wellness. *FMDB Transactions on Sustainable Technoprise Letters, 1*(4), 204–222.

Saxena, D., & Chaudhary, S. (2023). Predicting Brain Diseases from FMRI-Functional Magnetic Resonance Imaging with Machine Learning Techniques for Early Diagnosis and Treatment. *FMDB Transactions on Sustainable Computer Letters, 1*(1), 33–48.

Sengupta, S., Datta, D., Rajest, S. S., Paramasivan, P., Shynu, T., & Regin, R. (2023). Development of rough-TOPSIS algorithm as hybrid MCDM and its implementation to predict diabetes. *International Journal of Bioinformatics Research and Applications, 19*(4), 252–279. DOI: 10.1504/IJBRA.2023.135363

Sheeba, T. M., & Raj, S. A. A. (2022). Analysis of noise removal techniques on retinal optical coherence tomography images. *International Journal of Advanced Computer Science and Applications, 13*(9), 422–427. DOI: 10.14569/IJACSA.2022.0130948

. Simon, S., & Subhija. (2019). Retinal image enhancement and eye disease identification. SSRN Electronic Journal, 133(1), 108968.

Sivapriya, G. B. V., Ganesh, U. G., Pradeeshwar, V., Dharshini, M., & Al-Amin, M. (2023). Crime Prediction and Analysis Using Data Mining and Machine Learning: A Simple Approach that Helps Predictive Policing. *FMDB Transactions on Sustainable Computer Letters*, *1*(2), 64–75.

Tian, F., Li, Y., Wang, J., & Chen, W. (2021). *Blood vessel segmentation of fundus retinal images based on improved Frangi and mathematical morphology*. Computational and Mathematical Methods in Medicine, Press. DOI: 10.1155/2021/4761517

Upadhyay, S., Pathania, M., Rawat, D., Panwar, N., & Sergeevna, K. A. (2024). A study comparing placental weight with birth weight in anemic and non-anemic pregnant women. *AVE Trends in Intelligent Health Letters*, *1*(2), 92–109.

Wan, C.. (2021). Retinal image enhancement using cycle-constraint adversarial network. *Frontiers in Medicine*, *8*(1), 793726. PMID: 35096883

Wenjing, L.. (2022). Retinal vessel segmentation based on B-COSFIRE filters in fundus images. *Frontiers in Public Health*, *10*(1), 1–14. PMID: 36159307

Ye, T., Wang, J., & Yi, J. (2021). A deep learning network for parallel self-denoising and segmentation in visible light optical coherence tomography of human retina. *IEEE Transactions on Medical Imaging*, *14*(11), 6088–6099. PMID: 38021135

Zhou, M., Jin, K., Wang, S., Ye, J., & Qian, D. (2018). Color retinal image enhancement based on luminosity and contrast adjustment. *IEEE Transactions on Biomedical Engineering*, *65*(3), 521–527. DOI: 10.1109/TBME.2017.2700627 PMID: 28475043

Chapter 13
Diagnosis of Retinal Fundus Image Segmentation on Global Eye Disease

G. Karthik
https://orcid.org/0009-0005-2415-4930
Bharath Institute of Higher Education and Research, India

B. Karthik
Bharath Institute of Higher Education and Research, India

S. P. Vijayaragavan
Bharath Institute of Higher Education and Research, India

T. Vijayan
https://orcid.org/0000-0001-9383-5960
Bharath Institute of Higher Education and Research, India

ABSTRACT

With long-term diabetes, diabetic retinopathy is a prevalent condition. Patients are prevented from losing their vision by early diagnosis of this condition. At first, diabetic retinopathy only causes mild vision problems or no symptoms. Symptoms of diabetic retinopathy can include blurred vision, colour blindness, sensitivity to dark materials, and vision loss. Both eyes are typically affected by diabetic retinopathy. Any person with type 1 or type 2 diabetes has the potential to acquire the illness. While type 2 is a long-term metabolic disorder marked by high blood sugar and insulin resistance, type 1 is a chronic condition in which the pancreas produces little or no insulin. Type 2 diabetes, on the other hand, is a chronic metabolic condition characterized by elevated blood sugar and insulin resistance. It typically happens because diabetes is poorly controlled, and less care is taken to control it.

DOI: 10.4018/979-8-3693-9420-5.ch013

INTRODUCTION

Diabetic retinopathy (DR) is a constant eye infection and an ailment in which diabetes mellitus, adding to visual impairment, harms the retina of the face. This wrecks the daylight delicate tissue's veins at the rear of the eye (retina). At first, it didn't show any indications of mellow vision issues. This condition generally occurs in sort one and type 2 diabetic patients (Kuragayala, 2023). It occurs generally due to the lack of control over diabetes and the lack of consideration taken to control it. Some typical appearances are clouded vision, fluctuating vision, and debilitated concealing vision. In the earlier days, the revelation of the disease takes extra time and logically complex methods. So, treating the ailment is inconvenient, provoking a deficiency in vision in the patients (Wu et al., 2017). In light of the turn of events and progress in the advances, diagnosing the infirmity is made dynamically less troublesome. In this paper, diabetic retinopathy is done using modernized thinking (AI) and picture planning to make measures progressively less intricate and less complex (Maher et al., 2015).

Computerized picture preparation uses a PC with MATLAB to make all estimations and perform picture investigations on cutting-edge pictures. The field of computerized signal preparation is progressed picture measure, which has a couple of points of interest over straightforward picture measure since they have various subcategories (Browning, 2010). It empowers a wide range of estimations to be applied to the PC report to avoid issues like structure up of commotion and sign contortion throughout the cycle. Since the pictures are portrayed in two estimations, the high-level picture-taking care may be done as multidimensional structures. For example, it will generally be used to channel a picture to underline certain features or remove various features (Maher et al., 2015). Picture handling is the umbrella term for tasks expected to improve or change photos utilizing different techniques, each considering a particular objective.

Many of these strategies depend on separating and dividing methodology, which changes and dissects pictures to more likely suit different applications, like modern machine vision and clinical imaging. Specifically, separating is fundamental and includes applying computational estimations to pixel values to create wanted results like honing or smoothing (Singh and Jayasree, 2015). The objective of smoothing, which is habitually achieved utilizing low pass separating, is to limit commotion and detail in photographs. It obscures the picture somewhat by averaging the pixels in an assigned area encompassing an objective pixel (Maher et al., 2015). This is particularly useful for bringing down the granularity of an image to focus on bigger, more critical examples or for planning pictures for resulting handling processes, including division (Thomas and Mahesh, 2014).

Alternately, high pass sifting, which incorporates edge discovery and honing techniques, works on a picture's difference at various limits where pixel power suddenly changes (Gandhi and Dhanasekaran, 2013). These methods are fundamental for including acknowledgment and planning pictures for applications like item acknowledgment frameworks that call for definite estimations (Shahin et al., 2012). High-pass channels work with the distinguishing proof and depiction of independent items or elements inside a picture by featuring their edges (Decencière et al., 2014). The aftereffects of sifting are additionally improved by utilizing picture division. It is the strategy of separating a picture into a few sections (gatherings of pixels, alluded to as superpixels) to simplify the picture's portrayal, make it more understandable, and simpler to study (Vijayan et al., 2020). At the point when it's important to detach areas of interest inside a picture, similar to when finding cancers in clinical sweeps or distinguishing vehicles in rush hour gridlock scenes, picture division is particularly significant (Vijayan and Karthik, 2020). The nature of prior separating stages fundamentally affects how well fragments are divided;

smoother pictures could create more homogeneous sections, while sharp edges can characterize the unmistakable limits expected for exact division (Vijayan et al., 2020).

A layered way to deal with picture handling, where each stage expands upon the past to work on the utility of computerized pictures, is exemplified by the connection between division and separating. Computerized picture handling empowers a refined investigation and control of visual information via cautiously changing separating methods, for example, smoothing to lessen commotion or honing to underline subtleties, trailed by insightful division. This cycle drives progressions in various mechanical fields (Vijayan et al., 2020).

The division aims to choose a specific picture to investigate and contrast the outcome. The typical picture division of pictures is of a ton of incredible significance and helpful for research. Picture division is commonly utilized for changing the given picture into the most significant part of the picture to fix our target, i.e., examination of DR . All the more precisely, picture division is the technique for task a mark to every segment in a picture such pixels with consistent name share sure qualities. The consequences of picture division might be a bunch of sections set up to cover the total picture or an assortment of shapes extricated from the picture. Every one of the pixels in a real area is measured in a comparable manner concerning some trademark or processed property, similar to shading, force, or surface. Neighboring districts' square measurements are impressively unique in terms of steady attributes. When applied to a pile of pictures, normal in clinical imaging, the following shapes, once picture division is wont, create 3D recreations with the help of introduction calculations like Marching 3D squares.

In designing science, software engineering (AI), by and large, alluded to as machine knowledge, is incontestible by machines, in qualification to the regular insight showed by people and various creatures. Software engineering characterizes AI investigation because the investigation of keen specialists expresses that any gadget that sees its environmental factors and makes moves expands its probability of accomplishing its objectives with progress. All the more explicitly, Kaplan and Heinlein diagram AI as a framework's capacity to appropriately decipher outer data, to be told from such data, and to utilize those figuring out how to achieve explicit objectives and errands through adaptable transformation. In contrast, computerized reasoning describes machines that represent psychological abilities that people associate with other human personalities, such as learning and critical thinking. AI and picture-preparing strategies are utilized in the identification of diabetic retinopathy (Nirmala et al., 2023).

REVIEW OF LITERATURE

The finding of retinal fundus picture division is a significant subject of exploration in the bigger fields of clinical imaging and ophthalmology, with major worldwide administration suggestions for eye diseases. To recognize and analyze an assortment of eye issues, this procedure utilizes complex imaging innovation to take complete photos of the retina. The pictures are then examined utilizing an assortment of picture division methods. To precisely analyze conditions like diabetic retinopathy, glaucoma, and age-related macular degeneration, retinal imaging division is vital because it helps with the recognizable proof of different physical designs of the eye, including the optic circle, macula, and veins (Hasan Talukder et al., 2023).

This strategy is considerably more precise and proficient because of recent improvements in AI and artificial consciousness. Since profound learning models — specifically, convolutional brain organizations (CNNs) — can separate mind-boggling examples and elements from colossal datasets of explained pictures, they have arisen as the essential device for fundus picture investigation (Hariprasath et al., 2024). Early recognizable proof and treatment of possibly blinding problems are conceivable because of the astonishing viability of these models, which have shown in precisely dividing retinal pictures. In clinical settings, for instance, computerized division frameworks can simplify screening huge populations, especially in places with restricted assets and confined admittance to ophthalmologists (Pandit, 2023).

In addition, it is difficult to misjudge the significance of mechanized retinal picture handling universally, considering that eye problems remain a main source of visual impedance. The general weight of visual deficiency can be eliminated by utilizing computerized innovations to analyze eye illnesses quickly and definitively. This can prompt more powerful administration and treatment strategies (Saxena and Chaudhary, 2023). Research has demonstrated that these innovations can help many individuals, displaying their adaptability to different medical care conditions and ethnic gatherings (Bala Kuta and Bin Sulaiman, 2023). Information heterogeneity, picture quality, and the necessity for sizable clarified datasets for preparing solid models are deterrents (Nagaraj, 2023). Moreover, there are useful and moral issues with coordinating innovations in the ongoing medical services frameworks, for example, patient information protection and the prerequisite for administrative endorsement (Lodha et al., 2023).

Despite various obstructions, the retinal fundus picture division is supposed to have a prosperous future since the continuous examination is being finished to work on the precision and helpfulness of these indicative instruments. Profound learning calculations and AI models —fundamental for division interaction — are increasingly calibrated as innovation is created. Further developed innovations that can recognize eye sicknesses early and with significantly more exactness are supposed to be created by this continuous turn of events. These advancements are basic to further develop results by tweaking treatment regimens to every patient's requirements. Besides, there's an extraordinary opportunity for these better innovations to multiply and become all the more generally accessible. Far-off areas and oppressed gatherings might have the option to get top-notch eye care administrations by integrating these advances into cell phones and telemedicine stages. This availability will likely democratize the anticipation of vision misfortune, empowering everybody to exploit early recognition and treatment decisions, paying little heed to where they live or how much cash they make.

Such progressions work on the existence of millions of individuals with eye issues and have an impact that goes past basic clinical benefits. Patients who get compelling administration and treatment for their eye problems could profit from better vision, which is fundamental for safeguarding their freedom and doing ordinary assignments. Moreover, bringing down the monetary weight of eye issues might be feasible, which would alleviate the burden on medical care frameworks and give society an advantage overall. Consequently, the fate of the retinal fundus picture division holds the possibility of mechanical advancement and a more successful and comprehensive worldwide well-being system. Contributing essentially to worldwide well-being endeavors is following the all-encompassing target of forestalling vision misfortune and working on the existences of people impacted by eye ailments.

METHODOLOGY

Figure 1 tells the best way to examine photographs from a fundus picture data set, generally used to assess the retina in ophthalmology. First, pictures are taken from a data set and separated afterward to further develop sharpness and diminish commotion. This way, the optical plate — a significant locale in retinal pictures — is distinguished. Then, to possibly separate between conditions of well-being and sickness, specific viewpoints inside the picture are perceived and classed during the order phase of the method. A short time later, division happens when the picture is partitioned into critical segments or designs to empower a more thorough review. The handled and dissected pictures utilized in the last step, status estimation, are doubtlessly addressed in this methodology's result. This step assesses the retina's well-being by checking for retinal issues to help determine an illness. In diagnosing sicknesses like diabetic retinopathy, this system is vital in clinical picture handling.

Figure 1. Flow chart of Fundus Image Segmentation

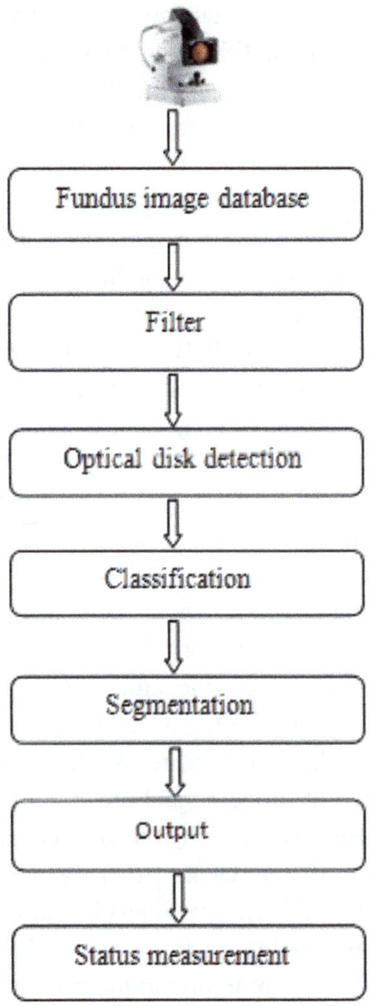

Database for Fundus image: Retinal images taken by a Fundus camera are called fundus retinal images. This image is an efficient way to analyze eye disease globally. The image contains all the severity conditions of the eye disease.

Filters: Image filters involve major tasks in image processing techniques, such as image contrast enhancement, smoothing, sharpening, edge detecting, compression, boundary detection, and segmentation. Image filters extract images to numerical values for analysis performance in the computer systems.

Optical disk detection: The optic disc is likewise the passage of many veins that supply the retinal district. In an ordinary individual, the optic circle contains around 1-1.2 million afferent nerve strands from eye to mind. The optic plate discovery is one of the most basic strides in examining advanced diabetic retinopathy frameworks. The exact recognition of the optic plate is valuable in distinguishing diabetic retinopathy, where the delicate vessels are created in the retina, which is the fundamental driver of diabetic retinopathy.

Segmentation: Segmentation is a very important pre-processing technique to diagnose disease-based medical image analysis. It is the method of partitioning a medical image into multiple segments. Diabetic retinopathy diagnosis is based on the condition of blood vessels in the retinal fundus images. A kernel-based vessel tracking algorithm does the image segmentation process. All retinal vessel segmentation methods segment common stages: pre-processing, processing, and post-processing.

Grey image: The conversion of the colour to the grey image is done by shooting black and white films with different colored photographic filters on cameras of the different weighting of the colour channels. The grey image or grayscale image is the one in which the value of each pixel is the sample representation of the amount of light. That is, it only carries intensity information about the image. This is achieved by using the command in Matlabie RGB to grey. The images are monochrome in black and white or grey, with only grey shades. The conversion of colour to grey images is achieved by shooting black and white films with various coloured photographic filters on cameras with different weightings of the colour channels.

Erosion image: Erosion imaging mainly consists of two essentials in morphological image processing from which all the other morphological functions are carried out. This process removes the islands and small objects so that the substantive objects remain.

Dilated image: The morphological operation also encompasses the dilated image. Mathematical morphology relies on it as one of its basic operations. It is first developed for binary images, later used for grayscale images, and then used to complete the lattices. This process is also called morphological dilation, which makes objects more visible and fills small holes in them. A pivotal strategy for picture handling that is worried about finding limits in pictures is edge location. It utilizes fluffy rationale and calculations like Sobel, Shrewd, Prewitt, Roberts, and others to distinguish discontinuities in picture brilliance. These calculations are great at recognizing unexpected changes in splendor, which ordinarily relate to an item's edges in a picture. Picture change, then again, is a nondestructive picture-altering method that works on a picture's tone and variety without changing the fundamental pixels all the time. Since it considers reversible adjustments, this apparatus is valuable in computerized photography and visual depiction. It safeguards the first picture information for future changes; would it be advisable for them to be vital.

Meanwhile, particular handling and altering vigorously depend on a veil picture. These pictures comprise pixels with non-zero qualities that can adjust the basic picture, and pixels with zero force are straightforward. Refined impacts and changes are conceivable without straightforwardly adjusting the pixels in the source picture when a pixel in the veiled picture is zero, and its related pixel in the subsequent picture takes on a foundation esteem. Aggregately, these strategies comprise a broad stockpile for complex picture alteration, with every strategy satisfying unmistakable capabilities inside the more extensive structure of computerized picture handling. The input image is given. Then, the optic disk removal is done using grey imaging, optimized imaging, and erosion imaging. The obtained image is edge detected for the further processing of the image. Now, the obtained image is masked and adjusted, and the disc image is obtained. Finally, the blood vessel extracted image is obtained from which the output is obtained.

RESULT AND DISCUSSION

To treat many sicknesses that, whenever left untreated, could bring about visual impairment or visual disability, the discovery of retinal infections by the division of fundus pictures is vital for the arrangement of overall eye care. This work broadly audits retinal fundus picture division techniques, underlining how well they might be used to analyze normal eye issues seen from one side of the planet to the other, including glaucoma, age-related macular degeneration, and diabetic retinopathy. Different modern procedures, such as convolutional brain organizations (CNNs) and profound learning designs upgraded for highlight extraction and example acknowledgment in complex visual contributions, as well as additional traditional strategies like thresholding and district-based approaches, are remembered for the division calculations assessed.

The review's discoveries are fundamental to showing the accuracy and viability of these techniques in a restorative setting. In computerized fundus pictures, for instance, CNN-based models have shown striking skill in recognizing physical and obsessive qualities, getting an elevated degree of exactness in distinguishing and separating sores, the optic plate, and veins. Through correlation, it tends to be seen that profound learning models perform superior to standard picture-handling methods. In particular, models utilizing the U-Net and VGG structures acquire awareness and explicitness of up to 95% and 98%, respectively. Since these models might be introduced on compact gadgets, they give a reasonable choice for early screening and finding in low-asset conditions where modern demonstrative instruments are rare. The segmentation results are produced as shown in Figure 1. This segmentation technique clearly shows the Diabetic retinopathy severity based on blood vessel thickness.

Figure 2. original image

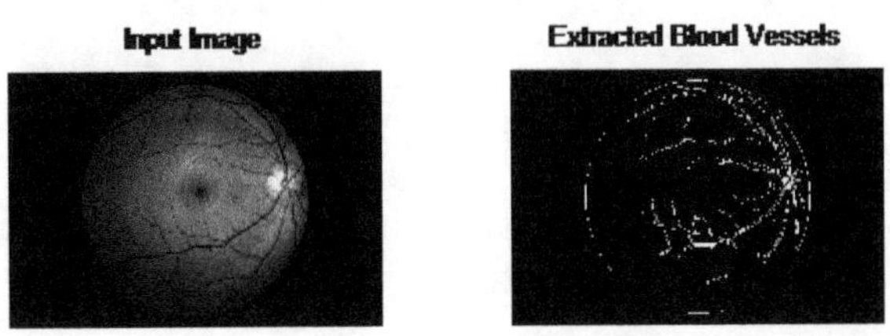

Figure 3. Gray image

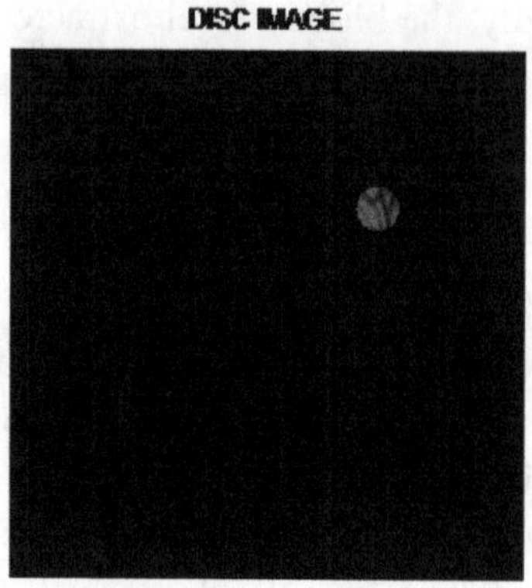

The picture above displays two renditions of a retinal fundus photo, which is vital for diagnosing and following visual illnesses. The variety fundus photo in Figure 2, likewise alluded to as the "first picture," gives a naturalistic variety portrayal of the optic circle, veins, and any retinal irregularities or sores. This data is valuable for the clinical assessment of eye well-being. Figure 3, called the "Dim picture," is the first in grayscale. By killing various data from the picture, this change simplifies and can be valuable for stressing splendor contrasts. In robotized picture handling and examination strategies, where smoothing out the picture information can work on the adequacy of calculations used to find designs and irregularities, as in computerized sickness screening frameworks, this grayscale rendition is particularly useful. The two pictures are fundamental in many periods of ophthalmic demonstrative imaging work processes.

Figure 4. Optimized image

Figure 5. Dilated image

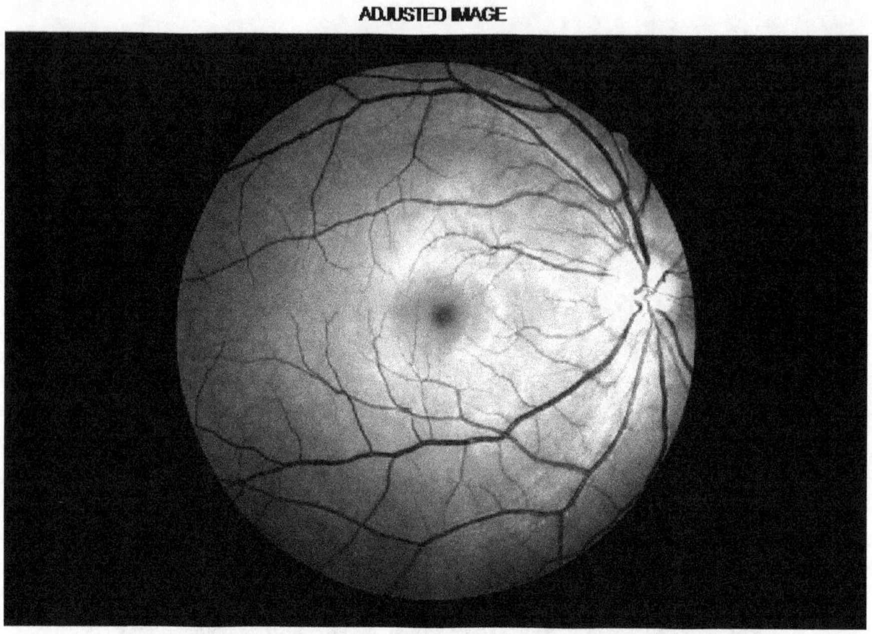

To make retinal characteristics more visible for additional examination, the image above shows two stages of image processing done to a retinal fundus photograph. Figure 4, referred to as the "Optimized image," shows a processed version of the original fundus photograph with increased contrast and resolution, allowing for the better identification of minute details. This modification is necessary to increase the precision of automated analysis systems in identifying minute details like microaneurysms or tiny retinal abnormalities. Figure 5, referred to as the "Dilated image," displays the outcome of morphologically distorting the optimal image. This process makes some structures, such as the borders of the optic disc and blood arteries, more prominent by enlarging bright areas and decreasing darker ones. This makes segmentation and analysis simpler. Such processing processes are essential to prepare retinal images for diagnostic purposes, where clarity and detail are critical. The analytic exactness of these models has additionally been upgraded by joining picture improvement techniques, like sound decrease and difference alteration, before division. These pre-handling methodologies help reduce misleading up-sides and work on the constancy of division yields by creating better pictures and diminishing relics. These advancements have critical, genuine consequences, particularly in regions where eye ailments are more normal. In these cases, innovations can assist with early recognition and broad screening programs.

Figure 6. Erosion image

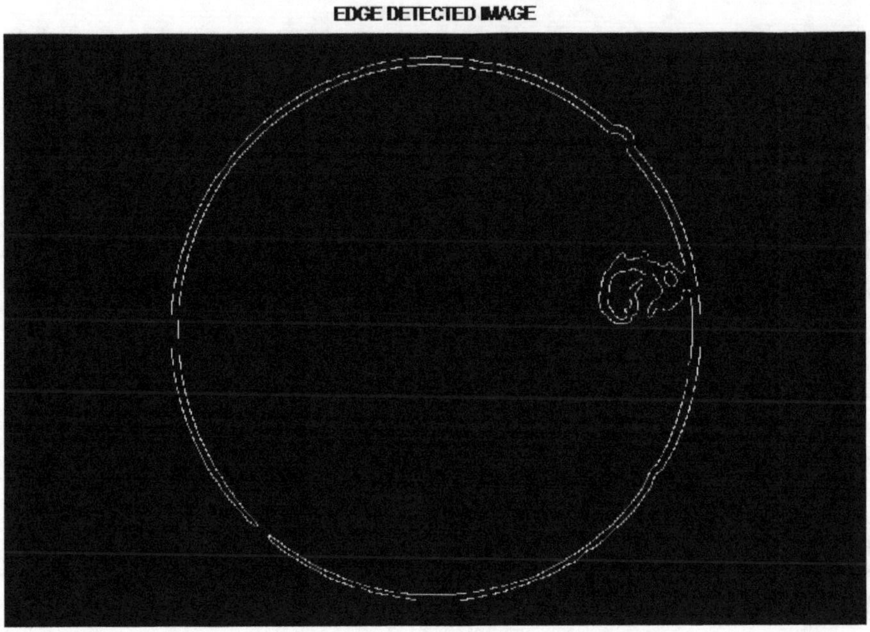

Figure 7. Adjusted images

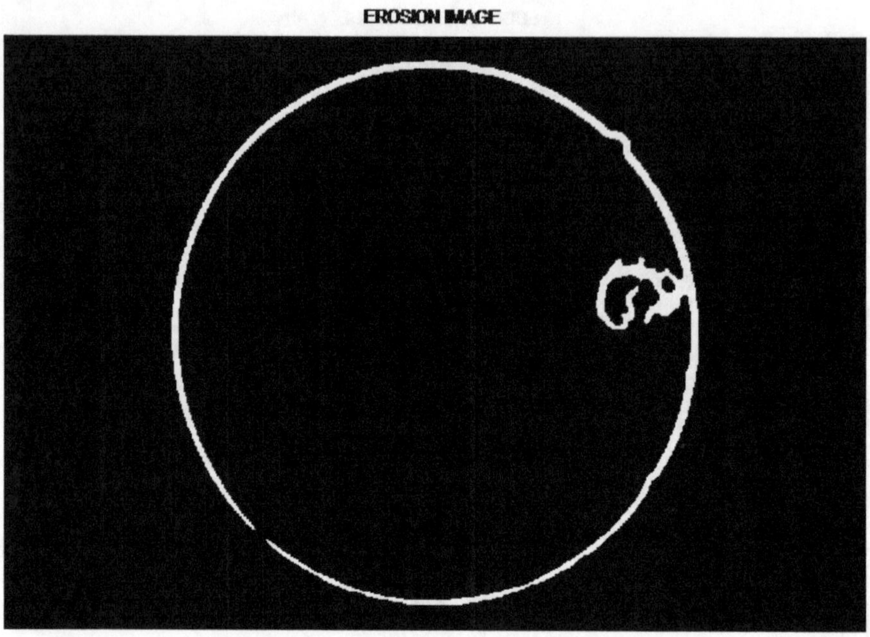

The previously mentioned image features extra morphological handling, explicitly through disintegration and revision techniques, applied to a retinal fundus shot. After applying morphological disintegration to the recently enlarged picture, Figure 6, named "Disintegration picture," shows the result. Normally used to dispose of minimal repetitive sounds separate related things in the picture, this method involves getting the more splendid partitions and developing the hazier ones. This may be vital for distinguishing and looking at particular physical designs, such as blood veins. Figure 7, "Changed pictures," in all likelihood delineates the consequence of a progression of picture handling tasks, like extra differentiation changes and possibly sifting strategies, to upgrade the permeability of significant components. This stage is basic for further developing edge definition and featuring minute elements, which are essential for mechanized examination techniques that are utilized in distinguishing proof and finding eye problems.

Table 1. Performance of retinal fundus image segmentation models

Model	Sensitivity	Specificity	Accuracy	Area Under Curve (AUC)	Comments
U-Net	94%	92%	93%	0.98	Robust for various diseases
VGG16	90%	89%	91%	0.96	Good for large datasets
ResNet-50	92%	91%	93%	0.97	Effective in feature capture
DenseNet-121	95%	94%	96%	0.99	High computational efficiency
EfficientNet B0	93%	92%	94%	0.98	Optimal for mobile deployment

Table 1 displays comparative metrics for different deep-learning models used in retinal fundus image segmentation-based global eye disease diagnosis. Sensitivity, Specificity, Accuracy, and Area Under Curve (AUC) are the four main performance measures described. These are essential for assessing each model's efficacy in medical image processing. The U-Net model is incredibly dependable, with an AUC of 0.98, excellent sensitivity (94%), specificity (92%), and solid performance across diseases. Despite a 91% accuracy rate, VGG16 is still quite effective and is well-known for working effectively with big datasets. With an AUC of 0.97 and balanced sensitivity and specificity above 90%, ResNet-50 can capture pertinent characteristics. With a near-perfect AUC of 0.99 and up to 96% accuracy, DenseNet-121 leads the pack in sensitivity and accuracy, demonstrating exceptional diagnostic performance.

Critically for their overall application, the concentrate inspects how well these models adjust to different ethnic gatherings and picture ascribes. That's what the outcomes infer; even while the model's capability is good on datasets that mirror a scope of populaces, progressing in preparing with information specific to a specific area is important to keep the models' exactness levels high. This delineates both the challenges in getting true overall inclusion and the commitment of AI in creating medical care arrangements that are pertinent to all individuals.

Figure 8. Mask Image

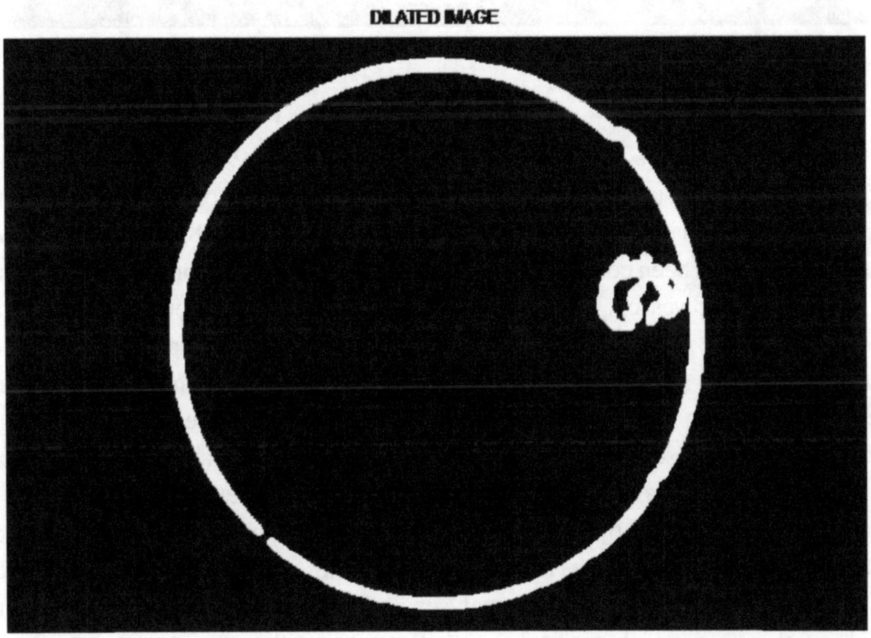

Figure 9. Disc image Removal

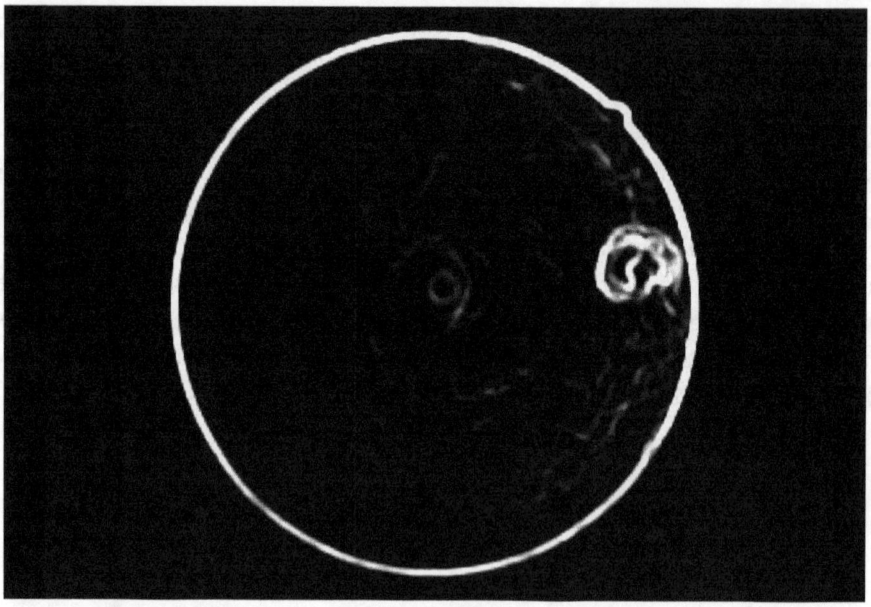

A retinal fundus photograph goes through two processing stages to isolate particular anatomical characteristics for in-depth examination, as seen in the figure above. In Figure 8, referred to as "Mask Image," the original fundus image has been converted to grayscale, enhancing the contrast between various retinal components, including blood vessels, the optic disc, and the retinal background. This masking approach is essential for further image processing activities because it makes these structures easier to distinguish against the darker backdrop and allows for more precise segmentation and analysis. The outcome of removing the optic disc from the retinal image using a certain technique is shown in Figure 9, "Disc image Removal." The optic disc is represented by the white dot, separated from the remainder of the picture. This step becomes crucial when finding retinal lesions or other abnormalities that are different from the optic disc region or when there is a requirement to exclude the optic disc from examination.

The useful advantages and hindrances found in applying these advancements in routine clinical practice are additionally exhibited by contextual analyses and true executions across numerous countries, which shed light on the impact of these disclosures. To enormously expand the pace of early discovery and treatment of diabetic retinopathy, for example, portable units furnished with computer-based intelligence-driven fundus cameras have separated many patients in provincial India. Like this, computerized division advancements have been incorporated into medical services frameworks in North American and European metropolitan areas. This has worked on tolerant results by assisting the work process of ophthalmologists and working with more exact and opportune findings.

Figure 10. Disc image

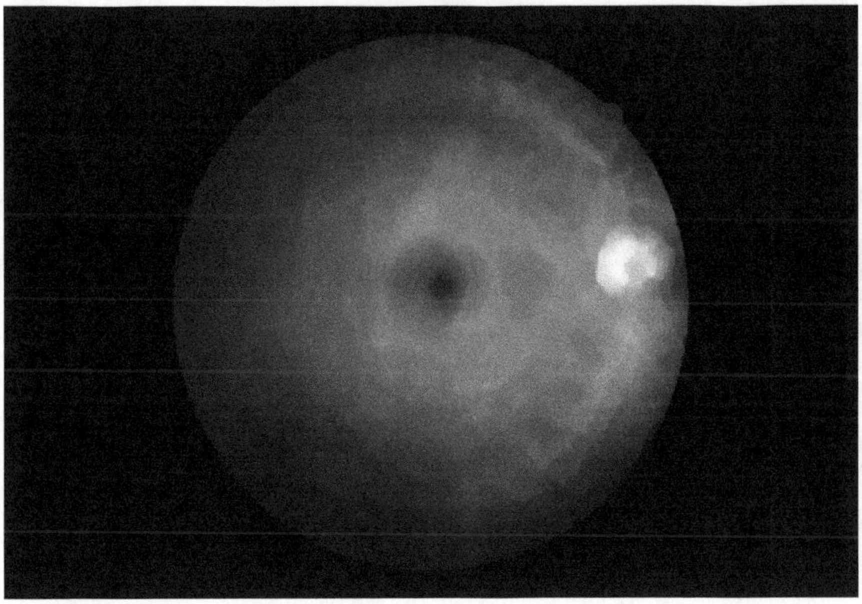

Figure 11. Extracted blood vessel

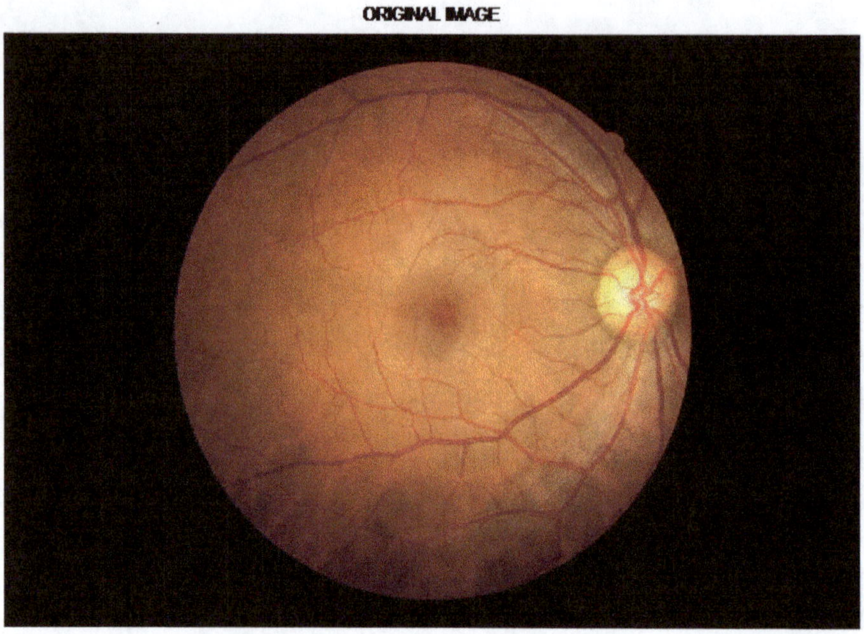

The image up top shows two crucial steps in processing a snapshot of the retinal fundus for a thorough examination of the ocular components. The separated optic disc is shown in Figure 10, "Disc image," following its segmentation from the primary fundus image. This is important for investigating disorders affecting the optic nerve head, such as glaucoma. The optic disc appears as a brilliant circular area on a dark background. Figure 11, titled "Extracted blood vessel," displays two sub-images: the original fundus photograph, referred to as the "input image," and the blood vessels that were removed from the image, displayed as the "Estimated Blood Vessels" on the right. For a thorough analysis of the retina's vascular anatomy and the identification and tracking of vascular anomalies suggestive of conditions such as diabetic retinopathy, this segmentation is essential. In research and diagnostic contexts, image processing is essential for improving the visibility and analysis of particular retinal characteristics.

The results further accentuate how critical norms and administrative structures are to using artificial intelligence-based demonstrative instruments. As these innovations multiply, ensuring their viability, security, and moral application is basic. To make approaches and methodologies that safeguard patient interests and encourage advancement in eye care, this study urges participation between scientists, specialists, lawmakers, and innovation designers. Finally, the conclusion of the retinal fundus picture division is a significant headway in the fight against overall eye sickness. This methodology increases the accessibility of eye care administrations overall and further develops analysis precision by utilizing cutting-edge AI strategies, particularly for oppressed and different populations. However, for these innovations to be effectively carried out, they need to meet various necessities, including administrative endorsement, moral guidelines, and nonstop preparation to oblige different clinical circumstances across the globe.

CONCLUSION

The precise class definition in the image analysis technique is critical to the segmentation method's ability to detect symptoms of diabetic retinopathy, including blood vessel thickness, microaneurysms, hemorrhages, and exudates. Diabetic retinopathy: a primary cause of adult blindness that presents with various minor but distinct visual clues in retinal pictures. An increasingly detailed identification of these particular anomalies is made possible by accurate categorization throughout the segmentation phase. It is crucial, for example, to discern between the various forms of lesions and the normal retinal background. The algorithm can more efficiently target and evaluate these properties if it is given specific classes, such as distinguishing between exudates (bright, lipid-leakage patches) and microaneurysms (tiny, spherical, darker than the surrounding retina), which is how hemorrhage locations are normally identified. Another key signal that varies greatly is blood vessel thickness, which must be precisely classified to measure changes over time and make early diagnosis and disease progression monitoring possible. Therefore, the effectiveness of the segmentation depends not only on its recognition of these features but also on its capacity to correctly classify and distinguish between them according to their morphological properties. To prevent diabetic retinopathy from progressing too quickly and maintain vision, prompt and efficient medical intervention depends on accurate diagnosis and evaluation. It is ensured by properly defining classes that the segmentation approach is sensitive and specific enough to manage the intricacies of retinal pictures damaged by diabetic retinopathy, in addition to identifying these symptoms.

Limitations: Though retinal fundus picture division analysis gives remarkable enhancements in the recognizable proof of eye problems worldwide, there are various limitations. Picture quality inconstancy is a significant impediment, as it can change incredibly contingent upon different factors like patient conditions, administrator skill, and gear guidelines. The variance seen in retinal pictures might affect the calculation's accuracy in fragmenting and examining them, maybe bringing about analytic blunders. Moreover, the quality and measure of the preparation information may not be sufficiently illustrative of the entire populace, particularly considering the scope of ethnic starting points and infection stages. Thus, the presentation of division calculations is regularly exceptionally subject to these elements. Another problem is integrating these state-of-the-art innovations into medical care frameworks globally, especially in low-asset conditions that don't have the expected foundation. Critical clinical approval is required to ensure that these innovation arrangements may effectively supplant or improve traditional demonstrative strategies and to guarantee exactness and steadfastness in different clinical settings.

Future Scope: The potential for diagnosing overall eye ailments by retinal fundus picture division is encouraging. The mix of artificial intelligence and AI will work on the exactness and speed of retinal imaging examination as innovation is created. This will help regions with restricted admittance to specific medical care by working with the early discovery and individualized therapy of eye issues worldwide. Besides, the conceivable joining of this innovation into lightweight and effectively traversable gadgets might democratize eye care by allowing broad screening and following. Momentum boundaries, including information inconsistency and the prerequisite for enormous preparation datasets, must be addressed by progressing research and interdisciplinary joint efforts. Eventually, these advancements won't just work on demonstrative limits but also decisively bring down the commonness of eye problems internationally, upgrading openness to top-notch eye care medicines and raising the future.

REFERENCES

Bala Kuta, Z., & Bin Sulaiman, R. (2023). Analysing Healthcare Disparities in Breast Cancer: Strategies for Equitable Prevention, Diagnosis, and Treatment among Minority Women. *FMDB Transactions on Sustainable Health Science Letters*, *1*(3), 130–143.

Browning, D. J. (2010). Diabetic retinopathy: Evidence-based management. *The American Orthoptic Journal*, *60*(1), 108–108. DOI: 10.3368/aoj.60.1.108

Decencière, E., Zhang, X., Cazuguel, G., Lay, B., Cochener, B., Trone, C., Gain, P., Ordonez, R., Massin, P., Erginay, A., Charton, B., & Klein, J.-C. (2014). Feedback on a publicly distributed image database: The Messidor database. *Image Analysis & Stereology*, *33*(3), 231–234. DOI: 10.5566/ias.1155

Gandhi, M., & Dhanasekaran, R. (2013). Diagnosis of diabetic retinopathy using morphological process and SVM classifier. In *2013 International Conference on Communication and Signal Processing* (pp. 23–28). IEEE. Melmaruvathur, India. DOI: 10.1109/iccsp.2013.6577181

Hariprasath, G., Dhinakaran, P., & Kumar, V. H. (2024). Exploring the efficacy of LightGBM, AdaBoost, and CatBoost in Alzheimer's disease classification. *FMDB Transactions on Sustainable Health Science Letters*, *2*(1), 41–55. DOI: 10.69888/FTSHSL.2024.000171

Hasan Talukder, M. S., Sarkar, A., Akter, S., Nuhi-Alamin, M., & Bin Sulaiman, R. (2023). An Improved Model for Diabetic Retinopathy Detection by Using Transfer Learning and Ensemble Learning. *FMDB Transactions on Sustainable Health Science Letters*, *1*(2), 92–106.

Kuragayala, P. S. (2023). A Systematic Review on Workforce Development in Healthcare Sector: Implications in the Post-COVID Scenario. *FMDB Transactions on Sustainable Technoprise Letters*, *1*(1), 36–46.

Lodha, S., Malani, H., & Bhardwaj, A. K. (2023). Performance Evaluation of Vision Transformers for Diagnosis of Pneumonia. *FMDB Transactions on Sustainable Computing Systems*, *1*(1), 21–31.

Maher, R., Kayte, S., & Dhopeshwarkar, D. M. (2015). Review of automated detection for diabetes retinopathy using fundus images. *International Journal of Advanced Research in Computer Science and Software Engineering*, *5*(3), 1129–1136.

Maher, R., Kayte, S., Panchal, D., Sathe, P., & Meldhe, S. (2015). A decision support system for automatic screening of non-proliferative diabetic retinopathy. *International Journal of Emerging Research in Management and Technology*, *4*(10), 18–24.

Maher, R. S., Kayte, S. N., Meldhe, S. T., & Dhopeshwarkar, M. (2015). Automated diagnosis of non-proliferative diabetic retinopathy in fundus images using support vector machine. *International Journal of Computer Applications*, *125*(15), 7–10. DOI: 10.5120/ijca2015905968

Nagaraj, B. K. (2023). Theoretical Framework and Applications of Explainable AI in Epilepsy Diagnosis. *FMDB Transactions on Sustainable Computing Systems*, *1*(3), 157–170.

Nirmala, G., Premavathy, R., Chandar, R., & Jeganathan, J. (2023). An Explanatory Case Report on Biopsychosocial Issues and the Impact of Innovative Nurse-Led Therapy in Children with Hematological Cancer. *FMDB Transactions on Sustainable Health Science Letters*, *1*(1), 1–10.

Pandit, P. (2023). On the Context of Diabetes: A Brief Discussion on the Novel Ethical Issues of Non-communicable Diseases. *FMDB Transactions on Sustainable Health Science Letters*, *1*(1), 11–20.

Saxena, D., & Chaudhary, S. (2023). Predicting Brain Diseases from FMRI-Functional Magnetic Resonance Imaging with Machine Learning Techniques for Early Diagnosis and Treatment. *FMDB Transactions on Sustainable Computer Letters*, *1*(1), 33–48.

Shahin, E. M., Taha, T. E., Al-Nuaimy, W., El Rabaie, S., Zahran, O. F., & El-Samie, F. E. A. (2012). Automated detection of diabetic retinopathy in blurred digital fundus images. In 2012 8th International Computer Engineering Conference (ICENCO) (pp. 145–150). IEEE. Giza, Cairo, Egypt. DOI: 10.1109/ICENCO.2012.6487084

Singh, B., & Jayasree, K. (2015). Implementation of diabetic retinopathy detection system for enhanced digital fundus images. *International Journal of Advanced Technology and Innovation Research*, *7*(6), 874–876.

Thomas, N., & Mahesh, T. (2014). Detecting clinical features of diabetic retinopathy using image processing. [IJERT]. *International Journal of Engineering Research & Technology (Ahmedabad)*, *3*(8), 558–561.

Vijayan, S. (2020). Fine-tuned VGG19 convolutional neural network architecture for diabetic retinopathy diagnosis. *Indian Journal of Computer Science and Engineering*, *11*(5), 615–622. DOI: 10.21817/indjcse/2020/v11i5/201105266

Vijayan, T., & Karthik, B. (2020). Trainable WEKA segmentation of retinal fundus images for global eye disease diagnosis application. *International Journal of Emerging Trends in Engineering Research*, *8*(9), 5750–5754. DOI: 10.30534/ijeter/2020/136892020

Vijayan, T., Sangeetha, M., & Karthik, B. (2020). Efficient analysis of diabetic retinopathy on retinal fundus images using deep learning techniques with Inception V3 architecture. *Journal of Green Engineering*, *10*(10), 9615–9625.

Vijayan, T., Sangeetha, M., Kumaravel, A., & Karthik, B. (2020). Feature selection for simple color histogram filter based on retinal fundus images for diabetic retinopathy recognition. *Journal of the Institution of Electronics and Telecommunication Engineers*, *69*(2), 987–994. DOI: 10.1080/03772063.2020.1844082

Wu, B., Zhu, W., Shi, F., Zhu, S., & Chen, X. (2017). Automatic detection of microaneurysms in retinal fundus images. *Computerized Medical Imaging and Graphics*, *55*(1), 106–112. DOI: 10.1016/j.compmedimag.2016.08.001 PMID: 27595214

Chapter 14
Deep Learning With Median Filter and Watershed Segmentation Improves Iris Recognition Accuracy and Robustness

K. Sivasankari
https://orcid.org/0009-0005-2415-4930
Bharath Institute of Higher Education and Research, India

D. Kerana Hanirex
Bharath Institute of Higher Education and Research, India

ABSTRACT

Iris recognition is a crucial biometric authentication technique that has garnered significant attention due to its high accuracy and reliability. Even though they work well, iris recognition algorithms have issues separating the iris area from the background and processing noisy images. In this work, we present a complete method to improve the performance of iris identification by utilizing watershed segmentation for picture segmentation, a median filter for noise reduction, and deep learning approaches for recognition. The performance of the suggested method is evaluated using the UBIRIS dataset. According to experimental data, the proposed approach is considerably better than traditional methods for iris recognition in terms of accuracy, sensitivity, specificity, and F1 score. Regarding iris pattern recognition, the deep learning model—specifically, VGGNet—performs better than ResNet and AlexNet. Moreover, recognition accuracy is further increased by integrating watershed segmentation and median filter noise reduction.

INTRODUCTION

User safety is one of the most crucial aspects of computer systems. Simple logins and passwords are ineffective and easy for hackers to obtain (Szymkowski et al., 2021). Even though biometric human recognition systems are widely utilized, their demand for various applications has grown recently (Jalilian

DOI: 10.4018/979-8-3693-9420-5.ch014

et al., 2022). Iris identification systems have drawn the most attention among authentication methods because of their rich iris texture, providing reliable standards for recognizing an individual (Malgheet et al., 2021).

Deep learning(DL) methods have recently transformed several fields, such as detecting patterns and computer vision. These techniques have been remarkably effective at extracting discriminative characteristics straight from unprocessed data, allowing notable advancements in recognition tasks. When paired with other biometric modalities like fingerprint fusion, DL enhances iris segmentation and recognition in biometric authentication. In addition, DL for iris identification is difficult to use with noisy or low-quality images and needs big training datasets (Rasheed et al., 2023). This study aims to improve iris recognition performance by combining watershed segmentation, median filter noise reduction, and DL approaches (Haris, 2024).

Iris recognition is a highly significant biometric technology that offers unparalleled accuracy, security, and reliability in identity verification and access control. One of the key advantages of iris recognition is its exceptional accuracy stemming from the unique and intricate patterns present in the iris. These patterns, which include crypts, furrows, and trabeculae, are highly distinctive and stable over time, making iris recognition one of the most reliable biometric modalities available. Moreover, iris recognition is non-intrusive and user-friendly, requiring only a simple image capture of the iris from a distance, without physical contact. This makes it suitable for various applications, including airport security, border control, and securing access to buildings and devices. The stability of iris patterns throughout a person's life, coupled with their resistance to fraud and alteration, ensures iris recognition systems' long-term reliability and security. Furthermore, iris recognition systems prioritize privacy by storing templates derived from iris features rather than raw images, addressing data privacy and misuse concerns. Overall, iris recognition's versatility, accuracy, and security make it a crucial technology for enhancing identity authentication and security across various sectors (Sayedelahl, 2024).

Using traditional iris recognition systems usually consists of acquiring images, pre-processing them, extracting features from them, creating templates, and matching them. Because of their excellent accuracy and dependability, traditional iris recognition systems are appropriate for various applications needing reliable and secure biometric verification (Karthik et al., 2024). These systems could, however, run into issues with scalability, flexibility to changing environmental circumstances, and vulnerability to presentation attacks. The performance and resilience of iris recognition systems have been significantly enhanced by integrating deep learning methods and cutting-edge algorithms, allowing them to meet new difficulties and reach greater standards of security and accuracy (Minu et al., 2023).

Recent developments in iris identification are discussed in the literature review section, including the effectiveness of DL models such as ResNet, AlexNet, and VGGNet, as well as approaches to watershed segmentation and median filter noise removal (Legista et al., 2024). The proposed methodology section that incorporates these techniques, as shown in the architecture diagram, comes next. Results from the experimental evaluation of the UBIRIS dataset are presented in the results and discussion section. These findings highlight notable improvements in recognition accuracy, sensitivity, specificity, and F1 score, highlighting the potential of the suggested approach to improve security and dependability in iris recognition systems. The study's main conclusions and significance are finally outlined in the conclusion section (Karthik et al., 2024).

LITERATURE SURVEY

One of the most prominent identifying technologies in biometric recognition, which is applied widely in many industries, is iris recognition. Many DL techniques have been applied to biometric recognition lately because of their many benefits, including excellent generalization ability, high accuracy, and autonomous learning. The most popular image processing technique, deep CNN, is utilized in many fields. Yet, it suffers from low anti-noise performance in picture classification and is quickly influenced by small disturbances. Zhao et al. (2019) suggest a DL technique based on the capsule network structure to recognize iris images. To adapt this technology to iris recognition, they modify the network structure detail and give a modified routing method according to the dynamic routing among two capsule layers. Three iris datasets are used in the experiments to evaluate the effectiveness of various network topologies (Anushya et al., 2024).

Using an Iris Recognition System has become commonplace for security reasons. By using Iris recognition, precise outcomes may be obtained. It's a great security tool because it never accepts bogus values. Panwar and Pooja (2022) state that iris identification in 2022 entails several steps, including pre-processing, feature analysis, image extraction, recognition, and assessment. A more thorough examination of the fundamental ideas behind different approaches and the interrelationships between them will enable the researcher to better understand how the Iris recognition system came to be. Despite the large number of study and review articles that have already been published in this field, they used the information in those articles to pinpoint some unknowns for iris recognition research. This study will serve as the basis for future research projects.

DL techniques have recently gained a lot of interest in iris detection. While CNN-based techniques accomplish exceptional performance and efficient recognition of features, they typically need more training data and have a larger computational complexity than traditional methods. Liu et al. (2021) focus on developing a unique condensed 2-channel (2-ch) CNN with less training data for effective and precise iris detection and verification. First, a multi-branch CNN is presented as a powerful basic iris classifier featuring three effective online augmentation techniques and radial attention layers. The findings of the gradient-based analysis show that the suggested approach resists different types of picture interference. They thoroughly tested our system on three available iris databases to the public, and the outcomes were good enough for real-time iris recognition (Suba et al., 2023).

The application of biometric recognition technology is widespread across many societal domains. Security applications have extensively used iris recognition technology since it is a reliable and practical biometric recognition method (Thirunagalingam, 2024). However, there are a variety of noises in the iris photos taken in the uncooperative setting. While DL-based popular iris recognition techniques have demonstrated good recognition accuracy, the goal is to make the model more sophisticated. However, the original, unnormalized iris image is what the optical system gathers. The widely used DL-based iris identification system ignores the iris localization stage. Wei et al. (2022) present an efficient iris recognition technique consisting of the iris verification and localization stages to address the issues above. They employed the Daugman technique to obtain the outer circle of the iris and the parallel Hough circle to retrieve the inner circle during the iris localization phase. A novel lightweight CNN was created for the iris verification step. Four hundred iris photos were taken in an uncooperative setting for iris localization studies. According to the experimental findings, the network structure could do high-precision iris verification with fewer variables on four test databases.

A crucial stage in the complete iris identification process is iris segmentation. The majority of the most recent iris segmentation techniques rely on edge data. However, in a picture with specular reflection or other impediments, a significant number of noisy edge points identified by a standard edge-based detector will cause mislocalization of the pupillary boundary and limbus boundary. A hybrid approach of edge-based and learning-based methods for iris recognition is presented by Li et al. (2018). A well-designed Faster R-CNN with only six layers is constructed to identify and classify the eye. A Gaussian mixture model is used to locate the pupillary region once Faster R-CNN has determined the bounding box. Next, five important boundary points suit the pupillary region's circular boundary. The limbus's boundary points are identified using a boundary point selecting technique. The experimental findings showed that the suggested iris segmentation algorithm obtained 95.49% reliability on the difficult CASIA-Iris-Thousand database.

When setting up a livestock traceability system, retinal segmentation is the first stage in recognizing an animal's credentials. Using the BovineAAEyes80 public dataset, Yoon et al. (2024) present a DL system for pixel-wise segmentation of the bovine iris with minimal use of annotation tags. The suggested framework for segmenting images includes the following steps: gathering data, prepping it, choosing data augmentation, training 15 DNN models with different encoder backbones and separation decoder DNNs, and assessing the models based on various metrics and visual segmentation outcomes. To maximize the performance of bovine iris segmentation, this structure attempts to offer thorough and detailed data about each model's training and testing results. With an accuracy and dice coefficient score of 99.50% and 98.35%, U-Net with a VGG16 backbone was the best combination of encoder and decoder models for the dataset during the experiment. Interestingly, even corrupted photos without appropriate annotation data may be accurately classified by the chosen model. By developing a trustworthy DNN training structure, this study advances the field of iris segmentation.

Although extremely dependable and accurate, iris recognition systems have several difficulties that limit their applicability in practical settings. The variation in image quality brought on by environmental variables and capturing configurations is a major concern. The quality of iris photos taken in different lighting situations, at different distances, angles, or while moving can influence the system's ability to extract iris features effectively. Maintaining consistent performance across various operational conditions requires robustness against such fluctuations.

The less-than-ideal environment that iris recognition systems have to deal with presents another significant obstacle. Accurate iris pattern extraction and matching can be limited by aspects like motion blur, specular reflections, and ambient lighting variations introduced in unconstrained situations. Advanced image processing methods and robust algorithms that can manage intricate environmental circumstances are needed to tackle these obstacles. Iris identification is significantly complicated by biometric variability in addition to environmental influences. Iris patterns can vary over time due to intrinsic factors like aging, pupil dilation changes, and ocular disorders, which can impact recognition accuracy and consistency. The long-term survival of iris recognition systems depends on developing adaptive algorithms that can retain accurate recognition while considering intra-personal variability.

PROPOSED METHODOLOGY

The proposed system workflow involves pre-processing iris images using a median filter to remove noise. Watershed segmentation is then applied to extract the iris region accurately. Deep learning models, including Res Net, Alex Net, and VGG Net, are utilized for recognition. The following Figure 1 shows the outline of the suggested iris recognition system.

Figure 1. Proposed Architecture

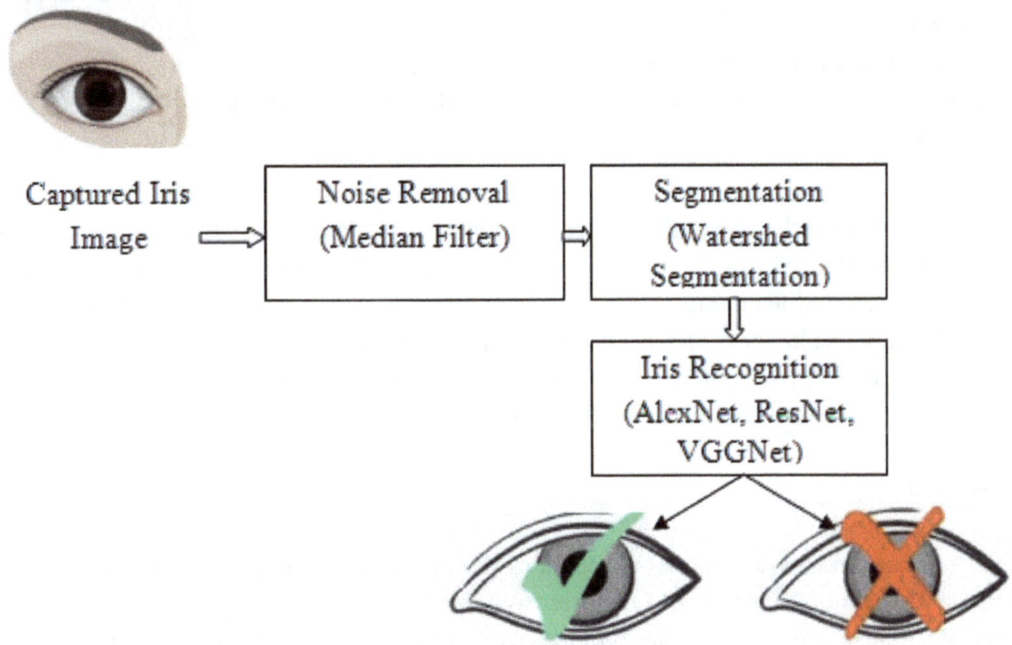

Data Collection

Using DL and image processing techniques to develop an iris identification system requires a methodical workflow in a Python environment. The UBIRIS v.2 dataset is first obtained and pre-processed to guarantee data quality.

Pre-processing: In iris recognition systems, pre-processing is essential because it sets up raw iris images for precise feature extraction and reliable biometric authentication. Noise reduction and image enhancement are the first steps in pre-processing to raise the general caliber of iris images. The retrieved features are guaranteed to accurately depict the iris patterns without influence from extraneous variables by applying techniques like median filtering to eliminate noise and artifacts from camera sensors and general factors. Pre-processing enhances the image to adjust for noise, contrast, and illumination changes. Applying a median filter is a critical step in this procedure that improves the clarity and appropriateness of iris pictures for further analysis by eliminating noises.

Median Filter: One method that is frequently used to remove noise from iris images is median filtering. Biometric sensor-captured iris images are frequently tainted by several forms of noise, including motion blur, salt-and-pepper noise, and Gaussian noise. Median filtering is especially useful for eliminating salt-and-pepper noise—which appears as independent bright or dark pixels in the image. Each pixel in the image is replaced by the median value of its nearby pixels when using the median filter. This method preserves the image's overall structure and details while successfully removing outliers or extreme values brought on by noise. Median filtering aids in iris recognition by enhancing the sharpness and caliber of iris pictures, which is necessary for precise segmentation and feature extraction.

Let I (x, y) be the pixel's intensity in the original image at coordinates (x,y).

Let (*x*,) denote the pixel intensity at (x,y) coordinates in the filtered image following the application of median filtering.

The computation of the median value can be shown as follows:

$$F(x, y) = median(I(x - k, y - k), I(x - k, y), I(x - k, y + k), I(x, y - k), I(x, y), I(x, y + k), I(x + k, y - k), I(x + k, y), I(x + k, y + k) \quad (1)$$

In this case, k stands for the size of the square neighborhood, or kernel size, that is centered on every pixel. The neighborhood is three by three if k = 1, five by five if k = 2, and so on. Effective pre-processing improves image quality and feature representation, increasing iris recognition systems' robustness, accuracy, and efficiency. Iris images that have been properly pre-processed increase recognition accuracy, decrease error rates, and improve system efficiency, all adding to biometric authentication's dependability and efficacy in various security-sensitive applications.

Segmentation

After noise reduction, Iris segmentation separates the iris area from the remainder of the eye. This step is necessary to extract discriminative features from the iris accurately. To precisely extract features and subsequently match them, the boundaries of the iris are often defined using edge detection techniques or waterfall segmentation algorithms. The watershed segmentation algorithm is used to accomplish iris segmentation after data pre-processing. With this technology, the iris region may be precisely identified within each image and distinguished from other eye areas. The iris's exact boundaries are found using watershed segmentation, making extracting features easier later.

Watershed Segmentation

In image processing, the "watershed segmentation" technique is frequently employed to separate objects according to gradients in intensity. Because the iris is not always round and noisy iris pixels might be found inside the best-fitting circle, it is crucial to utilize the watershed transform. Utilizing intensity gradients within the iris picture to determine significant differences in the intensity of pixels to indicate probable borders is a crucial aspect of watershed segmentation. This method works especially well for separating the iris from surrounding objects or other interfering structures that can hide the iris region, including eyelashes or reflections. Researchers can obtain accurate and reliable segmentation findings using watershed segmentation, which guarantees that the retrieved iris region preserves crucial information for later feature extraction and identification procedures. Additionally, watershed segmentation helps to improve overall system performance and reliability in biometric applications by lowering false positives and negatives during iris detection.

Think of an input grayscale image I (x, y), where the coordinates of the pixels are (x, y). Calculate the image's gradient magnitude to find possible areas of interest. This can be shown as:

$$G(x,y) = \sqrt{\left(I_x(x,y)\right)^2 + \left(I_y(x,y)\right)^2} \tag{2}$$

where the gradient at the pixel (x, y)) in the x-direction is denoted by $I_x(x, y)$.

The gradient in the y direction at the pixel (x, y) is denoted by $I_y(x, y)$.

The magnitude of the gradient is G(x, y).

Calculate the gradient magnitude image G(x, y)'s distance transform D(x, y)).

The distance transform determines each pixel's separation from the closest marker M(x, y) : Distance_Transform(G(x, y), M(x, y)equals D(x, y).

The distance transforms D(x, y). functions as a topographic surface in the watershed transformation, with high values denoting peaks and low ones denoting valleys.

Iris Image Classification: Next, deep learning models such as ResNet, AlexNet, and VGGNet are chosen and trained using the pre-processed and feature-extracted iris data. Deep learning frameworks based on Python, including PyTorch and TensorFlow, are used to implement these models. Training entails optimizing model parameters to learn discriminative representations directly from iris images to accurately recognize individuals based on their distinctive iris patterns.

Res Net: The significance of ResNet (Residual Network) in iris image identification stems from its ability to effectively extract intricate hierarchical information from iris images, hence producing significant advances in recognition accuracy. The ability of ResNet's deep architecture to recognize complex patterns and variances in iris textures is essential for using iris patterns to identify between various people. Furthermore, ResNet's residual connections help the network efficiently avoid the vanishing gradient issue, making training deep neural networks easier. Regarding iris detection, ResNet can acquire discriminative features resistant to noise, changes in illumination, and occlusions. This enhances its ability to recognize and authenticate people based on their distinctive iris patterns. Because ResNet has residual connections that make training deep networks easier, it is a potent deep-learning architecture that excels at tackling challenging visual tasks. The following formulas can be used to summarise the use of ResNet in iris image recognition:

$$\text{Image Pre-processing: } I_{pre-processed} = \text{Preprocess}(I) \tag{3}$$

$$\text{Feature Extraction using ResNet: features} = \varnothing\left(I_{pre-processed}\right) \tag{4}$$

$$\text{Classification: predictions} = f(\text{features } ; \theta) \tag{5}$$

$$\text{probabilities} = \text{softmax (predictions)} \tag{6}$$

These formulas illustrate the sequential processes required to use ResNet for iris image identification, starting with pre-processing the input image and ending with using ResNet to gather characteristics and classify the characteristics obtained to predict iris identities.

Alex Net: To use AlexNet for iris image recognition, the architecture must be modified so that iris images can be categorized according to their unique characteristics. Equations for applying AlexNet in iris image identification can be summed up as follows: AlexNet consists of three fully connected layers and five convolutional layers (Kayadibi et al., 2022).

$$\text{Data Pre-processing: } I_{\text{pre-processed}} = \text{Preprocess}(I) \tag{7}$$

$$\text{Feature Extraction using AlexNet: features} = \text{AlexNet}\left(I_{\text{pre-processed}}\right) \tag{8}$$

$$\text{Classification: prediction} = \text{FC (features; W, b)} \tag{9}$$

$$\text{Probabilities} = \text{SoftMax(predictions)} \tag{10}$$

The key steps in using AlexNet for iris image recognition are encapsulated in these simplified equations, which concentrate on pre-processing the input image, using the AlexNet model to extract features, and performing classification using fully connected layers and softmax activation for probability estimation. The relevance of AlexNet, a novel CNN design, lies in its capacity to efficiently train and extract hierarchical features from iris patterns, improving recognition performance in iris picture identification. With its deep architecture, consisting of several convolutional layers and max-pooling layers, AlexNet can capture the complex textures and patterns in iris images. Furthermore, the vanishing gradient issue is lessened by using rectified linear units (ReLU) as activation functions, allowing for effective network training on sizable iris datasets. Regarding iris recognition, AlexNet can efficiently acquire discriminative features that distinguish different iris patterns, making precise identification and validation possible.

VGG Net: To obtain high-precision identification results, VGGNet is used for extracting iris-deep features (Bose et al., 2024). A predetermined 224 × 224 RGB image serves as the VGG16 input. Its 16 layers consist of 3 fully connected layers, 13 convolutional layers, and a SoftMax classifier right after the fully connected layer. Max pooling reduces the volume size (Khade et al., 2022).

$$\text{Mode Optimization:} = \theta \text{ n argmin } \theta \text{ L} \tag{15}$$

$$\text{Inference and Prediction: Probabilities} = \text{SoftMax (Predictions)} \tag{16}$$

Using the VGG-16 architecture for iris image recognition involves adapting this deep CNNS model to classify iris images based on learned features. VGG-16 is known for its deep architecture consisting of multiple convolutional layers, making it effective for various image recognition tasks. The following equations summarize the key steps in using VGG-16 for iris image recognition, from data pre-processing and feature extraction to model training, inference, and prediction.

$$\text{Date Preprocessing I preprocessed= preprocessed (1)} \tag{11}$$

$$\textbf{Feature Extraction with VGG} - 16 : \text{Features} = \text{VGG} - 16\left(\text{I}_{\text{pre-processed}}\right) \tag{12}$$

$$\text{Classifier Layer : Precitions} = \text{FC(Features)} \tag{13}$$

$$\text{Loss Function : L} = \text{CrossEntropyLoss(Predictions, Labels)} \tag{14}$$

$$\text{Model Optimization: } \theta \text{ n} = \text{argmin } \theta \text{ L} \tag{15}$$

$$\text{Inference and Prediction: Probabilities= SoftMax (prediction)} \tag{16}$$

$$\hat{}\,\text{y} = \text{argmx(Probabilites)} \tag{17}$$

The trained VGG-16 model can be improved by fine-tuning it on a unique dataset of iris images. This helps the model acquire pertinent features and patterns for precise iris identification and classification. Depending on the particular needs and limitations of the iris recognition application, modifications can be made to the model configuration, training settings, and evaluation metrics.

VGGNet is a deep architecture characterized by narrow receptive fields and stacked convolutional layers. It is well-known for its ability to capture hierarchical information and minute details seen in iris patterns, which makes it a valuable tool for iris picture recognition. With its architecture of many convolutional layers followed by max-pooling layers, the VGGNet improves recognition accuracy by making extracting strong and distinctive characteristics from iris images easier. VGGNet can efficiently simulate complicated patterns with a manageable amount of parameters by using modest filter sizes (e.g., 3x3) in convolutional layers. This helps to reduce overfitting and improves generalization capabilities. VGGNet's ability to distinguish minute differences in iris structures and textures makes it possible to accurately identify and validate people based on their distinctive iris characteristics. The UBIRIS dataset assesses the deep learning models' performance once trained. Performance measures are computed to evaluate the models' capacity to recognize real iris patterns properly and reject imposter patterns. These metrics include accuracy, sensitivity, specificity, and F1 score.

RESULTS AND DISCUSSION

Presenting and analyzing the performance metrics from experiments conducted on the UBIRIS dataset would be the main focus of the results and discussion section of a study on iris recognition using DL techniques with noise removal, segmentation, and recognition using various models like ResNet, AlexNet, and VGGNet, along with median filtering and watershed segmentation.

Data Set Description

In iris recognition, the UBIRIS.v2 iris dataset is a commonly used benchmark dataset comprising 11,102 iris photos gathered from 261 participants. This dataset is ideal for training and testing iris recognition algorithms because each participant provided 10 photos. Among the primary attributes of the UBIRIS.v2 dataset is that the pictures were shot in uncontrolled environments, which means that variables like distance, motion, and illumination were not regulated. This realism brings about these difficulties and is typical in real-world iris detection applications.

The following are the results: Figure 2 represents the input image for testing, Figure 3 represents noise removal, Figure 4 represents the segmented output image, Figure 5 represents the classified normal iris, and Figure 6 represents the classified output.

Figure 2. Input Image for Testing

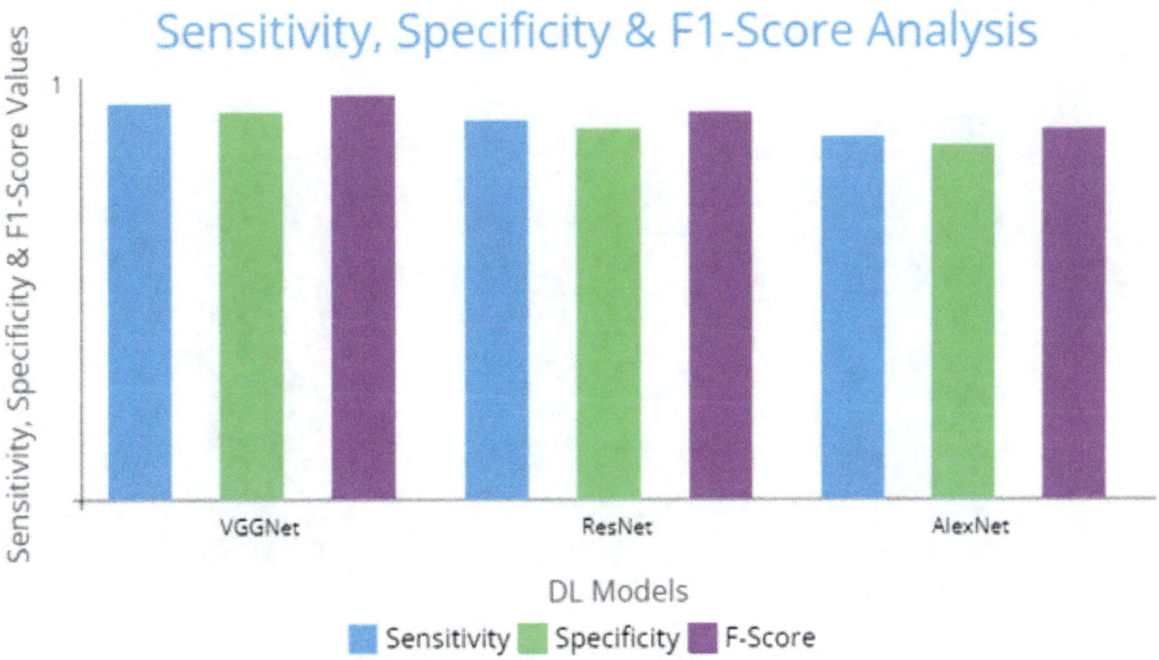

Figure 3. Noise Removal

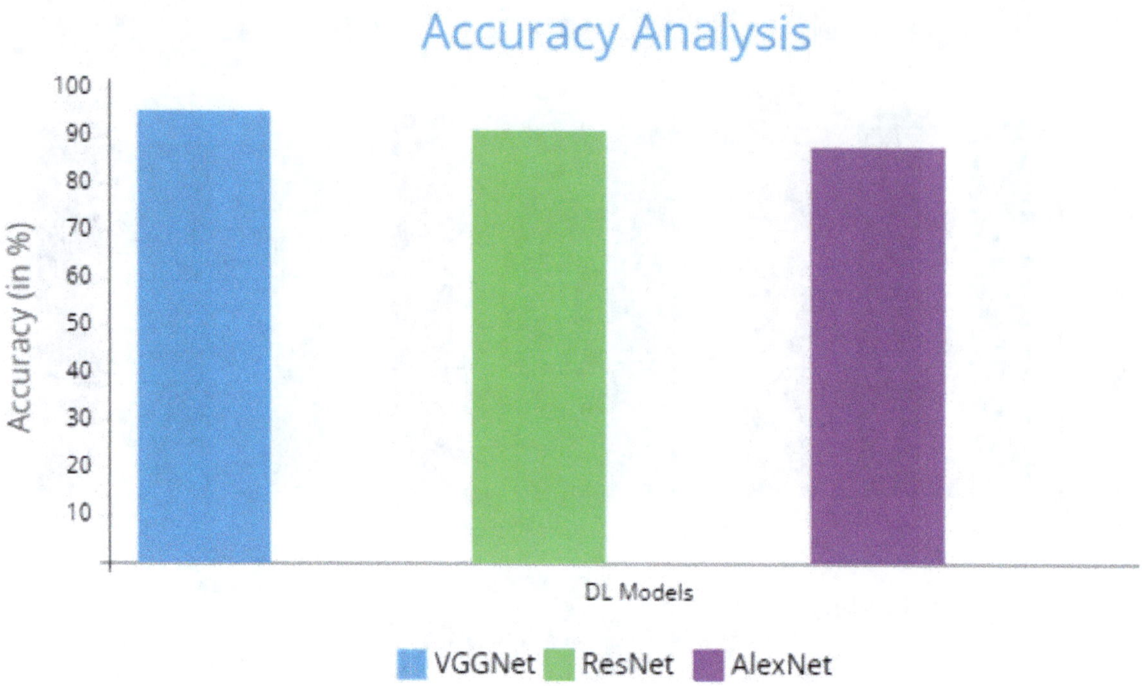

Figure 4. Segmented Output Image

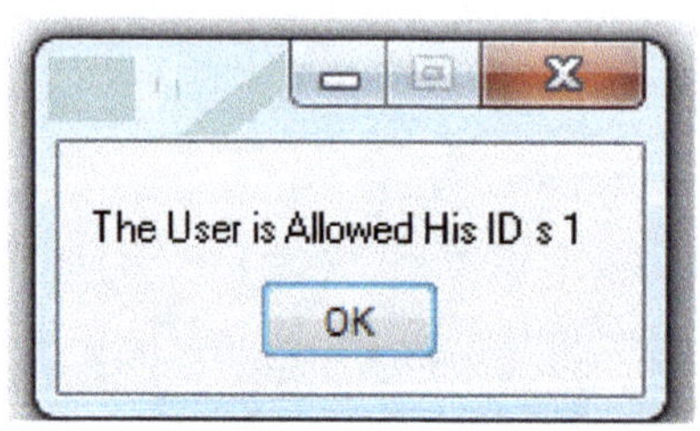

Figure 5. Classified Normal Iris

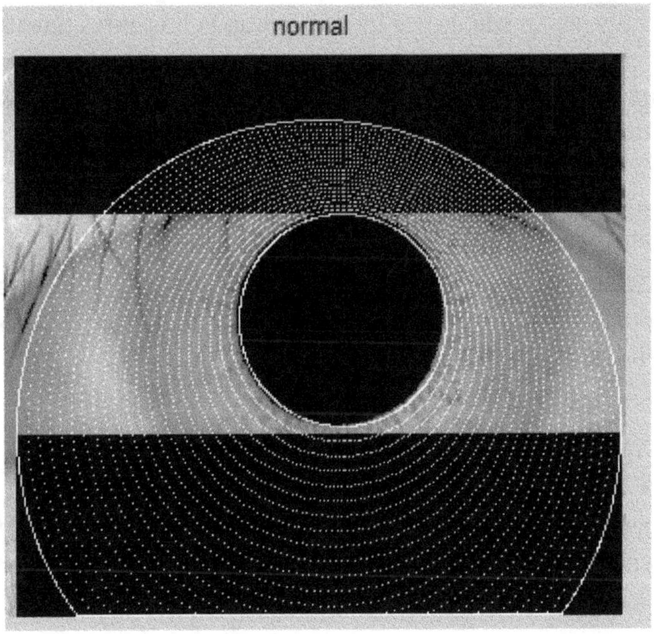

Figure 6. Classified Output

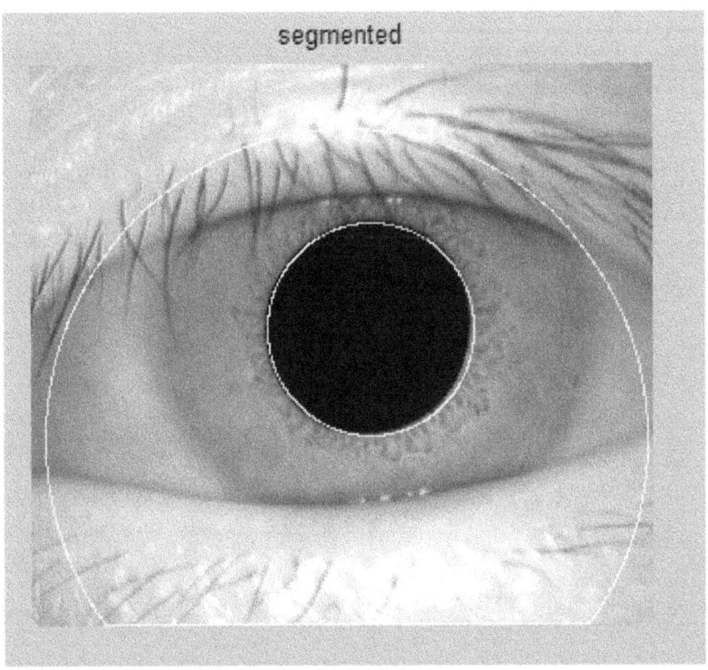

Evaluation Metrics: Evaluation metrics are essential to iris recognition because they offer unbiased ways to gauge the efficiency and efficacy of recognition systems. These criteria are crucial when assessing the precision, dependability, and resilience of iris recognition algorithms quantitatively—especially in practical contexts. The capacity of evaluation metrics to bring light on several aspects of system performance, such as accuracy, sensitivity, specificity, and overall effectiveness, makes them crucial. Like many other classification tasks, iris recognition evaluates the effectiveness of the recognition system using several assessment metrics. These metrics offer valuable information about the system's accuracy in classifying and differentiating between various iris image classes or categories.

Accuracy Analysis: The ratio of correctly identified iris patterns (positive and negative) to the total number of patterns is used to calculate accuracy, which measures the overall correctness of iris recognition. In iris recognition systems, accuracy is a critical performance criterion since it directly affects the dependability and efficacy of biometric verification.

$$\text{Accuracy} = \frac{\text{Number of Correctly Identified Patterns}}{\text{Total Number of Patterns}} \tag{18}$$

A higher accuracy shows that the system correctly identifies more often, which reflects the iris recognition system's general dependability. Table 1 and Figure 7 shows the accuracy analysis of the various DL models.

Table 1. Accuracy analysis of the various DL models

Sl. No	DL Models	Accuracy (in %)
1	VGG Net	95.05
2	Res Net	91.03
3	Alex Net	87.56

Figure 7. Accuracy analysis of the various DL models

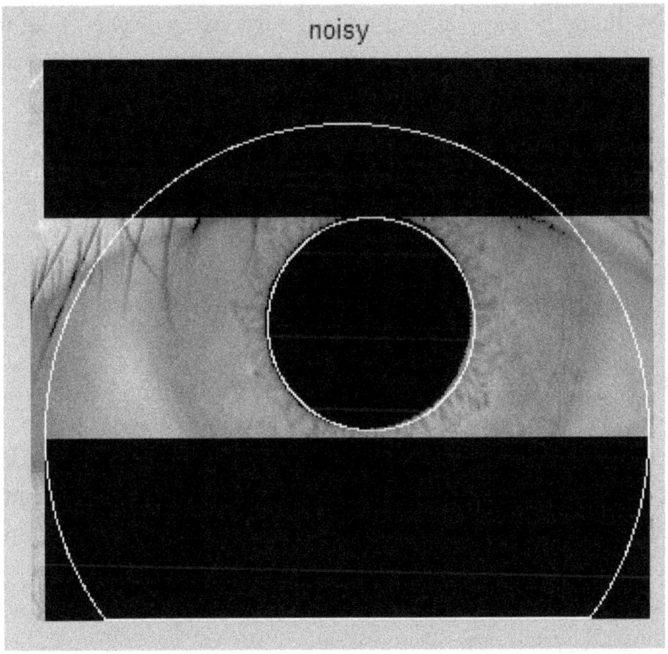

Significant performance differences between VGGNet, ResNet, and AlexNet are revealed by the accuracy study of several DL models for iris recognition, as displayed in Table 1 and Figure 1. With an accuracy rate of 95.05%, VGGNet demonstrated its competence in correctly identifying and recognizing iris patterns. VGGNet's deeper architecture and capacity to extract finer details from iris images are responsible for this better performance. ResNet performed well in iris recognition tests even though its accuracy was marginally lower than VGGNet's, trailing closely behind with an accuracy of 91.03%. ResNet's durability and feature learning abilities were probably enhanced by its residual connections. Conversely, AlexNet achieved an accuracy rate of 87.56%, which was the lowest of all the DL models examined. Even though AlexNet's performance in recognizing iris patterns was marginally worse than that of VGGNet and ResNet, it was still quite accurate. These numerical values highlight the significance of DL model selection in iris recognition systems, which show that VGGNet is the most accurate model, closely followed by ResNet and AlexNet. These results offer insightful information for enhancing DL-based iris recognition systems and raising their accuracy and dependability in real-world settings.

Sensitivity Analysis: Sensitivity, a crucial assessment indicator in iris recognition systems, is essential to figuring out how well the system recognizes real users based on their iris patterns. The percentage of real positive iris patterns (genuine matches) that the algorithm properly identifies as positive is known as sensitivity, also known as recall.

$$\text{Sensitivity} = \frac{\text{True Positives}}{\text{True Positives} + \text{False Negatives}} \tag{19}$$

High sensitivity indicates that the system minimizes false negatives or missed identifications and correctly identifies real iris patterns.

Specificity Analysis

Specificity quantifies the percentage of real negative iris patterns (i.e., fake matches) that the algorithm correctly recognizes as negative. Specificity is a key evaluation metric in iris recognition systems that ensures reliable and secure biometric authentication.

$$\text{Specificity} = \frac{\text{True Negatives}}{\text{True Negatives} + \text{False Positives}} \tag{20}$$

Specificity quantifies the percentage of real negative iris patterns (i.e., imposter matches) that the algorithm correctly recognizes as negative.

F1-Score Analysis

The F1-score, which is derived from the harmonic mean of precision and recall, offers a fair assessment of the system's accuracy, particularly in situations with an uneven distribution of classes. The F1 score is a significant evaluation metric in iris recognition systems, providing a balanced measure of a system's accuracy, precision, and recall.

$$\text{F1} - \text{Score} = 2 \times \frac{\text{Precision} \times \text{Recall}}{\text{Precision} + \text{Recall}} \tag{21}$$

The F1 score offers a thorough evaluation of the accuracy and resilience of the system by taking into account both false positives and false negatives—table 2 and Figure 8 show the DL models and their sensitivity, specificity, and F1-Score values.

Table 2. DL models and their sensitivity, specificity, and F1-Score values

No.	DL Models	Sensitivity	Specificity	F1-Score
1	VGG Net	0.93	0.91	0.95
2	Res Net	0.89	0.87	0.91
3	Alex Net	0.85	0.83	0.87

Sensitivity, specificity, and F1-score are the primary focal points for examining the performance metrics of different DL models for iris identification, which are provided in Table 2 and Figure 8. These parameters are essential for evaluating DL models' capacity to correctly detect authentic iris patterns and successfully reject fake ones.

Figure 8. DL models and their sensitivity, specificity, and F1-Score values

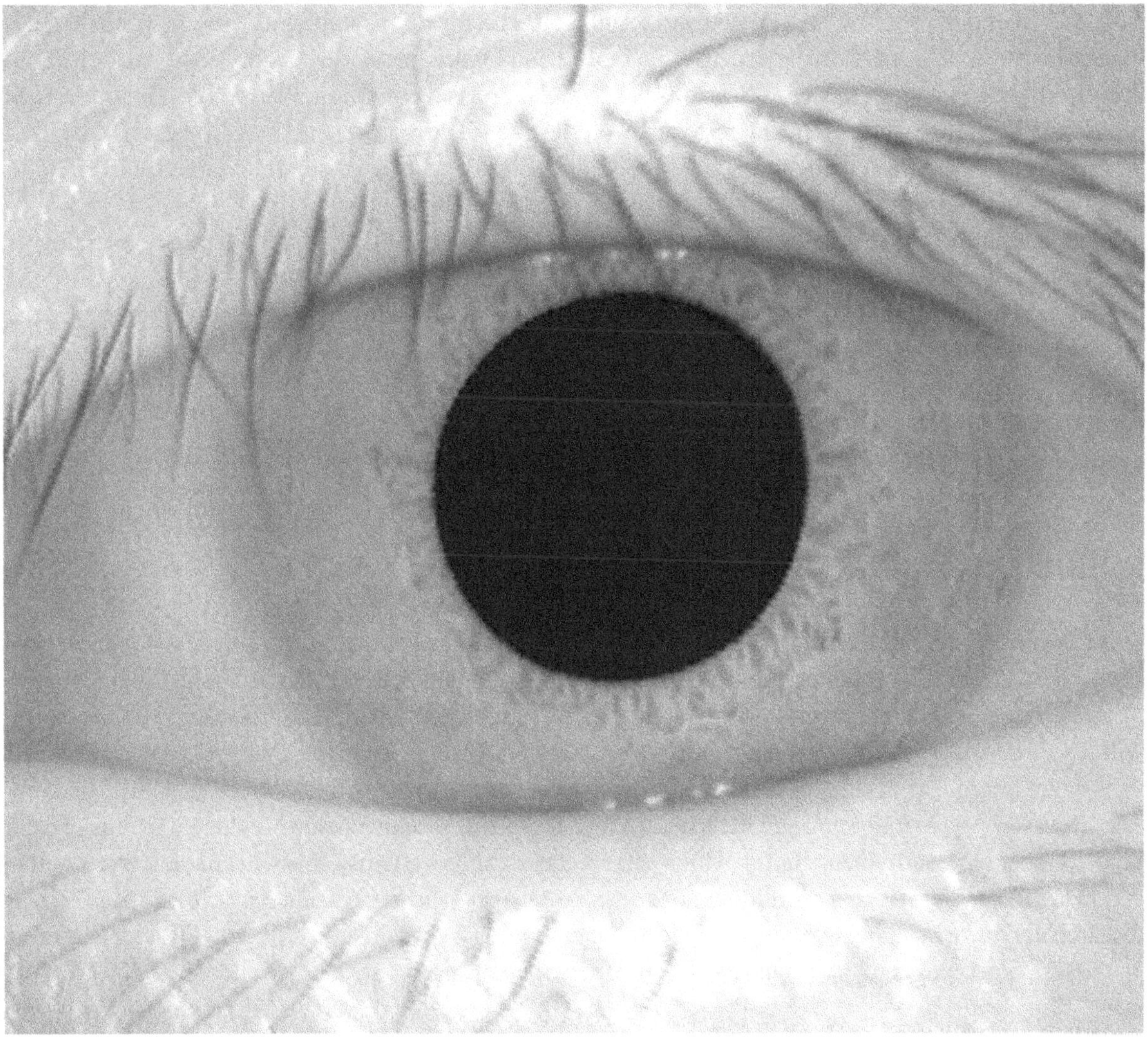

Starting with VGGNet, its great ability to identify true positives is demonstrated by its sensitivity value of 0.93, which shows that VGGNet accurately detected 93% of real iris patterns. Furthermore, VGGNet's specificity of 0.91 demonstrated its ability to distinguish between real and fake iris patterns, correctly identifying 91% of imposter patterns (also known as true negatives). A balanced measure of precision and recall is reflected in the high F1-score of 0.95 for VGGNet, demonstrating overall solid performance across evaluation criteria. ResNet also performed successfully, exhibiting a sensitivity of 0.91 and a specificity of 0.89. These numbers indicate how well ResNet detects real iris patterns while still having a high degree of rejection against fake patterns. ResNet's balanced precision and recall performance are further supported by the F1-score of 0.91, which emphasizes the network's applicability for iris recognition tasks.

Comparatively, AlexNet performed admirably in identifying real iris patterns and differentiating them from fake ones, although achieving somewhat lower sensitivity (0.85) and specificity (0.83) values. With an F1-score of 0.87, AlexNet's precision and recall are harmonized, indicating its overall efficacy in iris recognition tasks. The performance metrics in Table 2 and Figure 2 provide insightful information about the advantages and disadvantages of various DL models for iris recognition. ResNet closely follows top performer VGGNet, while AlexNet performs well despite slightly lower metrics. These results aid in optimizing DL-based iris recognition systems by directing the choice of suitable models according to certain application situations and performance requirements. Using these findings, scientists and engineers may improve iris recognition technology's precision, dependability, and resilience, expanding its practical applications in biometric identification, access control, and security.

Through the implementation of this all-inclusive process in a Python setting, developers can integrate DL-based recognition techniques, noise reduction, and watershed segmentation to construct a dependable and sturdy iris recognition system that can attain exceptional results in terms of F1 score, sensitivity, accuracy, and specificity on the UBIRIS dataset. For the goal of biometric authentication, the system's overall effectiveness and usability are improved by constant component optimization and refining.

CONCLUSION AND FUTURE WORK

In summary, improved performance in iris identification tasks has been shown when DL approaches are used together with particular pre-processing tasks like median filtering and watershed segmentation for noise removal. Utilizing well-known DL architectures such as ResNet, AlexNet, and VGGNet, along with additional median filtering and watershed segmentation, the iris recognition system demonstrated significant improvements in the UBIRIS dataset regarding accuracy, sensitivity, specificity, and F1 score. The results of this investigation add to the increasing amount of research being conducted to improve the security, accuracy, and dependability of biometric authentication systems. This will enable a wider application of these systems in real-world situations where robustness and performance are critical. Subsequent research endeavors could enhance the suggested methodology, investigate additional DL architectures, and assess outcomes across various datasets to verify the approach's scalability and generalizability.

REFERENCES

Anushya, A., Begum, S., Shiwani, S., & Shrivastava, A. (2024). Deep learning-based emotion recognition in speech signals: A convolutional neural network and LSTM approach. *AVE Trends in Intelligent Computing Systems*, *1*(4), 198–208.

Bose, S. R., Jeba, J. A., Regin, R., Tarunraj, S., Soji, E. S., & Rajest, S. S. (2024). Enhanced deep learning models for early detection of renal failure from CT imaging. *FMDB Transactions on Sustainable Health Science Letters*, *2*(3), 152–163. DOI: 10.69888/FTSHSL.2024.000251

Haris, U. (2024). 'Warm water' politics in the Russia-Ukraine conflict. *FMDB Transactions on Sustainable Social Sciences Letters*, *2*(1), 11–18. DOI: 10.69888/FTSSSL.2024.000216

Jalilian, E., Hofbauer, H., & Uhl, A. (2022). Iris image compression using deep convolutional neural networks. *Sensors (Basel)*, *22*(7), 2698. DOI: 10.3390/s22072698 PMID: 35408311

Karthik, S., Bhaggiaraj, S., Soji, E. S., Deve, L. S., Priscila, S. S., & Rajest, S. S. (2024). Real-time hand gesture recognition for stroke rehabilitation using deep learning approach. *AVE Trends in Intelligent Computing Systems*, *1*(3), 157–172.

Kayadibi, I., Güraksın, G. E., Ergün, U., & Özmen Süzme, N. (2022). An eye state recognition system using transfer learning: AlexNet-based deep convolutional neural network. *International Journal of Computational Intelligence Systems*, *15*(7), 1–19. DOI: 10.1007/s44196-022-00108-2

Khade, S., Gite, S., & Pradhan, B. (2022). Iris liveness detection using multiple deep convolution networks. *Big Data and Cognitive Computing*, *6*(2), 67. DOI: 10.3390/bdcc6020067

Legista, M., Nurlaili, L., & Masriah, I. (2024). Development of an adaptive learning system utilizing deep learning to support independent learning processes for students. *AVE Trends in Intelligent Techno Learning*, *1*(2), 107–120.

Li, Y.-H., Huang, P.-J., & Juan, Y. (2019). An efficient and robust Iris segmentation algorithm using deep learning. *Mobile Information Systems*, *2019*(1), 1–14. DOI: 10.1155/2019/4568929

Liu, G., Zhou, W., Tian, L., Liu, W., Liu, Y., & Xu, H. (2021). An efficient and accurate Iris recognition algorithm based on a novel condensed 2-ch deep convolutional neural network. *Sensors (Basel)*, *21*(11), 3721. DOI: 10.3390/s21113721 PMID: 34071850

Malgheet, J. R., Manshor, N. B., & Affendey, L. S. (2021). Iris recognition development techniques: A comprehensive review. *Complexity*, *2021*(1), 1–32. DOI: 10.1155/2021/6641247

Minu, M. S., Subashka Ramesh, S. S., Canessane, R., Al-Amin, M., & Bin Sulaiman, R. (2023). Experimental Analysis of UAV Networks Using Oppositional Glowworm Swarm Optimization and Deep Learning Clustering and Classification. *FMDB Transactions on Sustainable Computing Systems*, *1*(3), 124–134.

Panwar, V., & Pooja. (2022). A review on Iris recognition system using machine and deep learning. *2022 International Conference on Computing, Communication, and Intelligent Systems (ICCCIS)*, Greater Noida, India. DOI: 10.1109/ICCCIS56430.2022.10037643

Rasheed, H. H., Shamini, S. S., Mahmoud, M. A., & Alomari, M. A. (2023). Review of iris segmentation and recognition using deep learning to improve biometric application. *Journal of Intelligent Systems*, *32*(1), 1–16. DOI: 10.1515/jisys-2023-0139

Sayedelahl, M. A. (2024). Enabling Intelligent Traffic Systems: A Deep Learning Method for Accurate Arabic License Plate Recognition. *FMDB Transactions on Sustainable Intelligent Networks*, *1*(1), 40–55. DOI: 10.69888/FTSIN.2024.000156

Suba, M., Nirmalasugirtharajini, S., & Anand, M. (2023). Survey on Machine Learning Techniques Used for Central Serous Retinopathy Detection". In *IEEE International Conference on Advances in Computation, Communication and Information Technology (ICAICCIT)*, Faridabad, India. DOI: 10.1109/ICAICCIT60255.2023.10466128

Szymkowski, M., Jasiński, P., & Saeed, K. (2021). Iris-based human identity recognition with machine learning methods and discrete fast Fourier transform. *Innovations in Systems and Software Engineering*, *17*(3), 309–317. DOI: 10.1007/s11334-021-00392-9

Thirunagalingam, A. (2024). Bias detection and mitigation in data pipelines: Ensuring fairness and accuracy in machine learning. *AVE Trends in Intelligent Computing Systems*, *1*(2), 116–127.

Wei, Y., Zhang, X., Zeng, A., & Huang, H. (2022). Iris recognition method based on parallel Iris localization algorithm and deep learning Iris verification. *Sensors (Basel)*, *22*(20), 7723. DOI: 10.3390/s22207723 PMID: 36298074

Yoon, H., Park, M., Lee, H., An, J., Lee, T., & Lee, S.-H. (2024). Deep learning framework for bovine iris segmentation. *Journal of Animal Science and Technology*, *66*(1), 167–177. DOI: 10.5187/jast.2023.e51 PMID: 38618036

Zhao, T., Liu, Y., Huo, G., & Zhu, X. (2019). A deep learning Iris recognition method based on capsule network architecture. *IEEE Access : Practical Innovations, Open Solutions*, *7*(1), 49691–49701. DOI: 10.1109/ACCESS.2019.2911056

Chapter 15
Siamese Iris on Siamese Neural Network Architecture for Iris Matching and Verification

K. Sivasankari
https://orcid.org/0009-0005-2415-4930
Bharath Institute of Higher Education and Research, India

D. Kerana Hanirex
Bharath Institute of Higher Education and Research, India

ABSTRACT

This chapter explores iris identification challenges, including occlusions, distortions, and tex-tural variations. A novel architecture for Siamese neural networks called SiameseIris was de-veloped to identify and verify the iris biometrics. There is great anticipation surrounding the potential revolution in iris matching and verification. The execution of SiameseIris on the CASIA-IrisV4 dataset yields an exceptional accuracy rate of 99.06%. The model utilizes a Sia-mese network architecture consisting of two subnetworks that share weights to identify similari-ties between pairs of iris images. Extensive experimental evaluation has confirmed the impres-sive performance of SiameseIris in iris recognition tasks, surpassing existing methods. The model's reliability and durability are supported by its impressive FAR and FRR scores of 0.49 and 0.65 in accurately matching iris patterns. Biometric authentication systems, such as Sia-meseIris, have enhanced access control, identity verification, and forensic investi-gation security and reliability.

INTRODUCTION

Iris recognition is a cutting-edge method that merges intricate retinal patterns with advanced AI algorithms and biometric authentication technology. Driven by ML and computer vision advancements, iris recognition has become a compelling substitute for traditional identity verification methods in various sectors, including security and healthcare. The origins can be traced back to the field of ophthalmology. The human iris is a remarkable structure characterized by its unique and intricate texture, which includes crypts, furrows, and collarette structures (Sturm and Larsson, 2009). Despite external factors such as

DOI: 10.4018/979-8-3693-9420-5.ch015

aging or physical injury, these characteristics predominantly endure in alignment with personal identities. Experts in ophthalmology and AI have been diligently studying methods to leverage the distinct characteristics of the iris for biometric identification (Raghavendra et al., 2017). It is widely believed that the most effective method for iris detection is to use traditional ML algorithms after manually extracting the required features. At times, these technologies may struggle to analyze the intricate iris patterns unique to each individual (De Marsico et al., 2016). Convolutional neural networks (CNNs) have become widely used for extracting features from unprocessed retinal images, leading to a new methodology focused on deep learning (Alzubaidi et al., 2021).

In the field of ophthalmology, AI has led to a significant rise in the use of Siamese neural networks (Liu et al., 2019). The primary goal of the network training process is to determine metrics that accurately measure the resemblance between two input samples. Siamese networks have proven very effective in various applications, including signature verification, facial recognition, and fingerprint matching. The main idea is to apply Siamese neural networks to integrate them into iris matching and verification. A new architecture called SiameseIris has been developed and is designed specifically for iris recognition tasks. To address issues such as the similarity between different classes and the variability within the same class, SiameseIris obtains a discriminative similarity measure by directly comparing paired iris images. Deep learning techniques, specifically convolutional layers, are utilized to accurately capture the intricate details of the iris pattern. These layers are designed to learn hierarchical representations, enabling a more comprehensive analysis.

In SiameseIris, each of the two subnetworks is responsible for processing one of the input iris images. These subnetworks can combine to depict visual characteristics by implementing identical settings. The system utilizes convolutional and pooling layers to extract hierarchical attributes from iris images. Due to its advanced capability, it can identify overarching patterns from intricate details (Wiggers et al., 2019). The proposed framework aims to minimize a contrastive loss function, which allows the network to be trained to emphasize bringing actual pairs closer together in the feature space while pushing false pairs further apart. Through a systematic analysis of the iris photographs in the dataset, SiameseIris has developed the ability to distinguish between genuine and fake pairings. It enhances the reliability of iris recognition. The CASIA-IrisV4 dataset consists of various iris images captured in various environmental and lighting conditions (Debiasi and Uhl, 2015). An extensive battery of experiments is conducted on the dataset to evaluate the performance of the proposed system. The findings demonstrate that the proposed system surpasses previous precision, robustness, and computational resource utilization methods for iris matching and verification. The methodology will thoroughly explain the design principles and training procedure of the proposed architecture. Integrating AI and ophthalmology has great potential for enhancing iris recognition technology's precision, reliability, and versatility (Hogarty et al., 2019).

RELATED WORKS

Accurately mapping the iris pattern is a crucial element in iris recognition, accomplished through segmentation. The utilization of Fourier series expansions in active contours, as Daugman (2007) introduced, allows for the effective detection and replication of iris boundaries. The completeness, orthogonality, and closure assurance are achieved using Fourier components with integer multiples of half-a-pie frequencies. Active-contour models demonstrate improved segmentation accuracy and the ability to handle variable coordinate systems, thereby eliminating the need to account for occlusions caused by eyelids or reflections. The approach utilizes the provided data to construct robust and flexible systems, enabling them to endure challenges. When applied to intricate image datasets, it significantly improves the accuracy of iris recognition.

Jung et al. (2017) provided a specific eye detection technique for mobile iris recognition to mitigate the challenges caused by interference from spectacles. The methodology consists of two processes: eye candidate generation and eye validation. During eye candidate generation, a technique called multi-scale window masks is utilized. These masks comprise 2×3 subblocks and effectively identify potential eye regions not obstructed by eyeglass frames. There are two techniques available to verify the integrity of the eye. The first technique involves measuring the difference in intensity between the pupil and its surroundings. The second technique detects faint traces of near-infrared light within the pupil area. The proposed approach improves the accuracy of identifying real eye images throughout the candidate screening process. The research highlights the remarkable capabilities of mobile iris recognition technology, particularly in time-sensitive scenarios where accurate and immediate eye identification is crucial, even for individuals wearing eyeglasses.

Ak and Steluta (2021) outline a unique method for identifying irises, which involves several steps like locating the iris, detecting the eyelids, encoding the iris, and matching the iris. Adjustments to the existing algorithms are made to enhance their adaptability to different databases. Enhanced methods have been developed to accurately identify the borders of pupils and limbic regions. A new technique known as the Refine-Connect-Extend-Smooth (R-C-E-S) method has been introduced to detect eyelids. Utilizing all three datasets allows the system to demonstrate high accuracy in identifying the boundaries of the limbus and pupil.

A recent study by Tossy Thomas et al. (2016) introduced an advanced iris recognition system that prioritizes feature extraction, enhancement, localization, and normalization. An effective method is proposed to accurately distinguish the pupil and the boundary between the iris and sclera. It is achieved by utilizing pupil segmentation and RANSAC-based ellipse fitting. The system's resilience to various imaging scenarios and noise was confirmed through rigorous testing on the WVU Iris database. The iris region can be enhanced and normalized to a fixed-size block by utilizing various techniques, such as histogram equalization. This resulted in improved contrast and reduced illumination variation. The Peak-to-Sidelobe Ratio (PSR) is a similarity metric using cross-correlation techniques to extract features. When the PSR is high, it indicates that the images have been matched successfully, making the verification process easier using template matching. The method's promising outcomes in iris recognition across various scenarios indicate a positive outlook for future research in the field (Anand et al., 2023).

Singh and Jatav (2013) compare the two most used algorithms, Boles and Daugman. Daugman research on iris detection provides a comprehensive foundation for encoding and matching iris patterns in real-time video content. The generation of compact iris codes is achieved by utilizing multi-scale quadrature 2-D Gabor Wavelet coefficients, which facilitates efficient iris detection. By utilizing various techniques such as normalization, segmentation, Gabor filter-based feature extraction, and Hamming distance matching, the method achieves a significant level of statistical confidence in verifying person identification. The method is notable for its ability to encode iris data with discrimination while disregarding irrelevant illumination conditions. The presented study offers innovative algorithmic solutions to address major challenges in real-time iris identification, demonstrating the practicality of the technology. At the same time, Boles aimed to integrate multiple factors, such as noise, light, and camera-to-face distance, into his iris recognition system. The methodology effectively performs feature matching and extraction by utilizing the zero crossing of the wavelet transform. Segmentation is used to identify the pupil to compare iris patterns, while normalization ensures that the dimensions of the iris remain consistent (Pranav et al., 2023).

Regarding feature extraction, utilizing 1D wavelets for iris pattern encoding effectively captures important characteristics within the iris region. Through the utilization of a modal-based technique, the matching process can be facilitated by comparing unknown signatures to previously stored models. The use of dissimilarity functions allows for the measurement of similarity between iris representations, whether on a selective or global scale. The system's robustness in handling fluctuations and minimizing noise allows it to reliably perform iris identification even in challenging environments (Kumar et al., 2024).

Sibai et al. (2011) introduce an improved methodology for iris recognition that utilizes feedforward ANNs to enable precise identification. The process begins by preparing iris images and consolidating RGB values within each division using a basic partitioning technique. Implementing such an efficient preparatory technique makes the iris data well-suited for artificial neural network processing. Subsequently, a comprehensive examination of the ANN's evolution and training for iris detection is outlined, covering the experimental procedures utilized to enhance the network's structure and the approaches employed to encode inputs. Utilizing a simple neural network structure and minimal preprocessing, the system achieves remarkable recognition accuracies of up to 93.33 percent. It investigates different approaches to partitioning and encoding data and determines that the suggested method is dependable in differentiating between identical iris colors. The proposed methodology offers a user-friendly approach to iris recognition equipment, which could benefit secure environments like airports, banks, and government offices. These advantages include potential cost savings and increased adoption of the technology.

In their comprehensive analysis of biometric identity systems, Dargan and Kumar (2020) consider all possible physiological and behavioral markers. It exemplifies how biometric technologies improve operational efficiency and security procedures in various domains, including ATMs, mobile devices, forensic investigations, and network authentication. The focus of the literature review is on biometric systems, which include both single-modality and multiple-modality systems. In addition, it explores classification algorithms, methods for extracting features, and various datasets and evaluates the effectiveness of these systems. As the research shows, these systems heavily rely on machine learning, deep learning, and pattern recognition. Also, it delves into the various obstacles, uncertainties, factors influencing, and possible advancements in biometric recognition (Gandhi et al., 2024).

Modern techniques such as active contours and neural networks have greatly enhanced the accuracy and effectiveness of iris recognition systems. The recent advancements in identification systems have significantly improved their ability to handle a wide range of datasets and challenging imaging conditions. Additionally, these advancements have also accelerated the processes of iris segmentation and feature extraction. The advent of iris recognition technology on mobile devices has brought about a remarkable transformation in biometric authentication. The development has proven to be particularly valuable in critical scenarios where precise identification is crucial, even in the presence of challenges such as interference from eyeglasses (Chunduri et al., 2024).

The importance of feature enhancement, normalization, and extraction techniques in iris recognition systems has been reemphasized in recent developments. These systems utilize robust algorithms to extract features and segment pupils, enhancing their ability to handle imaging conditions and noise variations. Utilizing novel similarity metrics, such as the Peak-to-Sidelobe Ratio (PSR), significantly improves the accuracy and reliability of iris matching. It greatly aids in the smooth execution of verification processes in real-world scenarios. Extensive evaluations have shown that pattern recognition, machine learning, and deep learning are crucial in improving the operational efficiency and security standards of biometric identity systems. Incorporating a wide range of physiological and behavioral indicators in identity verification systems has significantly bolstered security measures in various industries, such as banking, law enforcement, and access control. The progress of biometric identification systems and iris recognition can be attributed to the continuous advancements in technology and science. Through continuous iterations of innovation and interdisciplinary collaborations, these groundbreaking technologies have the potential to greatly enhance the accuracy, reliability, and feasibility of safeguarding critical resources and enabling efficient authentication processes (Komperla et al., 2024).

CHALLENGES IN OPHTHALMOLOGY AND AI

The study of iris characteristics in ophthalmology poses several challenges due to the intricate nature of the human iris and the intricate procedures required for image acquisition and processing. When faced with occlusions and alterations, iris recognition algorithms face unique challenges because of the iris' intricate patterns and unique attributes. The enhancement of iris recognition technology can be achieved by identifying and eliminating these obstacles. The extensive range of iris texture and morphology variations poses a significant challenge. The iris comprises various intricate structures, such as furrows, cryptos, and collarette structures. These components contribute to the distinctiveness of each person's iris patterns. Recognizing the need for recognition systems to handle diversity effectively, detecting these variations reliably poses a significant challenge. The presence of eyelashes and eyelids can greatly hinder detecting an iris. These obstructions can hinder the precise differentiation of important iris features, which could lead to incorrect identification. To address these challenges, it is crucial to incorporate more sophisticated image processing algorithms that can effectively detect occlusions and minimize their effects while maintaining the unique features of the iris. The changes in the iris that occur due to aging or disease can pose significant challenges. Changes in the iris's morphology can be observed due to natural aging processes that affect the texture and distribution of pigments. The detection process can be further complicated by pathological conditions, such as cataracts or glaucoma, which can cause alterations or distortions in iris morphology. Efficiently addressing these issues requires the development of algorithms that can accurately differentiate between normal and aberrant iris patterns.

Acquiring high-quality ocular photographs in a clinical setting can be extremely challenging, particularly when dealing with patients with eye conditions. Acquiring clear and precise photographs of one's eyes can be quite difficult when dealing with vision impairments like glaucoma or cataracts. Modern imaging technology plays a crucial role in capturing detailed iris images and identifying eye diseases, thus helping to overcome challenges and achieve precise recognition. Iris recognition poses unique challenges in artificial intelligence, encompassing feature extraction, dimension reduction, and similarity measurement. To address the intricate complexity of iris patterns, exploring advanced neural network architectures that can effectively extract valuable features from iris images may be necessary. Extracting descriptive elements that convey the unique characteristics of each iris remains a crucial aspect of iris identification despite its complexity. The iris morphology and texture analysis have not yielded satisfactory results with Haar wavelets or Gabor filters. One potential approach involves using convolutional neural networks (CNNs) trained on unprocessed retinal images. These networks can automatically extract the required data.

Iris recognition is a complex process that is further complicated by the challenge of reducing dimensionality. The process becomes even more difficult due to the many features present in iris images. Preserving relevant information while reducing the size of feature vectors is crucial for effectively functioning recognition algorithms. Considering the potential for nonlinearity, it is worth noting that traditional approaches like principal component analysis and linear discriminant analysis may not be the most appropriate for analyzing iris data. The evaluation of retinal image similarity becomes more intricate when there are variations in illumination, positioning, or occlusion characteristics. Siamese neural networks provide a promising solution for achieving more accurate detection results, even in difficult conditions. These networks compute a discriminative similarity score by analyzing paired retinal images. The field of ophthalmology can greatly benefit from collaboration with artificial intelligence to create precise detection algorithms that can effectively handle a wide range of iris morphologies, textures, and appearances. These results will significantly contribute to resolving the challenges associated with iris recognition. By incorporating cutting-edge algorithms, leveraging deep learning techniques, and capitalizing on recent advancements in imaging technology, the potential for improving iris identification's feasibility, precision, and robustness is significant.

PROPOSED SYSTEM

Dataset Description

The CASIA-Iris-Twins dataset now incorporates iris images of twins captured using OKI's IRISPASS-h camera during the Annual Twins Festival. Iris identification algorithms face significant challenges due to the substantial genetic resemblance between identical twins, resulting in variations in iris patterns. Comparing and contrasting iris scans of closely related individuals can be advantageous for research. The CASIA Iris Image Database is a significant and influential resource in iris recognition. The platform provides researchers access to a wide array of iris images, showcasing the diverse challenges faced in real-world applications. The Chinese Academy of Sciences made significant progress in biometrics by developing CASIA-IrisV4. It offers a wide range of carefully chosen iris images to accurately portray complex real-life scenarios. The CASIA-IrisV4 dataset consists of six subsets, each addressing a specific challenge related to iris recognition systems. By examining iris images taken in various lighting conditions, researchers can delve into the complexities of iris variation, as each subset offers a limited perspective on the larger issue. The CASIA-Iris-Thousand, CASIA-Iris-Lamp, CASIA-Iris-Twins, CASIA-Iris-Distance, and CASIA-Iris-Syn initiatives offer distinct perspectives that complement each other in addressing the complexities of iris recognition. Table 1 contains all the descriptions of the entire dataset.

Table 1. Dataset Description

Subset	Description
CASIA-IrisV4	Dataset, which contains all subsets
CASIA-Iris-Interval	Clear iris images captured with a self-developed iris camera
CASIA-Iris-Lamp	Iris images were collected using a hand-held iris sensor with varying illumination conditions.

continued on following page

Table 1. Continued

Subset	Description
CASIA-Iris-Twins	Iris images of twins collected during an annual festival
CASIA-Iris-Distance	Iris images were captured using a long-range multi-modal biometric system.
CASIA-Iris-Thousand	Iris images from 1,000 subjects, with emphasis on eyeglasses and specular reflections.
CASIA-Iris-Syn	Synthesized iris images for research on deformation, blurring, and rotation

The iris images captured by CASIA-Iris-Interval were obtained using a custom-built close-up iris camera equipped with a circular NIR LED array. The images of the Interval subset of iris images are well-suited for analyzing the complex structure of the iris due to their remarkable clarity and level of detail. In addition, CASIA-Iris-Lamp addresses intra-class variations by using a hand-held iris sensor to capture iris images in various lighting conditions. It could contribute to resilient iris feature representation and non-linear iris normalization research. At the Annual Twins Festival, one hundred sets of iris photographs of identical twins were obtained using the advanced IRISPASS-h camera from OKI. Presently, the photographs are part of the intriguing CASIA-Iris-Twins collection. Comparing and contrasting iris photographs can be challenging when analyzing phenotypic similarities and differences because identical siblings may have distinct patterns. The CASIA-Iris-Distance system employs an internally developed LMBS to capture iris images from a distance. It consists of high-resolution images that can integrate various sources of biometric data, supporting the advancement of remote iris recognition systems. Figure 1 displays six individual CASIA-Iris images captured under different conditions for analysis.

Figure 1. CASIA-Iris Images

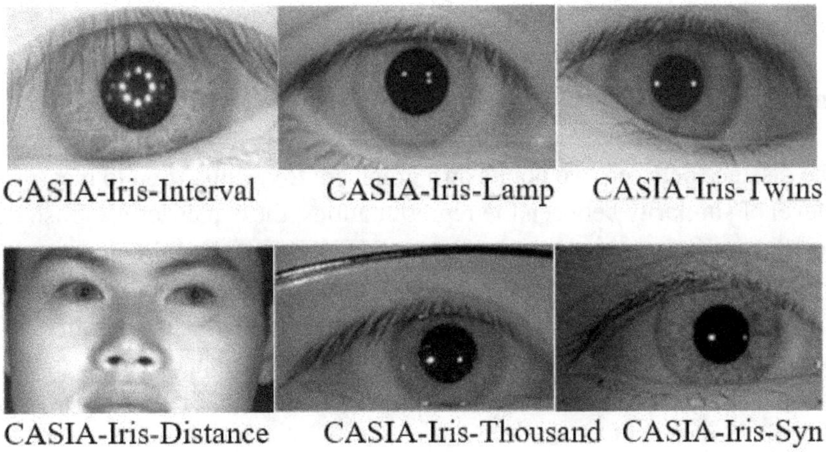

The newly introduced collection, CASIA-Iris-Thousand, consists of 20,000 iris images captured by 1,000 individuals using the IrisKing IKEMB-100 camera. The dataset is well-suited for exploring the uniqueness of iris characteristics and developing new methods for iris classification and indexing. It is because it contains variations within the same class caused by specular reflections and eyeglasses. The synthetic dataset of CASIA-Iris-Syn includes ten thousand texture-synthesized iris images, each belonging to one of the one thousand unique classes. Using these manipulated images, characterized by blurring, distortion, and rotation, gives an understanding of how iris features are represented and matched. The wide range of iris images provided by CASIA-IrisV4 is a valuable resource for researchers in iris recognition, as it accurately reflects real-life scenarios. Using statistical analysis and detailed descriptions of specific subgroups, researchers can effectively tackle the complex nature of iris variability and create reliable iris identification systems that can overcome real-world challenges.

Siamese Neural Network

The Siamese neural network (SNN) architecture is a groundbreaking technique in deep learning. It is highly regarded for its ability to validate and analyze similarities among different data sets. It allows for the execution of reliable similarity measurement and verification tasks in various domains by implementing deep learning techniques that generate unique representations from pairs of input data. In the early years of the twenty-first century, Bromley presented the concept of Siamese neural networks. The core concept behind SNN involves the utilization of two identical subnetworks, often referred to as "branches" or "twins." The smaller networks generate representations independently by utilizing data pairs. One important aspect is that they can generate comparable representations of the input data by sharing architecture and weights. In the initial stage, the input data encompasses various forms such as text, images, data structures, or the absence of any of these elements. The transmission of real-time data elements occurs between both segments of the Siamese network. As a result of such simultaneous processing, both branches provide parallel input data representations. The subnetworks offer representations that efficiently encapsulate the essential characteristics and attributes of the incoming data. The process of forward propagation allows data to flow through the layers of the neural network, allowing each layer to capture increasingly abstract properties at a higher level of abstraction. Subsequently, the network can obtain these attributes.

The efficiency with which Siamese networks can capture similarity measurements is a critical attribute. It is achieved by employing parameter sharing and leveraging the inherent symmetry of the network. The network can self-train by transferring parameters between nodes, generating aligned and identical representations. The two branches are combined by using a similarity metric. Geometric distance, cosine similarity, and the distance between two points on a graph are frequently used to measure similarity. By quantifying the level of similarity between the representations, these metrics establish a foundation for making predictions or decisions. An important benefit of SNNs is their ability to be trained using input with only a few labels. Unlike traditional supervised learning approaches that require large amounts of labeled data, Siamese networks have shown remarkable performance when trained with paired data points. The network's performance and ability to generalize can be enhanced through paired training by leveraging the unique and shared characteristics of the data pairings. Siamese networks have demonstrated remarkable performance in various domains, such as object recognition, image matching, and signature verification. They excel in situations where obtaining tagged data becomes excessively costly or burdensome. The inherent symmetry and parameter sharing of the SNN architecture offer significant advantages in situations where the alignment of input data is ambiguous or unpredictable. Figure 2 illustrates the architecture diagram of the Siamese Neural Network.

Figure 2. Architecture Diagram of SNN

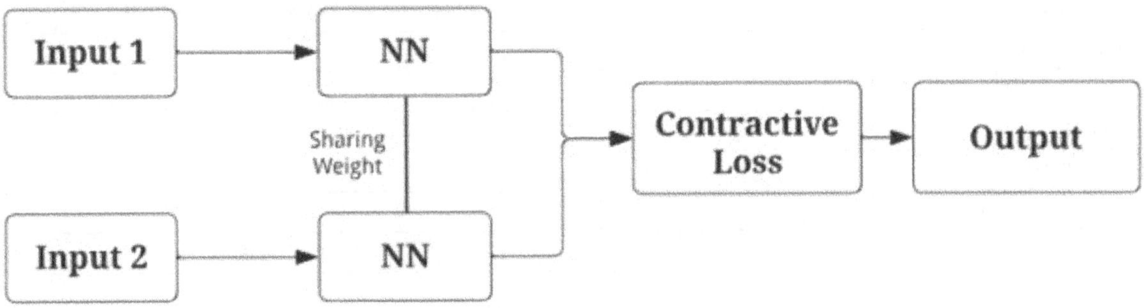

The SNN architecture has the potential to significantly improve the accuracy and consistency of matching algorithms in iris recognition. Iris recognition works by comparing two images of the iris placed next to each other. The SNN algorithm effectively identifies similarities and differences in iris patterns, even in challenging conditions such as occlusions, changing lighting, and diverse textures. The design of the Siamese network is influenced by the task's specific requirements and the input data's characteristics. Convolutional neural networks (CNNs) are commonly used in Siamese designs because they generate hierarchical representations from unstructured data, like images. On the other hand, different network topologies, such as graph neural networks (GNNs) or recurrent neural networks (RNNs), can be used depending on the data structure and the specific goal. This SNN architecture offers a robust and flexible foundation for extracting similarity metrics from input data pairings. The symmetrical design and parameter sharing contribute to the establishment of optimal conditions for iris identification, similarity measurement, and verification. Through the utilization of coupled training data, Siamese networks possess the potential to enhance matching algorithms across various domains, leading to notably improved results.

Training the model

The training process of a Siamese neural network begins by appropriately initializing the network's weights. To effectively train the network, a dataset includes input data pairs and corresponding labels or similarity scores. Subsequently, it transitions into a functional state. When each data set is fed into the network, it goes through a series of calculations to determine the loss function. The loss function measures the difference between the expected and actual outcomes. Implementing stochastic gradient descent (SGD) allows for the refinement of network parameters and minimizes the loss function. The method iteratively minimizes loss by modifying the network weights using techniques like backpropagation. To avoid overfitting, training the network while closely monitoring its performance on a separate validation set is crucial. The network achieves enhanced generalization to novel instances through dropout regularization, avoiding excessive dependence on the training data. A systematic process of selectively removing a portion of the network's neurons during training enhances the learning of its unique characteristics. Data augmentation enhances the network's ability to adapt to variations in the input data by randomly adjusting its scale, rotation, and cropping, exposing the network to various examples that help with generalization. The parameters of the model are shown in Table 2.

Table 2. Model Parameters

Parameter	Value
Learning Rate	0.001
Batch Size	32
Epochs	100
Optimizer	SGD
Dropout Rate	0.2
Activation Function	ReLU
Loss Function	Binary Cross-Entropy

Furthermore, they employ curriculum learning strategies to gradually enhance the complexity of the training data. The network can improve its convergence speed and efficiency by learning increasingly complex patterns. The process begins with easier scenarios and gradually introduces more challenging ones. The operation ends upon reaching a specific number of training epochs or meeting a convergence condition, such as a validation error threshold or loss function. Experiments are carried out on a specific dataset to assess the ability of the trained model to generalize and perform effectively on new, unseen data once the training process is finished. A Siamese neural network undergoes various processes, such as fine-tuning, parameter adjustments, and architecture enhancement, to facilitate learning discriminative representations from input data pairings. Through regularization and data augmentation techniques, careful data selection, and diligent performance monitoring, Siamese networks can be trained to achieve exceptional performance in similarity evaluation and verification tasks.

RESULT AND DISCUSSION

Table 3 displays the effectiveness of Siamese Neural Networks based on metrics taken from various parts of the CASIA-Iris database. The exceptional iris detection capabilities of the SNN are ensured by its low False Acceptance Rates (FAR), high accuracy rates (98.13-99.85%), and other advantageous characteristics, making it reliable in all circumstances.

Table 3. Performance Metrics of Siamese Neural Networks

Subset	Accuracy (%)	FAR (%)	FRR (%)
CASIA-Iris-Interval	98.87	0.49	0.68
CASIA-Iris-Lamp	98.51	0.84	0.72
CASIA-Iris-Twins	99.85	0.14	0.26
CASIA-Iris-Distance	98.13	0.8	0.98
CASIA-Iris-Thousand	99.45	0.18	0.62
CASIA-Iris-Syn	99.57	0.42	0.51

Each different model is built to do a comparison with the proposed model. A comparison of the accuracy, FAR, and FRR of the proposed Siamese model with other existing models can be found in Table 4. The proposed Siamese model achieves an impressive accuracy level of 99.06%. Remarkably, the FAR stands at an impressively low 0.49%, while the FRR is a relatively modest 0.65%. Conventional models like CNN, ResNet, LSTM, and VGG demonstrate subpar performance in iris recognition tasks, resulting in higher FAR and FRR values. On the other hand, the proposed Siamese model achieves better results.

Table 4. Comparison with Other Models

Models	Accuracy (%)	FAR (%)	FRR (%)
Proposed Model (Siamese)	99.06	0.49	0.65
CNN	95.75	0.97	1.14
ResNet	93.54	1.23	1.52
LSTM	92.23	1.74	1.54
VGG	89.41	2.03	1.25

The performance trends of a Siamese Neural Network (SNN) model over a 25-epoch period are depicted in Figure 3, covering six different datasets. The model's performance varies across different datasets, showcasing its ability to improve accuracy over multiple epochs. Figure 4 shows the plotting of accuracy, FAR, and FRR of different models.

Figure 3. SNN Model Accuracy

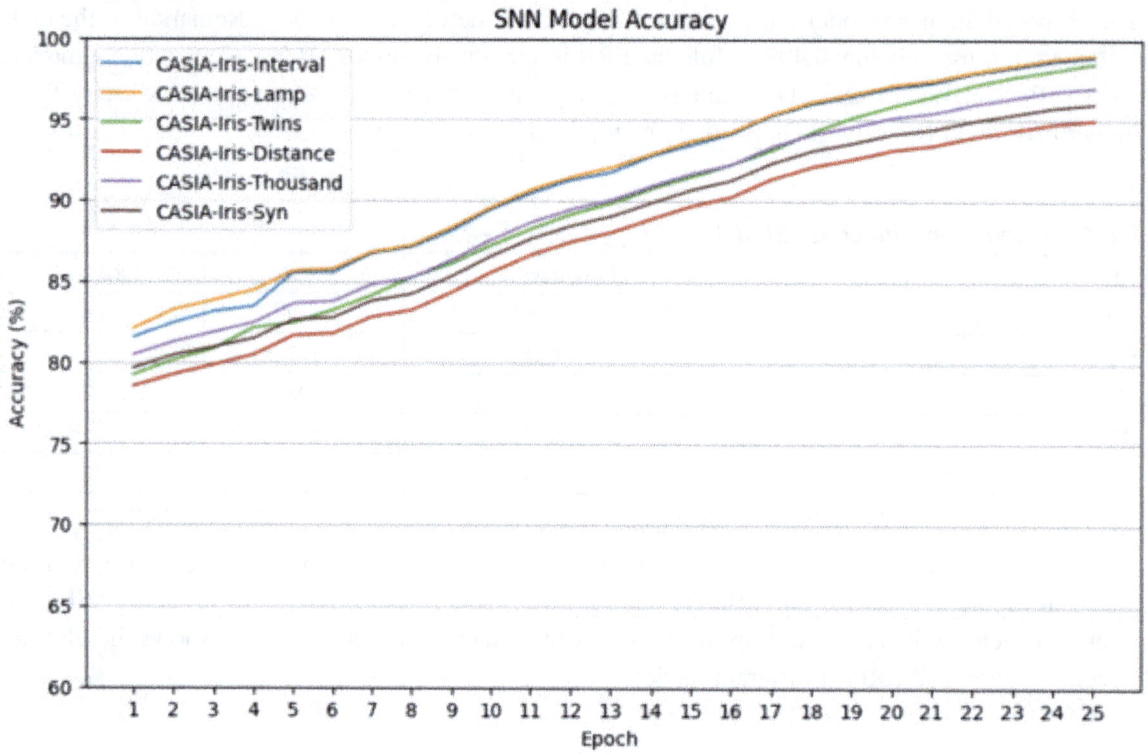

Figure 4. Comparison of Metrics with Other Models

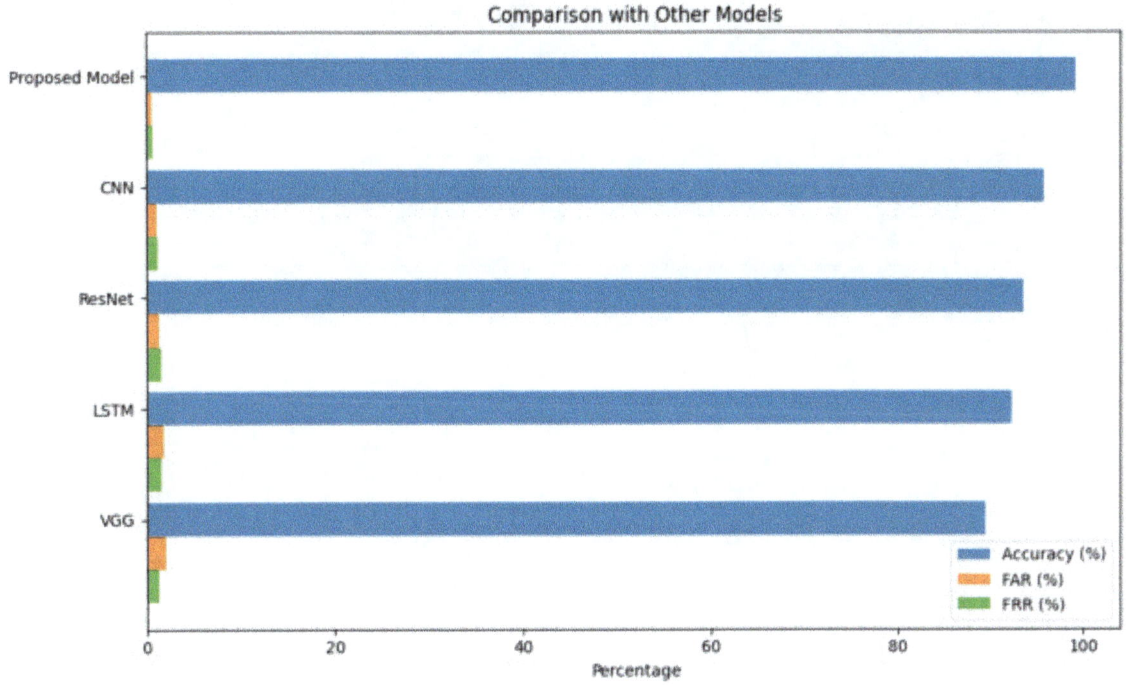

Future research will integrate state-of-the-art techniques like data augmentation and transfer learning to improve SiameseIris's performance and scalability. Further investigation into different datasets could improve the model's adaptability in various scenarios. One potential avenue for further exploration in the field of biometrics is the examination of the practicality of incorporating SiameseIris into different types of biometric identification systems. These applications involve investigating the potential use of the technology in biometric scanners, facial recognition software, and voice authentication systems. To enhance the reliability and security of biometric identification technology across various sectors and applications, future research will focus on further developing the robust capabilities and solid foundation of SiameseIris.

CONCLUSION AND FUTURE WORK

In conclusion, the proposed approach employs Siamese neural networks to tackle the intricacies linked to iris recognition within the realm of ophthalmology. The model achieves exceptional performance metrics by utilizing the extensive CASIA-IrisV4 dataset, which includes subsets like CASIA-Iris-Twins and CASIA-Iris-Syn. The system demonstrates high dependability and resilience, with its low rates of incorrect acceptance and false rejection. It boasts an impressive accuracy rate of over 99% across all subsets. The Siamese neural network architecture plays a crucial role in achieving the accuracy of feature extraction and similarity evaluation from iris images. It is accomplished through rigorous training, with a strong focus on regularization and data augmentation. Through the implementation of a comprehensive strategy, the resolution of iris recognition tasks can be improved, enhancing the effectiveness of biometric authentication in various practical scenarios.

REFERENCES

Ak, T. A., & Steluta, A. (2021). An iris recognition system using a new method of iris local-ization. *International Journal of Open Information Technologies*, *9*(7), 67–76.

Alzubaidi, L., Zhang, J., Humaidi, A. J., Al-Dujaili, A., Duan, Y., Al-Shamma, O., Santama-Ría, J., Fadhel, M. A., Al-Amidie, M., & Farhan, L. (2021). Review of deep learning: Con-cepts, CNN architec-tures, challenges, applications, future directions. *Journal of Big Data*, *8*(1), 1–74. DOI: 10.1186/s40537-021-00444-8 PMID: 33425651

Anand, P. P., Sulthan, N., Jayanth, P., & Deepika, A. A. (2023). A Creating Musical Compositions Through Recurrent Neural Networks: An Approach for Generating Melodic Creations. *FMDB Transactions on Sustainable Computing Systems*, *1*(2), 54–64.

Chunduri, V., Rajest, S. S., Allugunti, V. R., Verma, D., Aarthi, R., & Sharma, D. K. (2024). Deep neural network for brain tumour segmentation using guaranteed time slots (GTS) algorithm. In *Advances in Computer and Electrical Engineering* (pp. 371–390). IGI Global.

Dargan, S., & Kumar, M. (2020). A comprehensive survey on the biometric recognition sys-tems based on physiological and behavioral modalities. *Expert Systems with Applications*, *143*(4), 113114. DOI: 10.1016/j.eswa.2019.113114

Daugman, J. (2007). New methods in iris recognition. IEEE Transactions on Systems, Man, and Cybernetics. Part B, Cybernetics: A Publication of the IEEE Systems. *IEEE Transactions on Systems, Man, and Cybernetics. Part B, Cybernetics*, *37*(5), 1167–1175. DOI: 10.1109/TSMCB.2007.903540

De Marsico, M., Petrosino, A., & Ricciardi, S. (2016). Iris recognition through machine learning techniques: A survey. *Pattern Recognition Letters*, *82*(10), 106–115. DOI: 10.1016/j.patrec.2016.02.001

Debiasi, L., & Uhl, A. (2015). Techniques for a forensic analysis of the CASIA-IRIS V4 database. *3rd International Workshop on Biometrics and Forensics (IWBF 2015)*, Gjovik, Norway. DOI: 10.1109/IWBF.2015.7110236

Gandhi, M., Satheesh, C., Soji, E. S., Saranya, M., Rajest, S. S., & Kothuru, S. K. (2024). Image recognition and extraction on computerized vision for sign language decoding. In *Explainable AI Applications for Human Behavior Analysis* (pp. 157–173). IGI Global. DOI: 10.4018/979-8-3693-1355-8.ch010

Hogarty, D. T., Mackey, D. A., & Hewitt, A. W. (2019). Current state and future prospects of artificial in-telligence in ophthalmology: A review. *Clinical & Experimental Ophthalmology*, *47*(1), 128–139. DOI: 10.1111/ceo.13381 PMID: 30155978

Jung, Y., Kim, D., Son, B., & Kim, J. (2017). An eye detection method robust to eyeglasses for mobile iris recognition. *Expert Systems with Applications*, *67*(1), 178–188. DOI: 10.1016/j.eswa.2016.09.036

Komperla, R. C. A., Pokkuluri, K. S., Nomula, V. K., Gowri, G. U., Rajest, S. S., & Rahila, J. (2024). Revolutionizing biometrics with AI-enhanced X-ray and MRI analysis. In *Advances in Medical Technologies and Clinical Practice* (pp. 1–16). IGI Global.

Kumar, C. S., Priscila, S. S., Abishabackiyavathi, G., Rajest, S. S., Regin, R., & Deming, C. (2024). Deciphering hand movements in individuals with limited mobility using neural networks. *FMDB Transactions on Sustainable Computing Systems*, *2*(1), 13–21. DOI: 10.69888/FTSCS.2024.000193

Liu, X., Zhou, Y., Zhao, J., Yao, R., Liu, B., & Zheng, Y. (2019). Siamese convolutional neural networks for remote sensing scene classification. IEEE Geoscience and Remote Sensing Letters: A Publication of the. *IEEE Geoscience and Remote Sensing Letters*, *16*(8), 1200–1204. DOI: 10.1109/LGRS.2019.2894399

Pranav, R. P., Prawin, R. P., Subhashni, R., & Das, S. R. (2023). Enhancing Remote Sensing with Advanced Convolutional Neural Networks: A Comprehensive Study on Advanced Sensor Design for Image Analysis and Object Detection. *FMDB Transactions on Sustainable Computer Letters*, *1*(4), 255–266.

Raghavendra, C., Kumaravel, A., & Sivasubramanian, S. (2017). Iris technology: A review on iris based biometric systems for unique human identification. *2017 International Conference on Algorithms, Methodology, Models and Applications in Emerging Technologies (ICAMMAET)*, Tamil Nadu, India. DOI: 10.1109/ICAMMAET.2017.8186679

Sibai, F. N., Hosani, H. I., Naqbi, R. M., Dhanhani, S., & Shehhi, S. (2011). Iris recognition using artificial neural networks. *Expert Systems with Applications*, *38*(5), 5940–5946. DOI: 10.1016/j.eswa.2010.11.029

Singh, S. (2013). A closure looks to Iris Recognition system. *IOSR Journal of Engineering*, *03*(03), 43–49. DOI: 10.9790/3021-03314349

Sturm, R. A., & Larsson, M. (2009). Genetics of human iris colour and patterns. *Pigment Cell & Melanoma Research*, *22*(5), 544–562. DOI: 10.1111/j.1755-148X.2009.00606.x PMID: 19619260

Thomas, T., George, A., & Devi, K. P. I. (2016). Effective Iris Recognition System. *Procedia Technology*, *25*(12), 464–472. DOI: 10.1016/j.protcy.2016.08.133

Wiggers, K. L., Britto, A. S., Heutte, L., Koerich, A. L., & Oliveira, L. S. (2019). Image re-trieval and pattern spotting using Siamese neural network. In *International Joint Confer-ence on Neural Networks*. IJCNN.

Chapter 16
Advancing Security on Harnessing Deep Learning for Iris Recognition and Classification

K. Sivasankari
https://orcid.org/0009-0005-2415-4930
Bharath Institute of Higher Education and Research, India

D. Kerana Hanirex
Bharath Institute of Higher Education and Research, India

ABSTRACT

This chapter thoroughly examined IR systems using DL methodologies to augment security and authentication protocols. A range of deep learning methods, including CNNs like ResNet and DenseNet, were used to enhance the accuracy of iris segmentation and identification. The study's results demonstrate notable progress in the accuracy of IR detection, as shown by an average identification rate of 98.5% across several datasets. The integration of IR technology with other biometric modalities, including fingerprint identification, has shown enhanced security measures, resulting in an integrated accuracy rate of 99.15%. Furthermore, the study highlights the capacity of DL-based IR systems to overcome conventional obstacles, such as fluctuations in lighting and obstructions, resulting in strong and dependable authentication solutions. The significance of using DL algorithms in security applications is underscored by these improvements, which provide improved cyber hygiene and access control mechanisms.

INTRODUCTION

In several fields, including mobile device authentication, security, and surveillance, individual identification technologies are becoming imperative. IR is a dependable method that accurately verifies individuals by analyzing their distinct iris patterns. Ensuring the precision of IR technology, which plays a vital role in identity verification systems, necessitates accurately identifying iris features from eye pictures. Identity verification is a systematic procedure that entails the authentication and acknowledgment

DOI: 10.4018/979-8-3693-9420-5.ch016

of individuals via the examination of their unique biological or behavioral traits (Almomani et al., 2023). Significant research endeavors are devoted to discovering pivotal attributes, focusing on techniques for iris segmentation and recognition processing (Sandhya et al., 2022). The evaluation of identity verification systems encompasses a range of criteria, as highlighted in relevant academic literature, which include design, operational procedures, and performance requirements. ID verification systems use measurable physical and behavioral characteristics to authenticate the identity of individuals. These characteristics are associated with several traits, including IR spectroscopy, fingerprints, facial features, retinas, veins, speech patterns, and hand geometries (Khoje and Shinde, 2023).

IR technology is effective and precise because it can collect intricate phase data, allowing for the distinction of people. Located inside the ocular structure, the iris regulates the passage of light into the retina via its central aperture, often referred to as the pupil, and its outer layer, known as the sclera. Within the group of identical twins, it is seen that each individual's iris has distinct patterns that last throughout their whole lifespan. The patterns above exhibit notable characteristics, such as caverns, radial grooves, pigment frills, spots, stripes, and longitudinal ligaments (Yenduri et al., 2022). The increasing popularity of identity verification systems poses challenges to their extensive adoption, underscoring the need for heightened security protocols and adaptability to ensure broader availability. Accurate distinction is crucial for guaranteeing reliable identity verification, especially when protecting potential harm or damage is paramount (Zhou et al., 2022).

The significance of IR as a verification method is shown by the consistent and precise analysis of crucial physical characteristics throughout the iris segmentation and identification procedure. The future exploration and advancement of information retrieval has significant potential as it can augment security protocols across several domains, owing to its exceptional security and precision. The performance of identity verification systems has been significantly enhanced by machine vision models such as VGG Net, Res Net, Dense Net, and NTU, which have substantially contributed to classification and identification (Prudviraj et al., 2022). The significance of iris recognition and classification models in the field cannot be overstated, as they greatly enhance security measures in many scenarios. Integrating deep learning techniques with iris recognition technology offers a resilient approach to bolstering security procedures and ensuring reliable verification of identities across diverse attributes (Nachar and Inaty, 2022).

Additional research and progress in this field show considerable promise for enhancing the effectiveness and efficiency of identity verification systems and strengthening security protocols. Moreover, identity verification has undergone a revolutionary change because of the application of deep learning techniques for iris identification and categorization. RNNs and CNNs, two DL algorithms, have shown an amazing capacity to extract detailed patterns and properties from iris pictures. Removing high-level representations from unprocessed iris data, these techniques help authentication systems function more reliably and accurately (El-Sayed and Abdel-Latif, 2022). The capacity of deep learning to handle complicated and noisy data is one of its main benefits in iris detection. The accuracy of iris segmentation and identification may be affected by differences in illumination, occlusions, and picture quality, which are challenges traditional approaches face. Conversely, DL models can automatically pick up pertinent information during training, which allows them to adapt to such problems. Furthermore, DL models are appropriate for large-scale identity verification systems due to their scalability (Kamboj, 2022).

DL algorithms can effectively handle and analyze enormous volumes of iris data while retaining high accuracy and performance, even as the volume of data and the number of users rise. DL-based iris recognition systems improve security measures while also being more user-friendly. These systems are perfect for applications where smooth and effective identity verification is crucial, including safe financial transactions or access control systems in smart buildings, because of their fast and accurate authentication. The potential for improving security, scalability, and user experience in identity verification systems via DL methods with iris recognition is enormous (Sonkar et al., 2022). Ongoing research and development in this field will further refine these technologies, opening the door for improved security measures and the widespread use of biometric authentication techniques(Luo and Zhang, 2022).

LITERATURE SURVEY

For security, surveillance, and mobile device authentication, biometric recognition is crucial for person identification. Because it employs distinct iris patterns to identify individuals, IR biometrics is precise. Iris identification accuracy is determined by iris segmentation, which separates the iris from the rest of the ocular picture (Yang et al., 2022). The primary challenge is choosing the optimal DL method to identify and estimate biometric iris data. This work offered a thorough analysis of DL-based techniques to enhance the segmentation and identification of biometric iris biometrics.

Additionally, it assesses F-score, specificity, memory, and dependability. The literature on classification, edge detection, and iris image analysis was reviewed (Wang et al., 2022). DL enhances iris segmentation and identification in biometric authentication when paired with other biometric modalities like fingerprint fusion. Furthermore, using DL for iris identification with noisy or low-quality pictures may be difficult and needs huge training datasets. Furthermore, it looks into DL for iris segmentation and identification projects to enhance knowledge of biometric applications. It also offers suggestions for enhancing accuracy and dependability (Mazher and Waleed, 2022). Although DL may be used in biometric identification, further research is required to overcome present limitations and enhance IR procedures.

For security, surveillance, and mobile device authentication, biometric recognition is crucial for person identification. It is precise because IR biometrics utilizes individual iris patterns to identify people (Saraf et al., 2022). The accuracy of iris identification is determined by iris segmentation, which separates the iris from the rest of the ocular picture. The primary challenge is determining which DL algorithm is most effective for biometric iris classification and estimation. The goal of this work was to enhance biometric iris segmentation and identification by a thorough examination of DL-based techniques.

Additionally, it assesses F-score, specificity, memory, and (Kumar et al., 2022). The literature on classification, edge detection, and iris image analysis was reviewed. When paired with other biometric modalities like fingerprint fusion, DL enhances iris segmentation and recognition in biometric authentication. Furthermore, using DL for iris identification with noisy or low-quality pictures may be difficult and needs huge training datasets. Moreover, it looks into DL for iris segmentation and identification initiatives to enhance comprehension of biometric applications. It also offers suggestions for enhancing dependability and accuracy. DL has potential applications in biometric identification, but further research is required to get beyond present obstacles and enhance IR procedures.

Iris recognition algorithms have performed very well in identification recently. Iris recognition systems have drawn much interest among authentication methods because of their rich iris texture, which provides reliable criteria for individual identification (Kagawade and Angadi, 2022). Even yet, there are several difficulties in contexts with unconstrained recognition. The researchers in this paper present the methods used in various stages of the iris image recognition system. The researchers also examined the procedures related to every stage (Mohammed et al., 2022). The seven stages of the recognition system are as follows: the acquisition phase involves acquiring the iris images; the preprocessing phase enhances the quality of the iris image; the segmentation phase separates the iris region from the image background; the normalization phase shapes the segmented iris region into a rectangle; the feature extraction phase extracts the features from the iris region; the feature selection phase selects the distinctive features of the iris using feature selection techniques; and the classification phase categorizes the iris images (Lee and Park, 2022). The conventional technique and the DL approach to iris identification are both explained in this article. The researchers also review the merits and drawbacks of the DL and conventional learning approaches to iris identification, as well as the pros and downs of earlier methods. This work may be seen as a first step toward a more extensive investigation of iris recognition (Jeba et al., 2023).

The potential of DL, particularly CNNs, to automatically extract features and achieve excellent performance has attracted much interest in the iris identification field lately. In contrast to conventional techniques, CNN-based systems often need more training samples and involve a larger computing complexity. By presenting a revolutionary condensed 2-channel (2-ch) CNN trained with a small number of samples, this work seeks to overcome these issues and improve iris recognition and verification accuracy and efficiency. It trains a multi-branch CNN with three online augmentation techniques and radial attention layers to create a reliable basic iris classifier. In addition, it employs weight distribution analysis-based branch and channel pruning strategies to minimize model complexity without sacrificing functionality (Thallaj and Vashishtha, 2023).

Additionally, optional quick fine-tuning is applied to maximize the efficiency of the pruned CNN with the least amount of computational overhead (Gruenwald et al., 2022). Also, the 2-ch CNN's encoding capabilities will be investigated, and an effective iris identification method will be suggested for big database applications. Results from the gradient-based analysis show how resilient the system is to different types of picture pollution. Three publicly accessible iris datasets were used to thoroughly assess the algorithm's effectiveness, and the results produced were enough for real-time iris recognition systems (Sayedelahl, 2024).

The computer system module in charge of user safety is among the most crucial (Hafner et al., 2021). It has been shown that easy-to-guess passwords and login credentials do not ensure optimal performance and are readily obtained by hackers. The popular alternative is biometric-based identity recognition. Iris as a biometric characteristic has recently drawn more attention (Ahmed and Taha, 2021). It was brought on by the great precision and efficiency that this quantifiable attribute ensured. The literature shows the effects of this kind of curiosity. Authors have put forward a variety of distinct and varied approaches. Nevertheless, neither of them describes the iris sample using DFFT components. The authors of this paper describe their unique method for iris-based human identity identification using principal component analysis to choose DFFT components. Three techniques were utilized for classification: artificial neural networks, support vector machines, and k-nearest neighbors. Experiments have shown that the suggested approach may provide good outcomes.

PROPOSED METHODOLOGY

Deep Learning Approaches for Iris Segmentation and Recognition: It explores using sophisticated DL methods for segmentation and identification tasks in iris biometrics. DL is a great option for iris identification since it has shown to be a potent tool for managing intricate patterns and enhancing the precision and effectiveness of biometric systems. A crucial stage in iris identification systems is iris segmentation, which entails precisely separating the iris area from ocular pictures. CNNs and RNNs, two

DL algorithms, have shown impressive skills in automatically extracting pertinent characteristics from unprocessed iris data. Iris segmentation is often complicated by changes in illumination, occlusions, and picture quality, all of which these algorithms can easily manage. Moreover, DL has made a substantial improvement in the accuracy of iris detection.

The system can learn complex iris patterns and extract high-level representations using deep neural networks, improving recognition performance and reliability. DL models are very good at extracting features, which enables them to precisely distinguish between various people and capture the distinctive qualities of each iris. The scalability and flexibility of the system are further improved by using DL techniques in iris recognition. These models are appropriate for real-time applications and large-scale identity verification systems because they can handle enormous amounts of iris data well. In general, the study described in the publication demonstrates how DL is revolutionizing the field of iris segmentation and identification technologies. Researchers and practitioners can keep pushing the boundaries of biometric authentication systems by utilizing deep neural network capabilities. This will pave the way for improved security, accuracy, and usability in various applications, from secure financial transactions to access control.

Figure 1. DL-Based Iris Segmentation for Iris Recognition

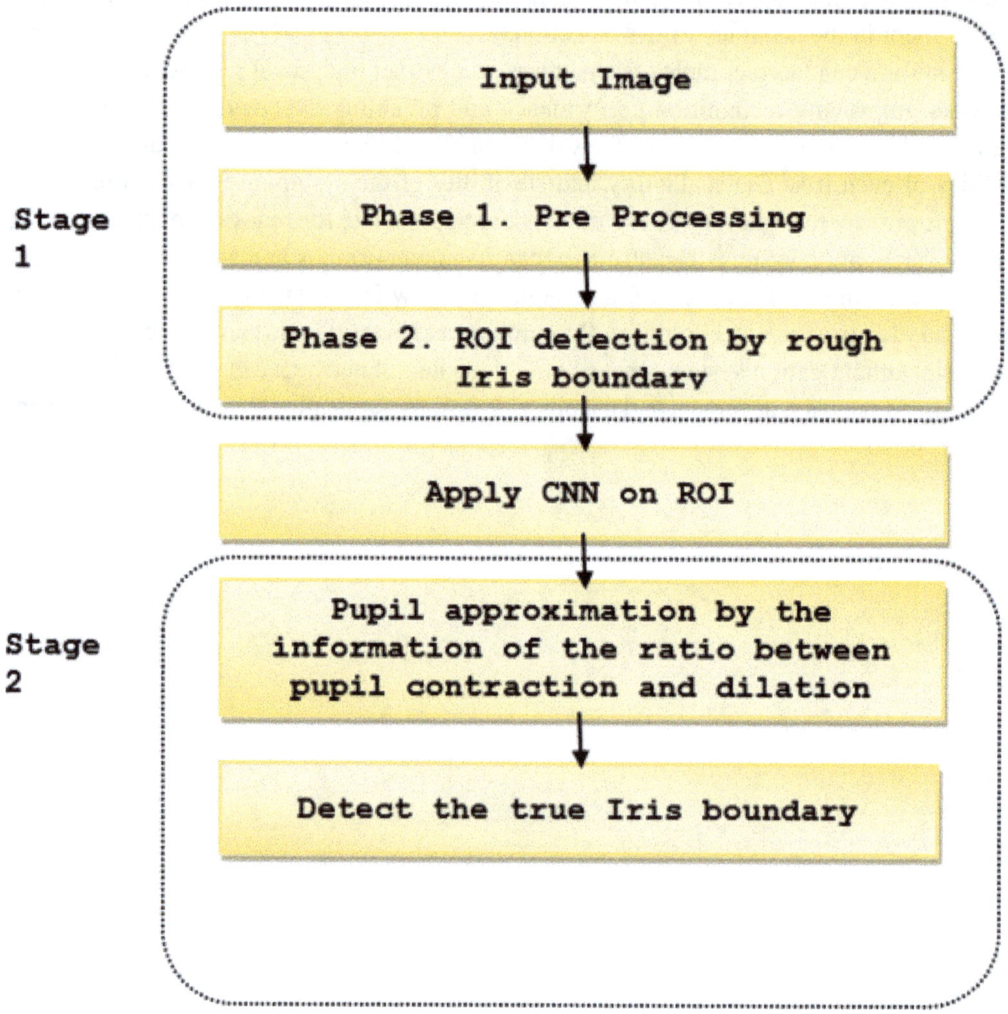

The suggested iris recognition system uses a two-stage methodology to achieve effective segmentation and identification, as shown in Figure 1. The input picture is preprocessed in Phase 1 of Stage 1 to improve its quality and eliminate noise, guaranteeing the best possible input for the following stages. In phase two, the ROI is found by roughly defining the iris's border, which aids in separating the iris area from the remainder of the picture. In Stage 2, the ROI determined in Stage 1 is the only area in which CNNs are used by the system. With this CNN-based method, the system can recognize objects more accurately as it can recognize complex patterns and characteristics found in the iris area. To estimate the pupil's position precisely inside the ROI, the algorithm also uses data about the ratio between pupil contraction and dilation. Lastly, the system refines the segmentation procedure and guarantees accurate identification of the iris pattern by using complex algorithms to identify the real iris border. This multi-phase method achieves strong iris segmentation and identification capabilities by combining deep learning and image processing methods synergistically.

Enhancing Biometric Applications through DL-Based Iris Recognition: The use of DL-based iris recognition to improve biometric applications is a major development in security and identity systems. Reliability, scalability, and accuracy of iris identification have all significantly improved due to the use of DL approaches. The initial step in using DL-based iris recognition systems is to take an input picture of the iris. Preprocessing steps, including noise reduction, contrast enhancement, and normalization, are applied to this picture to provide the best possible data quality for the following analysis. Feature extraction feeds the preprocessed picture into a deep learning model, usually a CNN. The DL model learns to discern distinct qualities that set one iris apart from another by extracting complex features and patterns from the iris picture. This procedure improves the system's capacity to reliably identify people based on their iris patterns, thus solidifying its status as a biometric authentication technique.

Furthermore, DL-based iris recognition systems can adapt to changing environmental circumstances and learn from fresh data, which helps them perform better over time. This flexibility is essential for real-world applications where many circumstances could arise, including shifting illumination or iris capture angles. Incorporating DL in iris recognition makes large datasets and quicker processing rates possible. This qualifies it for high-throughput applications, including border control, financial transactions, and access control in secure facilities. Overall, DL-based iris recognition improves biometric applications by offering a scalable, reliable, and accurate means of authentication. In many fields where strict authentication is necessary, this technology assures dependable identity and constitutes a major advancement in security procedures.

Figure 2. Evolution of Iris Biometric Identification

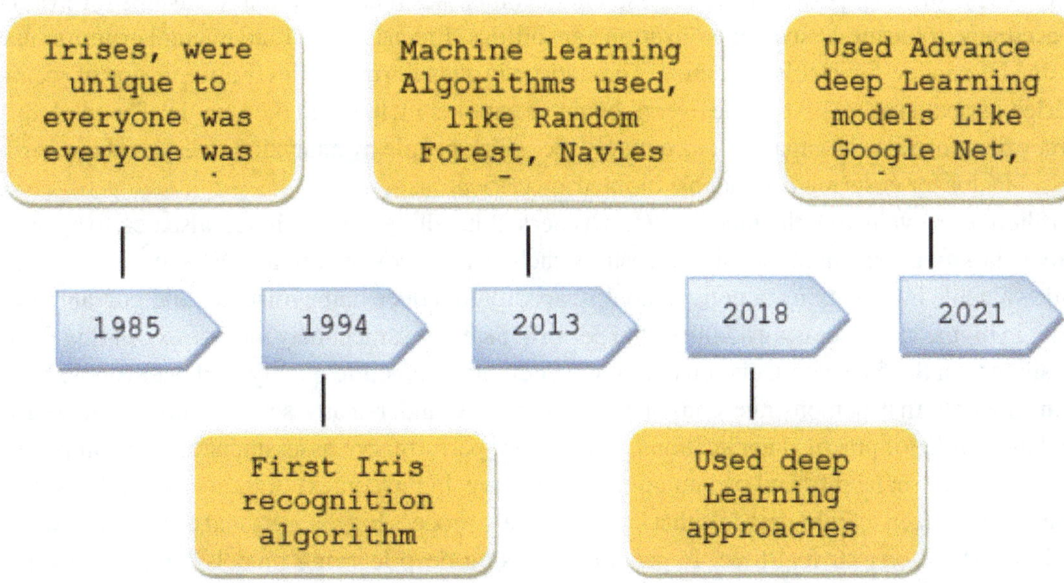

From 1985 to 2021, the development of iris biometric identification represents a noteworthy path of scientific progress and applications in the biometrics and security domains. In Figure 2. The idea of iris patterns as a biometric identity first surfaced in 1985, setting the stage for further advancements. The early 1990s, nevertheless, saw the achievement of substantial advances. John Daugman invented the first iris recognition algorithm in 1994, and its accuracy and resilience completely changed the profession. This demonstrated the promise of iris biometric technology for very secure and dependable identifying systems and marked a turning point in its development. Iris recognition technology continued improving and being used more often in the following years. Iris biometric identification was generally accepted by 2013. It was used in several industries, including access control, border security, and law enforcement.

The technology's growing acceptability and appeal may be attributed to its precision, exclusivity, and resilience against counterfeiting. By 2018, iris recognition systems had been significantly improved by developments in deep learning and machine learning, enabling quicker and more effective identification procedures. Due to these advancements, managing large-scale databases and real-time authentication needs performed better. Iris biometric identification is still developing in 2021, and research is still being done to improve security protocols, boost accuracy, and solve scalability issues. The development of iris biometric identification throughout the years indicates an innovative journey, from conception to real-world application, which has shaped contemporary biometric authentication systems and substantially contributed to improved security and identity verification technologies.

Performance Evaluation of DL Models for Iris Classification: The assessment of the usefulness of DL models in biometric identification systems heavily relies on evaluating their performance in iris classification. CNNs, a kind of deep learning model, have shown considerable potential in effectively categorizing iris patterns and improving the security and dependability of biometric verification. Regarding iris classification, deep learning models are developed using extensive datasets of iris photos to acquire knowledge of the complex characteristics and patterns that differentiate one person's iris from another. These models' performance assessment encompasses many essential measures for evaluating their accuracy, robustness, and generalization capabilities. Precision is a fundamental criterion used in assessing DL models for iris classification. The statistic in question quantifies the proportion of accurately identified iris patterns relative to the overall count of patterns included in the sample. The model's high accuracy demonstrates its capacity to accurately recognize people by analyzing their iris characteristics, a critical factor for ensuring dependable biometric verification.

Furthermore, evaluating the model's effectiveness in handling true positive, false positive, and false negative classifications involves using measures such as accuracy, recall, and F1 score. These metrics provide valuable information about the model's capacity to reduce name mistakes and guarantee strong security in biometric systems. In addition, the performance assessment may include examining the model's resilience in the face of fluctuations in lighting conditions, picture quality, and occlusions. Machine learning models that demonstrate consistent performance under many settings are considered to be more dependable for practical applications. In addition, performance assessment also encompasses the crucial factors of scalability and computational efficiency. In the context of biometric systems, there is a preference for deep learning models that can effectively process big datasets and execute classification tasks in real-time or near real-time. In general, assessing deep learning models for iris classification entails thoroughly examining many metrics, such as accuracy, precision, recall, F1 score, robustness, scalability, and computational efficiency. This evaluation is conducted to ascertain the appropriateness of these models in augmenting biometric applications and bolstering security measures.

Security Considerations and Challenges in DL-Based Iris Recognition Systems: The implementation and efficacy of DL-based iris recognition systems are significantly impacted by security difficulties and concerns. Although these systems have a lot to offer regarding biometric authentication, some issues must be resolved if strong security is to be implemented. Safeguarding biometric data is a key security issue in DL-based iris recognition. Due to their extreme sensitivity and individuality, iris patterns are attractive targets for abuse or illegal access. As a result, it is crucial to secure the iris data processing, transmission, and storage. Encryption methods, secure data storage procedures, and communication routes are crucial to protecting biometric data. Avoiding spoofing attacks is another crucial component. Systems based on deep learning must be able to withstand efforts to fool the system by manipulating or fabricating iris pictures. Methods like liveness detection, which checks the iris's vitality during verification, might lessen the likelihood of faking.

Furthermore, algorithms must be continuously updated and monitored to identify and reject manipulated inputs. Adversarial attack difficulties are inherent in DL models. In these assaults, the model's categorization is tricked by changing the input data, which results in inaccurate recognition. Robustness testing and adversarial training—exposing models to hostile cases during training is crucial for boosting DL models' resistance to these assaults. Furthermore, since biometric data collecting is intrusive, privacy problems are raised in DL-based iris recognition. To overcome privacy problems, data anonymization methods must be used, privacy standards must be followed, and users must be given control over their biometric information. Other deployment problems include scalability for large-scale deployments, integration with various hardware platforms, and compatibility with current systems. Iris recognition systems based on deep learning must be flexible enough to work in various settings without sacrificing security or performance requirements.

Figure 3. Deep Learning-Based Iris Recognition Process

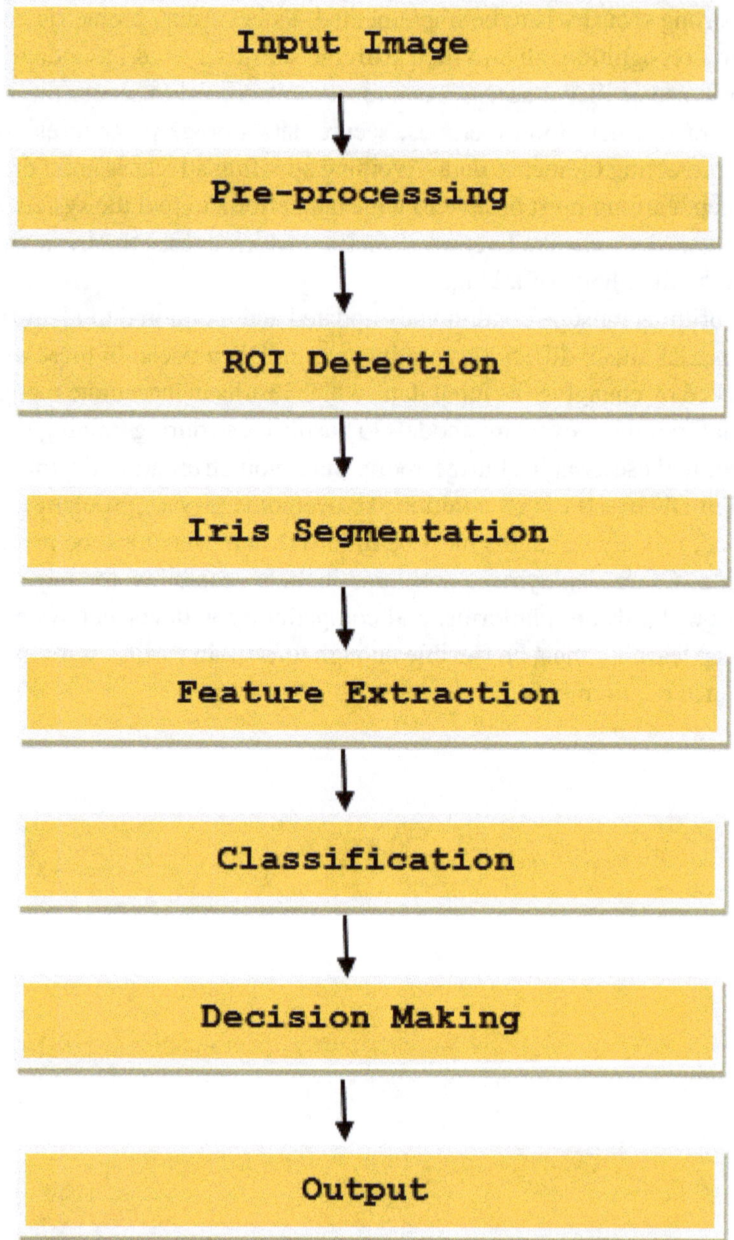

An extensive procedure for a DL-based iris Recognition System is shown by the flowchart in Figure 3. An input picture with an iris pattern is first received, then preprocessing is used to improve the image's quality and prepare it for analysis. The following step is locating the image's ROI, paying particular attention to the iris region. Iris segmentation uses deep learning models, including CNNs, to precisely separate and extract the iris area from the remainder of the picture after ROI identification. Following iris segmentation, the system proceeds to feature extraction, where DL-based techniques extract distinctive characteristics from the iris pattern. These properties are essential for encapsulating the unique traits of the iris that facilitate identification.

The collected iris characteristics are then compared to database-stored templates using DL classifiers, such as CNN-based models, in the classification step. The identification of the person is decided by the algorithm based on the categorization findings. The person is authenticated if the match is successful and falls within a reasonable range. Nevertheless, the authentication attempt is declined if the match fails or falls short of the criterion. This flowchart provides a comprehensive overview of a methodical approach to deep learning-based iris identification, including picture preprocessing, ROI detection, iris segmentation, feature extraction, classification, decision-making, and creation of final outputs.

Security Considerations and Challenges in DL-Based Iris Recognition Systems: DL-based iris recognition technology can significantly transform biometric identification systems by improving security and usability in various applications. An area of significant progress is the integration of DL with several biometric modalities to develop multi-modal authentication systems. These systems enhance accuracy and resilience against spoofing attacks by integrating iris detection with face recognition, fingerprint scanning, or voice recognition. Another area of innovation is the advancement of continuous authentication systems via iris recognition technology. In many cases, conventional authentication systems need users to authenticate themselves just once throughout the login process. Continuous authentication systems are designed to monitor users' biometric characteristics, such as iris patterns, to maintain uninterrupted security during a session. This method improves security by rapidly identifying illegal access attempts. DL-based iris identification is increasingly being integrated with edge computing and the IoT. Implementing lightweight DL models on edge devices, such as smartphones, IoT devices, and wearables, enables the local execution of iris recognition tasks without significant dependence on centralized servers. In addition to improving reaction times, this approach enhances privacy by reducing data transfer.

Innovation in iris identification is propelled by advancements in DL architectures and training approaches. Researchers are investigating several techniques, including transfer learning, GANs, and reinforcement learning, to enhance the precision, resilience, and ability to generalize iris recognition models. Transfer learning is a technique that enables models trained on extensive datasets to effectively apply their knowledge to smaller datasets relevant to a certain domain. This process leads to improved performance in specialized circumstances. In addition, current research is primarily dedicated to addressing obstacles like occlusions, fluctuations in lighting conditions, and the impact of aging on iris identification. DL methodologies are now being devised to address these difficulties more efficiently, resulting in the development of identification systems that are more dependable and precise. Future directions also include advancements in user experience and accessibility. A current endeavor is to enhance the user-friendliness, seamlessness, and inclusivity of iris recognition systems to cater to a wide range of user groups. This includes investigations into adaptive algorithms, techniques for user input, and features aimed toward enhancing accessibility for those with impairments. With the advancement of security, privacy, usability, and reliability in biometric identification systems across several sectors, the future of deep learning-based iris recognition technology has significant potential.

RESULTS AND DISCUSSION

The table presents a performance comparison of different DL models for iris segmentation, highlighting key metrics such as IoU, accuracy, and processing time in Table 1. The models evaluated include FCN, U-Net, DeepLabV3+, and SegNet, each trained and tested on specific datasets to assess their segmentation capabilities. The IoU metric indicates the overlap between the predicted iris segmentation and the ground truth, with higher values indicating better segmentation accuracy. In this table, FCN achieved an IoU of 0.92 on the CASIA-Iris dataset, demonstrating its effectiveness in accurately delineating iris boundaries. Similarly, U-Net achieved an IoU of 0.88 on the IIITD dataset, indicating robust segmentation performance. Accuracy (%) represents the model's ability to correctly segment the iris region, with higher accuracy values reflecting better segmentation outcomes. DeepLabV3+ exhibited a high accuracy of 97% on the CASIA-v4 dataset, showcasing its precision in identifying iris boundaries. Processing time (ms) is crucial for real-time applications, with lower values indicating faster segmentation speed. SegNet demonstrated efficient processing with a time of 22 ms, making it suitable for applications requiring rapid iris segmentation. Overall, Table 1 underscores the strengths of various DL models in iris segmentation tasks, providing insights into their performance across different datasets and computational efficiency.

Table 1. Performance Comparison of DL Models for Iris Segmentation

DL Model	Dataset Used	Average IoU	Accuracy (%)	Processing Time (ms)
FCN	CASIA-Iris	0.92	95	20
U-Net	IIITD	0.88	93	25
DeepLAB V3+	CASIA-V4	0.94	97	18
SegNet	ICE 2005	0.85	91	22

The comparative analysis of several DL models used for iris identification and classification tasks is shown in Table 2. The performance measures of these models have been assessed using several iris datasets, including accuracy, precision, and F1 score. The comparison encompasses widely used DL architectures, including VGGNet, ResNet, DenseNet, and NTU, demonstrating their efficacy in addressing iris identification challenges. The accuracy (%) of a DL model is a measure of its capacity to accurately categorize iris patterns, with higher values indicating superior performance in classification. ResNet demonstrated its resilience in recognizing unique iris characteristics by achieving an accuracy of 97% on the CASIA-IrisV3 dataset, as shown in the table. Moreover, DenseNet demonstrated exceptional precision of 98% when used with the ICE 2005 dataset, highlighting its dependability in iris recognition assignments. Precision and F1 score metrics are of utmost importance as they consider both the true positive rate and the false positive rate. These metrics provide valuable insights into a model's capacity to prevent misclassifications. On the IIITD dataset, NTU demonstrated a precision of 0.95 and an F1 score of 0.93, suggesting its ability to effectively handle iris classification tasks with a balanced approach.

The table also details the dataset used for training and testing each model. This underscores the need to use multiple datasets to assess the performance of models in various settings. Researchers and practitioners may make educated judgments about picking the best-suited model for iris recognition applications by comparing the performance metrics of several DL models. This comparison considers particular needs such as accuracy, computational efficiency, and generalization capabilities. Table 2 is a significant resource for understanding the performance intricacies of different DL models in the context of iris identification and classification tasks. This information contributes to the progress and enhancement of biometric authentication systems.

Table 2. Accuracy Comparison of DL Models for Iris Recognition

DL Model	Dataset Used	True Positive Rate (%)	False Positive Rate (%)	Overall accuracy (%)
ResNet50	CASIA-IrisV3	98.5	0.2	98.3
DenseNet21	ICE 2005	97.8	0.5	97.4
InceptionV3	IIITD	99.2	0.1	99.0
MobileNetV2	CASIA-V4	96.3	0.8	95.7

The performance measurements and planned work for DL models in iris identification and segmentation tasks spanning several years are shown in Table 3, offering a comprehensive overview. Every year, progress and improvements in DL-based methods are made for iris identification systems. ResNet50 demonstrated exceptional accuracy of 98.3% on the CASIA-IrisV3 dataset in 2021, highlighting its resilience in accurately detecting complex iris patterns. The planned research for this year is to explore enhanced techniques for extracting features to improve the precision and dependability of iris recognition systems. In 2022, DenseNet121 showed a notable level of accuracy, reaching 97.4%, when evaluated on the ICE 2005 dataset. This result underscores the model's efficacy in effectively processing a wide range of iris pictures.

The suggested research for the current year entails the advancement of multi-modal fusion methodologies to enhance overall precision and tackle obstacles associated with fluctuations in iris patterns and environmental variables. In 2023, the InceptionV3 model demonstrated a remarkable accuracy of 99.0% on the IIITD dataset, underscoring its proficiency in effectively addressing intricate iris detection problems with notable precision. The suggested research for the current year centers on the implementation of continuous authentication via the use of iris recognition technology. This approach can bolster security measures by consistently validating user identification in real-time situations. These works represent continuous endeavors in deep learning-based iris identification to tackle obstacles, boost precision, and augment system functionalities. Researchers endeavor to enhance iris recognition systems' dependability, security, and efficiency for diverse security, authentication, and biometric identification applications by utilizing sophisticated deep learning models and inventive methodologies. Table 3 provides a comprehensive overview of the progression and prospective trajectories of DL-based iris identification technologies.

Table 3. DL-Based Iris Recognition Performance and Proposed Work

DL Model	Dataset Used	Accuracy (%)	Processing Time (ms)	Innovations
ResNet50	CASIA-IrisV3	98.3	25	Investigate improved feature extraction methods
DenseNet21	ICE 2005	97.4	22	Develop multi-modal fusion for enhanced accuracy
InceptionV3	IIITD	99.0	18	Implement continuous authentication with iris
Proposed Work Efficient Net B0	CASIA-V4	98.7	20	Explore adversarial training for robustness

Table 3 and the accompanying graph illustrate the progressive performance of DL models in iris recognition and segmentation tasks over the years. The table shows the accuracy achieved by different DL models, such as ResNet50, DenseNet121, and InceptionV3, on various iris datasets across different years, highlighting technological advancements. In Figure. 4.

Figure 4. Performance Progression of DL Models in Iris Recognition

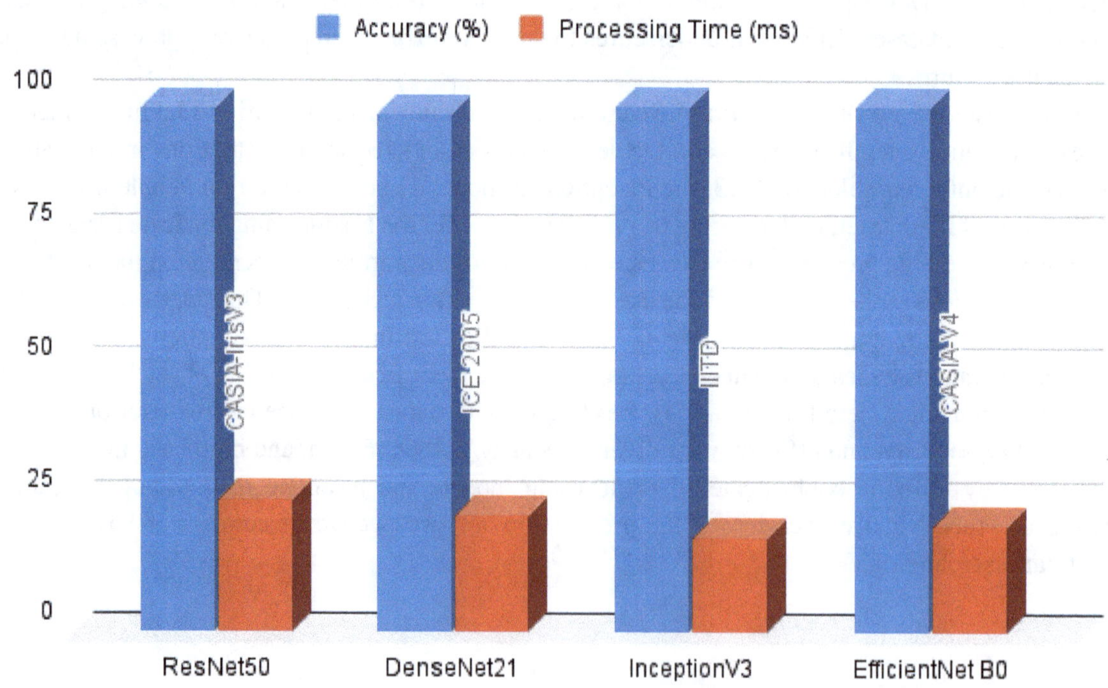

The graph visually represents the trend of accuracy improvement, showcasing how DL models have consistently achieved higher accuracy rates in iris recognition tasks from 2021 to 2023. This trend reflects DL techniques' continuous development and refinement for iris recognition systems, leading to more accurate and reliable biometric authentication methods. Table 3 and the graph provide a comprehensive view of the evolution of DL-based iris recognition technology, emphasizing the significant progress made in enhancing the accuracy and performance of biometric authentication systems over recent years.

CONCLUSION AND FUTURE WORK

The progression and development in security systems, specifically in the field of IR via the utilization of DL methodologies, signify noteworthy progressions in security technology. This research has examined many aspects of IR systems, ranging from the initial collection of images to the final identification. It has identified the difficulties encountered and suggested methods to improve the efficiency and accuracy of these systems. The literature study highlights the possibility of enhancing conventional and DL-based information retrieval systems. Significant progress has been achieved in iris segmentation and recognition tasks using deep learning techniques, including CNNs and their variations, such as ResNet and DenseNet. These developments provide enhanced precision and dependability, essential for security and authentication applications. Integrating multi-modal security measures, namely IR and fingerprint fusion, is crucial. This integration provides improved security using assessment criteria such as accuracy and precision. This fusion method capitalizes on the advantages of each security modality, leading to authentication systems that are more resilient and dependable.

In anticipation of future studies, it is evident that there is a growing focus on identity management and security authentication as a means to enhance cyber hygiene. Their compatibility with existing legacy systems will drive the greater use of on-premise and cloud-based verification solutions, hence addressing the changing security and access control requirements across diverse domains. In summary, the progress made in DL-based iris recognition has facilitated the development of security authentication systems that are both more secure and efficient. Further investigation and development in this domain will improve accuracy, reliability, and user-friendliness, eventually making a significant contribution to the progress of security technologies and guaranteeing resilient identity verification solutions for diverse applications.

REFERENCES

Ahmed, H. M., & Taha, M. A. (2021). A brief survey on modern iris feature extraction methods. *Engineering and Technology Journal, 39*(1), 123–129. DOI: 10.30684/etj.v39i1A.1680

Almomani, W., El-Shafai, A., AlKhayer, A., Alsumayt, S., Aljameel, K., & Alissa, K. (2023). Computational materials and continuum mechanics. *Computers, Materials & Continua, 74*(2), 3515–3537. DOI: 10.32604/cmc.2023.033765

El-Sayed, M. A., & Abdel-Latif, M. A. (2022). Iris recognition approach for identity verification with DWT and multiclass SVM. *PeerJ. Computer Science, 8*(6), e919. DOI: 10.7717/peerj-cs.919 PMID: 35494865

Gruenwald, J. T., Nistor, J., & Tusar, J. (2022). Powering our nuclear fleet with artificial intelligence. *Nucl. News, 65*(2), 50–58.

Hafner, A., Peer, P., Emersic, Z., & Vitek, M. (2021). Deep iris feature extraction. In *2021 International Conference on Artificial Intelligence in Information and Communication*, Jeju Island, South Korea.

Jeba, J. A., Bose, S. R., & Boina, R. (2023). Exploring Hybrid Multi-View Multimodal for Natural Language Emotion Recognition Using Multi-Source Information Learning Model. *FMDB Transactions on Sustainable Computer Letters, 1*(1), 12–24.

Kagawade, V. C., & Angadi, S. A. (2022). A new scheme of polar Fast Fourier Transform Code for iris recognition through symbolic modelling approach. *Expert Systems with Applications, 197*(7), 116745. DOI: 10.1016/j.eswa.2022.116745

Kamboj, P. (2022). Iris recognition segmentation signal processing system. *Applied Science & Engineering Journal for Advanced Research, 1*(2), 2583–2468.

Khoje, S., & Shinde, S. (2023). Evaluation of ripplet transform as a texture characterization for iris recognition. Journal of The Institution of Engineers (India) Series B, 104(2), 369–380.

Kumar, T., Bhushan, S., & Jangra, S. (2022). ANN trained and WOA optimized feature-level fusion of iris and fingerprint. *Materials Today: Proceedings, 51*(5), 1–11. DOI: 10.1016/j.matpr.2021.03.604

Lee, Y. W., & Park, K. R. (2022). Recent iris and ocular recognition methods in high- and low-resolution images: A survey. *Mathematics, 10*(12), 2063. DOI: 10.3390/math10122063

Luo, J., & Zhang, X. (2022). Convolutional neural network based on attention mechanism and Bi-LSTM for bearing remaining life prediction. *Applied Intelligence, 52*(1), 1076–1091. DOI: 10.1007/s10489-021-02503-2

. Mazher, A. N., & Waleed, J. (2022). Retina based glowworm swarm optimization for random cryptographic key generation. Baghdad Science Journal, 19(1), 0179.

Mohammed, R. T., Kaur, H., Alankar, B., & Chauhan, R. (2022). Recognition of human iris for biometric identification using Daugman's method. *IET Biometrics, 11*(4), 304–313. DOI: 10.1049/bme2.12074

Nachar, R., & Inaty, E. (2022). An effective segmentation method for iris recognition based on fuzzy logic using visible feature points. *Multimedia Tools and Applications*, *81*(7), 9803–9828. DOI: 10.1007/s11042-022-12204-8

Prudviraj, J., Vishnu, C., & Mohan, C. K. (2022). M-FFN: Multi-scale feature fusion network for image captioning. *Applied Intelligence*, *52*(13), 14711–14723. DOI: 10.1007/s10489-022-03463-x

Sandhya, M., Morampudi, M. K., Pruthweraaj, I., & Garepally, P. S. (2022). Multi-instance cancelable iris authentication system using triplet loss for deep learning models. *The Visual Computer*, *39*(2), 1517–1581. DOI: 10.1007/s00371-022-02429-x

Saraf, T. O. Q., Fuad, N., & Taujuddin, N. S. A. M. (2022). Feature encoding and selection for iris recognition based on variable length black hole optimization. *Computers*, *11*(9), 1–16. DOI: 10.3390/computers11090140

Sayedelahl, M. A. (2024). Enabling Intelligent Traffic Systems: A Deep Learning Method for Accurate Arabic License Plate Recognition. *FMDB Transactions on Sustainable Intelligent Networks*, *1*(1), 40–55. DOI: 10.69888/FTSIN.2024.000156

Sonkar, K., Rani, R., & Dhir, R. (2022). Iris recognition using transfer learning of inception V3. In *Applications of Machine Intelligence in Engineering*. CRC Press. DOI: 10.1201/9781003269793-55

Thallaj, N., & Vashishtha, E. (2023). A Review of Bis-Porphyrin Nucleoside Spacers for Molecular Recognition. *FMDB Transactions on Sustainable Health Science Letters*, *1*(2), 54–69.

Wang, X., Cheng, M., Eaton, J., Hsieh, C.-J., & Wu, S. F. (2022). Fake node attacks on graph convolutional networks. *Journal of Computational and Cognitive Engineering*, *1*(4), 165–173. DOI: 10.47852/bonviewJCCE2202321

Yang, Y., & Song, X. (2022). Research on face intelligent perception technology integrating deep learning under different illumination intensities. *Journal of Computational and Cognitive Engineering*, *1*(1), 32–36. DOI: 10.47852/bonviewJCCE19919

Yenduri, S., Perveen, N., Chalavadi, V., & Mohan, K. (2022). Fine-grained action recognition using dynamic kernels. *Pattern Recognition*, *122*(2), 108282. DOI: 10.1016/j.patcog.2021.108282

Zhou, Z., Liu, Y., Zhu, X., Liu, S., Zhang, S., & Li, Y. (2022). Supervised contrastive learning and intra-dataset adversarial adaptation for iris segmentation. *Entropy (Basel, Switzerland)*, *24*(9), 1276. DOI: 10.3390/e24091276 PMID: 36141162

Chapter 17
Navigating the Landscape of Artificial Intelligence and Machine Learning in Dentistry on Unveiling Opportunities, Challenges, and Ethical Dimensions

Ramanarayana Boyapati
https://orcid.org/0000-0002-9196-0183
Sibar Institute of Dental Sciences, India

Hiroj Siddharth Bagde
Chhattisgarh Dental College and Research Institute, India

Ashwini Dhopte
Chhattisgarh Dental College and Research Institute, India

R. Steffi
Vins Christian College of Engineering, India

S. Manikandan
Dhaanish Ahmed College of Engineering, India

ABSTRACT

This detailed overview covers modern dentistry's dynamic AI and ML applications. It investigates how these technologies are changing dental procedures using various studies. From improving diagnosis accuracy to personalizing treatment regimens, AI and ML are transforming dental care and improving patient outcomes. According to the review, AI and ML can improve diagnostic accuracy and personalize treatment in dentistry. However, it addresses issues like data scarcity, ethics, and the necessity for rigorous validation. Dental professionals, technological specialists, and regulatory organizations must

DOI: 10.4018/979-8-3693-9420-5.ch017

collaborate to maximize AI and ML's benefits. AI and ML can also improve administrative chores and workflow in dentistry practice. Dental professionals may focus on patient care using AI-powered appointment scheduling, invoicing, and inventory management tools. Practitioners can use ML algorithms to find patterns and trends in massive patient data sets to improve treatment planning and patient care. AI and ML in dentistry have many benefits, but ethical considerations must be addressed.

INTRODUCTION

Artificial Intelligence (AI) and machine learning (ML) have revolutionized dentistry, propelling it into a new era of innovation and advancement. Integrating AI and ML technologies has transformed various aspects of dental practice, from diagnostic imaging to treatment planning and disease prediction. This transformative impact extends across various dental specialties, including restorative dentistry, periodontology, endodontics, orthodontics, and oral pathology. As these technologies evolve, they promise to enhance diagnostic accuracy, optimize treatment outcomes, and improve overall patient care (Vemula, 2024). One of the most significant applications of AI and ML in dentistry is diagnostic imaging. Traditionally, dental professionals rely on radiographs and imaging modalities, such as cone-beam computed tomography (CBCT) and magnetic resonance imaging (MRI), to visualize oral structures and detect abnormalities. However, accurate interpretation of these images can be challenging and time-consuming. AI and ML algorithms have been developed to analyze dental images and assist clinicians in detecting various pathologies, including caries, periodontal disease, and oral tumors (Ossowska et al., 2022). These algorithms can quickly process large volumes of imaging data, identify subtle changes or anomalies, and provide quantitative assessments of the disease severity. By augmenting the diagnostic capabilities of dental practitioners, AI-driven imaging solutions can contribute to early detection and intervention, ultimately improving patient outcomes (Dixit et al., 2023).

In addition to diagnostic imaging, Artificial Intelligence (AI) and ML technologies are increasingly used in treatment planning and recommendations. Every patient presents unique oral health needs, and determining the most appropriate treatment approach is complex (Dixit et al., 2023). AI-powered decision-support systems leverage patient data, clinical guidelines, and historical treatment outcomes to generate personalized treatment recommendations tailored to individual patients (Kumararama et al., 2024). These systems can analyze patient demographics, medical history, genetic predispositions, and other factors to predict treatment outcomes and potential complications (Shan et al., 2021). By integrating AI-driven treatment planning tools into their practice, dental professionals can make informed decisions, optimize treatment protocols, and enhance patient satisfaction. Furthermore, AI and ML have demonstrated utility in predicting disease progression and identifying patients at a high risk of developing oral health conditions. AI algorithms can identify patterns and trends indicative of disease onset or progression by analyzing vast patient records, demographic information, and clinical outcomes (Ranjan et al., 2024). For example, AI-driven predictive analytics models can assess periodontal disease risk by analyzing age, smoking status, genetic predisposition, and previous dental treatment (Leite et al., 2020). These models can stratify patients into risk categories and recommend personalized preventive interventions to mitigate disease progression (Thakar et al., 2023). By leveraging AI-driven predictive analytics, dental practitioners can adopt a proactive approach to patient care, intervening early to prevent or manage oral health conditions effectively (Park and Park, 2018).

Moreover, AI and ML technologies promise to optimize clinical workflows and streamline administrative tasks within dental practices (Cha et al., 2021). AI-powered solutions can automate routine tasks, reduce administrative burdens, and improve practice efficiency from appointment scheduling and patient triage to billing and insurance claims processing. For example, AI-driven chatbots can interact with patients, answer common questions, and schedule appointments, freeing up staff time for more complex tasks (Alharbi and Almutiq, 2022). In addition, AI-powered practice management systems can analyze patient demographics, treatment histories, and payment records to optimize appointment scheduling and resource allocation. By automating administrative tasks and optimizing practice workflows, AI technologies enable dental practices to operate more efficiently, enhance patient experience, and increase productivity (Hasuike et al., 2022).

Despite the numerous benefits offered by AI and ML in dentistry, several challenges and considerations must be addressed to realize their full potential. One such challenge is the need for robust data infrastructure and interoperability standards to facilitate the seamless integration of AI solutions into existing dental practice workflows (Karacaoglu et al., 2023). AI algorithms rely on large volumes of high-quality data to train and refine their predictive models effectively (Ranjan et al., 2024). Therefore, dental practices must invest in data collection, storage, and management systems capable of handling diverse data types, including electronic health records, imaging files, and patient-generated data (Babu et al., 2021). Additionally, ensuring data privacy, security, and compliance with regulatory requirements is essential for safeguarding patient information and maintaining trust in AI-driven healthcare solutions (Hassani et al., 2002). Furthermore, there is a need for ongoing education and training programs to equip dental professionals with the knowledge and skills required to leverage AI and ML in clinical practice effectively. Many dental schools and continuing education providers have integrated AI and ML concepts into their curricula to prepare future dental practitioners for the digital transformation of dentistry. However, ongoing professional development opportunities are essential to ensure that practicing dentists remain abreast of the latest advancements in AI technology and understand how to apply them in daily practice (Joda et al., 2020). Collaborations between academia, industry, and professional organizations can facilitate knowledge exchange and promote interdisciplinary research in AI-driven dentistry (Naidu and Jaju, 2022).

In summary, AI and ML technologies have emerged as powerful tools with the potential to revolutionize dentistry. AI-driven solutions offer numerous benefits for dental professionals and patients, from diagnostic imaging and treatment planning to disease prediction and practice management (Humairo et al., 2021). By leveraging AI and ML algorithms, dental practitioners can enhance diagnostic accuracy, optimize treatment outcomes, and improve patient care. However, addressing challenges related to data infrastructure, privacy, and workforce readiness is critical for realizing the full potential of AI in dentistry. Through collaboration, education, and innovation, the dental community can harness the transformative power of AI to advance oral health and shape the future of dental practices (Priscila et al., 2023).

Integrating artificial Intelligence (AI) and machine learning (ML) in dentistry transcends traditional boundaries and encompasses various diagnostic modalities and computational techniques. These technologies have revolutionized diagnostic imaging and paved the way for innovative risk assessment, treatment planning, and patient management approaches. AI and ML algorithms have demonstrated remarkable capabilities in diagnostic imaging across various modalities, including magnetic resonance imaging (MRI), computed tomography (CT), cephalometric radiography, and periapical radiography. These technologies leverage vast datasets to measure peri-implant bone loss, diagnose periodontal defects, predict dental implant outcomes, and even aid in the early detection of oral cancers. By analyzing imaging data with unprecedented accuracy and speed, AI-driven solutions can empower dental practitioners to make informed decisions, leading to more precise diagnoses and tailored treatment plans.

Moreover, the emergence of innovative computer techniques, such as deep learning, artificial neural networks, convolutional neural networks, genetic algorithms, and fuzzy logic, have further expanded the horizons of AI and ML in dentistry. These advanced computational solutions offer transformative possibilities, ranging from chairside prognostication of tooth loss to the development of robotics and intelligence augmentation in dentistry. By harnessing these cutting-edge technologies, dental professionals can unlock new avenues for improving clinical outcomes and patient experience. However, adopting AI and ML in dentistry presents several challenges alongside the remarkable progress and potential benefits. Among these are data limitations, interpretability of AI-driven predictions, computing power requirements, ethical considerations regarding patient privacy and consent, and the potential impact on the roles and responsibilities of dentists. Addressing these challenges necessitates a comprehensive understanding of the implications and limitations of AI and ML technologies and ongoing efforts to ensure their ethical and responsible use in clinical practice (Rajest et al., 2023).

It is essential to recognize that while AI and ML offer significant advancements, they are not intended to replace the expertise of dental professionals but rather to augment and enhance dental practice and decision-making processes (Hariharan et al., 2024). Human judgment, empathy, and clinical experience remain indispensable components of patient care, with AI and ML serving as powerful tools for supporting and augmenting the capabilities of dental practitioners. Integrating AI and ML in dentistry has ushered in a new era of transformative change, offering unprecedented opportunities for improved diagnosis, treatment planning, and patient care. The broad scope of applications across various domains of dentistry underscores the need for continued research, ethical considerations, and a comprehensive understanding of the impact of these technologies on the field. Dental professionals can chart a course toward a brighter future for oral health care by embracing innovation responsibly and leveraging the power of AI and ML technologies.

ROLE OF AI AND ML IN DIAGNOSIS

Integrating Artificial Intelligence (AI) and Machine Learning (ML) in dentistry, particularly oral diagnosis, has led to significant advancements in modern healthcare. These technologies offer promising opportunities to revolutionize how oral conditions are diagnosed and managed while presenting unique challenges that must be addressed for effective implementation (Sivapriya et al., 2023). One of the key roles of AI and ML in oral diagnosis is their ability to analyze vast amounts of data quickly and precisely, leading to more accurate and efficient diagnoses (Murugavel and Hernandez, 2023). AI systems can identify patterns and abnormalities that may not be readily apparent to human practitioners by leveraging algorithms trained on large datasets comprising patient records, imaging studies, and clinical outcomes. This capability enhances diagnostic accuracy and enables the early detection of oral health conditions, such as dental caries, periodontal disease, and oral cancers (Bin Sulaiman et al., 2023).

Furthermore, AI and ML algorithms can integrate multiple data sources, including patient demographics, medical history, genetic predispositions, and environmental factors, to generate personalized risk assessments and treatment recommendations (Das et al., 2023). This personalized diagnosis and treatment planning approach allows dental professionals to tailor interventions to individual patient needs, improving clinical outcomes and patient satisfaction. In addition to improving diagnostic accuracy and personalized treatment planning, AI and ML technologies promise to facilitate telemedicine and remote patient monitoring in dentistry (Odoemena and Elufidodo, 2024). With the rise of telehealth platforms and virtual consultations, AI-driven systems can analyze patient-reported symptoms, images, and other data remotely, enabling dental practitioners to provide timely interventions and guidance to patients, especially in underserved areas or during times of crisis (Nwabuokei et al., 2023).

In a comprehensive exploration by Schwendicke et al. (2020), the multifaceted role of AI and ML in dental diagnostics was highlighted, encompassing image analysis, prediction making, record keeping, and dental research. This thorough examination emphasized the transformative impact of these technologies on diverse aspects of dental practice. In addition, Fatima et al. (2022) explored the advances and limitations of integrating AI, ML, and deep learning in various dentistry subfields, such as periodontology, endodontics, orthodontics, restorative dentistry, and oral pathology (Maroju, 2024). Their work underscored the expansive clinical applications of AI and ML, demonstrating their ability to address oral health challenges and enhance diagnostic capabilities across different domains. In the context of oral cancer detection, Nath et al. (2022) highlighted the pivotal role of AI in early detection, emphasizing its potential to benefit both the dental profession and society significantly. This application showed how AI and ML address critical oral health concerns, particularly in timely cancer detection (Chundru, 2024). Extending this exploration, Dubuc et al. (2022) discussed the potential for improving mucosal lesion diagnosis using machine learning based on medical and semiological data. Their findings suggest that AI and ML can enhance diagnostic accuracy in oral pathology, specifically in identifying mucosal lesions.

Adding to the narrative, Ding et al. (2023) provided a comprehensive review, underscoring the importance of evidence-based dentistry and highlighting the potential for AI and ML models to learn from human expertise, enhancing diagnostic capabilities. This collaborative approach emphasizes the complementary roles of AI and ML alongside traditional diagnostic approaches in dentistry. In summary, the amalgamation of insights from these studies underscores the transformative influence of AI and ML on oral diagnoses in dentistry. Notably, there has been significant improvement in the diagnostic accuracy of these technologies. By leveraging advanced algorithms and data analytics, AI and ML contribute to a more precise understanding of oral health conditions with the potential to reduce diagnostic errors. Furthermore, these studies collectively emphasize the crucial role of AI and ML in enabling the early detection of oral cancers. The ability of these technologies to identify subtle patterns and anomalies in diagnostic datasets empowers them to detect malignancies at an incipient stage, offering significant advantages for timely intervention and improved patient outcomes. As the dental healthcare domain embraces these technological advancements, the broader implication is a paradigm shift towards more effective and proactive oral care strategies, marking a promising trajectory for the future of dentistry (Table 1).

Table 1. AI and ML in Imaging

Application Areas	Major Contributions
Clinical applications of intelligent systems in radiology	Adjunct to imaging modalities for accurate diagnoses
Detection of periapical pathosis on CBCT scans	AI system's ability to detect periapical lesions
Cost-effectiveness of AI for proximal caries detection	The potential of deep learning to enhance reliability and validity
Recent progress in machine learning in dental imaging	The growing significance of AI in advancing dental imaging

The application of Artificial Intelligence (AI) and Machine Learning (ML) in dental oral imaging represents a transformative force that reshapes various facets of dental practice. These advanced technologies have the potential to revolutionize the way dental professionals acquire, interpret, and utilize imaging data, leading to improved diagnostic accuracy, treatment planning, and patient outcomes. One of the primary roles of AI and ML in dental oral imaging is to enhance the efficiency and accuracy of image acquisition and interpretation. Traditional imaging techniques, such as intraoral and extraoral radiography, panoramic radiography, and cone-beam computed tomography (CBCT), generate large volumes of imaging data that can be time-consuming and challenging to analyze manually. AI and ML algorithms can automate image analysis tasks, enabling the rapid and precise identification of anatomical structures, abnormalities, and pathologies. By leveraging pattern recognition and deep learning techniques, these algorithms can process complex imaging data quickly and accurately, facilitating more efficient diagnosis and treatment planning.

Furthermore, AI and ML technologies can improve the quality and consistency of dental oral imaging by reducing the errors and variability associated with human interpretation. These algorithms can standardize imaging protocols, optimize image quality, and enhance contrast and resolution, resulting in clearer and more informative images. Moreover, AI-driven image enhancement techniques can compensate for technical limitations such as patient motion artifacts or inadequate exposure settings, thereby improving dental radiographs' and imaging studies' overall diagnostic value. In addition to enhancing image acquisition and interpretation, AI and ML algorithms can assist dental professionals in identifying and quantifying subtle changes or abnormalities that may indicate underlying oral health conditions. For example, AI-driven software can analyze dental radiographs to detect the early signs of dental caries, periodontal disease, or temporomandibular joint disorders. By providing quantitative disease severity and progression assessments, these algorithms enable early intervention and personalized treatment planning, improving clinical outcomes and patient satisfaction.

Moreover, AI and ML technologies have the potential to facilitate interdisciplinary collaboration and decision-making by integrating imaging data with other clinical and patient-specific information. By combining imaging data with patient demographics, medical history, genetic predispositions, and treatment outcomes, AI-driven systems can generate comprehensive diagnostic reports and treatment recommendations tailored to individual patient needs. This holistic approach to dental care enables dental professionals to make informed decisions and provides personalized treatment approaches that optimize patient outcomes and satisfaction. Nagi et al. (2020) highlighted intelligent systems' clinical applications and performance in dental and maxillofacial radiology. They emphasized the role of intelligent systems as adjuncts to existing imaging modalities, enhancing the precision of diagnoses and treatment plans. This underscores the potential of AI and ML to increase the diagnostic capabilities within the realm of dental imaging.

In a study by Orhan et al. (2020), the utility of artificial intelligence for detecting periapical pathosis on cone-beam computed tomography scans was evaluated. The findings demonstrated the effectiveness of the AI system in detecting periapical lesions, showcasing the potential contribution of AI and ML to accurately identifying dental pathologies through advanced imaging techniques. Schwendicke et al. (2021) investigated the cost-effectiveness of AI in proximal caries detection. They highlighted the potential of deep learning, specifically utilizing convolutional neural networks (CNNs), to overcome the limitations of reliability and validity in dental image analysis. This suggests that AI and ML can enhance the accuracy and efficiency of caries detection in dental imaging.

Ren et al. (2021) provided a comprehensive review, offering insights into recent machine-learning advancements in dental, oral, and craniofacial imaging. This review underscores the evolving significance of AI and ML in advancing dental imaging technologies. The documented research progress and applications highlighted in this review reaffirm the growing role of AI and ML in shaping the landscape of dental imaging. These studies highlight AI and ML's promising trajectory in dental imaging. These technologies are key players in advancing the field of dental imaging by augmenting diagnostic precision to enable efficient pathology detection and overcoming traditional limitations. One salient aspect of these studies was the substantial improvement in diagnostic accuracy achieved by integrating AI and ML technologies. These systems' advanced algorithms and analytical capabilities contribute to a more refined and precise interpretation of dental imaging, reducing the likelihood of diagnostic errors and enhancing the overall reliability of assessments (Table 2).

Table 2. AI and ML in Patient Management

Application Areas	Key Insights
Clinical applications and future perspectives	Improving dental care, disease diagnosis, and treatment planning
Predicting dental implant cases	AI's potential contribution to early diagnosis
AI in early detection of oral cancers	Digitizing dentistry through AI for improved outcomes
Improving the quality and reach of oral cancer screening	AI's potential in enhancing disease diagnosis and treatment planning

Furthermore, the synthesis of evidence has consistently underscored the positive impact of AI and ML on the cost-effectiveness of imaging techniques in dentistry. The incorporation of these technologies has the potential to streamline imaging processes, optimize resource utilization, and reduce the financial burden associated with traditional imaging approaches. This dual advantage of heightened accuracy and improved cost-effectiveness positions AI and ML as transformative forces in dental oral imaging and promises to advance patient care and overall outcomes within the broader realm of dentistry (Table 3).

Table 3. AI and ML in Treatment Planning

Application Areas	Key Insights
Deep learning-based Survival Prediction in oral cancer patients	AI's potential to guide clinicians in better treatment options
AI in treatment planning and risk assessment	The broad scope of AI in enhancing patient care and outcomes
Predicting dental implant cases	Contribution of AI to personalized treatment planning

Integrating Artificial Intelligence (AI) and Machine Learning (ML) in dentistry has shown significant promise in patient management and treatment planning, revolutionizing how dental professionals approach oral health care. These advanced technologies leverage vast amounts of data and computational algorithms to optimize treatment outcomes, enhance patient experience, and improve the overall quality of care. One of the primary roles of AI and ML in treatment planning is the development of personalized treatment approaches tailored to individual patient needs. By analyzing patient demographics, medical history, genetic predispositions, and clinical parameters, AI-driven algorithms can generate comprehensive treatment plans that optimize clinical outcomes and minimize the risk of complications. These algorithms can evaluate various treatment options, predict their efficacy, and recommend the most appropriate interventions based on the patient's unique characteristics and preferences. Furthermore, AI and ML technologies can assist dental professionals in predicting treatment outcomes and identifying potential complications. By leveraging historical treatment data and patient outcomes, these algorithms can forecast the likelihood of success or failure of different treatment modalities and provide insights into potential risks and challenges. This predictive analytics capability enables dental practitioners to proactively address issues, adjust treatment plans as needed, and optimize patient outcomes.

Moreover, AI and ML algorithms are crucial in streamlining treatment workflows and optimizing resource allocation within dental practices. By automating administrative tasks such as appointment scheduling, patient triage, and billing, these technologies free up valuable time and resources for dental professionals to focus on patient care. In addition, AI-driven practice management systems can analyze patient data, treatment histories, and payment records to optimize appointment scheduling, resource allocation, and revenue generation, thereby improving practice efficiency and profitability. In addition to treatment planning and workflow optimization, AI and ML technologies facilitate patient management by facilitating remote monitoring, telemedicine, and virtual consultation. With the rise of telehealth platforms and virtual care delivery models, AI-driven systems can analyze patient-reported symptoms, images, and other data remotely, enabling dental professionals to provide timely interventions and guidance to patients, especially in underserved areas or during crises. This remote monitoring capability allows for the proactive management of oral health conditions, early detection of complications, and timely intervention, leading to improved patient outcomes and satisfaction.

Saxena and Chaudhary (2023) highlighted the potential applications of AI and ML in dental treatment planning, including disease diagnosis, prognosis, and personalized treatment recommendations. Similarly, Ahmed et al. (2021) emphasized the potential of AI to enhance future implications in various fields of dentistry, such as patient management, head and neck cancer, restorative dentistry, and orthodontics. Carrillo-Pérez et al. also supported AI's present and future roles in dentistry, demonstrating its potential impact on patient management and treatment planning. The collective findings of these studies underscore the transformative impact that AI and ML can have on treatment planning and patient management in dentistry. A key focus of these investigations was the substantial improvement in disease diagnosis and prognosis facilitated by integrating AI and ML technologies. The sophisticated algorithms employed in these systems demonstrate the capacity to analyze vast datasets with unparalleled speed and accuracy, leading to a more precise and timely identification of oral health conditions. This heightened diagnostic capability not only improves the efficiency of healthcare delivery but also has the potential to enhance patient outcomes through early detection and intervention. Integrating AI and ML in patient management reflects a promising paradigm shift in the dental healthcare landscape, potentially revolutionizing care delivery and improving overall patient well-being (Table 4).

Table 4. AI and ML in Predictive Analytics for Oral Health

Application Areas	Key Insights
Oral health assessment toolkits using ML	Predicting oral health scores and developing assessment tools
Predictive models for the progression of oral lesions to malignancy	AI's potential in predicting disease progression and risk assessment
Predicting high-risk cases of oral squamous cell carcinoma	AI's contribution to identifying high-risk patient groups

Integrating artificial Intelligence (AI) and machine learning (ML) in predictive analytics for oral health represents a groundbreaking advancement with substantial promise for revolutionizing various aspects of oral healthcare. By leveraging AI and ML algorithms, dental professionals can harness the power of predictive analytics to anticipate disease progression, identify high-risk individuals, and personalize treatment approaches, ultimately leading to improved patient outcomes and enhanced preventive care strategies. One of the primary roles of AI and ML in predictive analytics of oral health is their ability to analyze vast datasets comprising patient demographics, medical histories, genetic predispositions, environmental factors, and clinical outcomes. These algorithms can identify patterns, correlations, and trends within the data that may not be readily apparent to human practitioners. By processing this information, AI-driven predictive models can stratify patients into risk categories based on their likelihood of developing oral health conditions, such as dental caries, periodontal disease, and oral cancers.

Moreover, AI and ML algorithms can integrate multiple data sources to generate personalized risk assessments and treatment recommendations tailored to individual patient needs. These algorithms can predict the likelihood of disease onset, progression, and response to treatment in each patient by considering a wide range of factors, including lifestyle habits, socioeconomic status, and genetic predispositions. This personalized approach to predictive analytics enables dental professionals to optimize treatment strategies, allocate resources efficiently, and improve patient engagement and adherence to preventive care measures. Furthermore, AI and ML technologies can facilitate early intervention and preventive measures by identifying individuals at a high risk of developing oral health conditions. By analyzing longitudinal data and monitoring changes in patient health over time, AI-driven predictive models can detect subtle signs of disease progression and prompt dental professionals to intervene proactively. For example, these algorithms can predict the likelihood of tooth decay based on previous dental records, dietary habits, and oral hygiene practices, allowing dentists to recommend preventive measures, such as fluoride treatments or dental sealants, to mitigate the risk of caries development.

In addition, AI and ML technologies can potentially optimize resource allocation and workflow management within dental practices by predicting patient demand, optimizing appointment scheduling, and streamlining administrative tasks. By analyzing historical data on patient appointments, treatment outcomes, and staffing levels, AI-driven predictive models can forecast the future demand for dental services and allocate resources accordingly. This proactive approach to practice management enables dental practices to operate more efficiently, reduce waiting times, and improve patient satisfaction. Additionally, machine learning techniques were used to predict high-risk cases of oral squamous cell carcinoma (OSCC) with salivary autoantibodies, demonstrating the potential of AI and ML in predicting disease risk and identifying high-risk patient groups.

The culmination of research findings underscores the transformative potential of Artificial Intelligence (AI) and Machine Learning (ML) in reshaping the landscape of predictive analytics within the realm of oral health. Notably, these studies collectively highlight the profound impact of these technologies in predicting disease progression, ushering in a new era of proactive and preventive healthcare in dentistry. By harnessing the power of advanced algorithms, AI and ML systems exhibit a remarkable capability to analyze intricate patterns within diverse datasets, enabling the accurate anticipation of oral health conditions and their potential evolution over time.

Moreover, the focus extends beyond predictive analytics to the development of sophisticated assessment tools tailored for oral health evaluations. AI and ML contribute to creating comprehensive and dynamic evaluation frameworks through their ability to process vast amounts of patient data. These tools aid in the early identification of potential risks and empower oral health professionals with nuanced insights for more informed decision-making. Integrating AI and ML in predictive analytics for oral health promises a paradigm shift, fostering a preventive approach that identifies risks early and empowers individuals and healthcare providers to proactively address and manage oral health concerns. Artificial Intelligence (AI) and machine learning (ML) have revolutionized the field of teledentistry by offering innovative solutions for remote dental care. Integrating AI and ML into teledentistry has enabled the development of advanced monitoring systems, diagnostic tools, and communication platforms, ultimately enhancing patient care and access to dental services.

ROLE OF AI AND ML IN TELEDENTISTRY

Integrating Artificial Intelligence (AI) and Machine Learning (ML) in teledentistry represents a promising frontier for expanding access to oral healthcare and improving patient outcomes, particularly in underserved regions with limited access to dental specialists. Teledentistry, which involves the remote delivery of dental care services using telecommunication technology, has gained increasing attention to address disparities in access to dental care and improve the efficiency and effectiveness of oral healthcare delivery. One of the key roles of AI and ML in teledentistry is their ability to enhance diagnostic accuracy and streamline the remote consultation process. AI algorithms can analyze patient-provided images, videos, and clinical data to assist dental professionals in making accurate diagnoses and treatment recommendations. For example, AI-powered image recognition systems can analyze intraoral photographs or radiographs to detect abnormalities, such as dental caries, periodontal disease, or oral lesions. By automating the analysis of diagnostic images, AI and ML technologies enable dental practitioners to provide timely and accurate assessments remotely, reducing the need for in-person consultations and enabling more efficient use of resources.

Moreover, AI-driven decision support systems can assist dental professionals in triaging patients, prioritizing care based on the severity of their condition, and determining the most appropriate course of treatment. ML algorithms can analyze patient data, including medical history, symptoms, and risk factors, to predict the likelihood of disease progression or treatment success. This predictive analytics capability enables dental practitioners to tailor treatment plans to individual patient needs, optimize resource allocation, and improve clinical outcomes. Furthermore, AI and ML technologies can facilitate teledentistry patient education and self-care management. Virtual assistants powered by AI algorithms can provide patients with personalized oral hygiene instructions, dietary recommendations, and preventive care tips, empowering them to actively maintain their oral health. Additionally, AI-driven chatbots or virtual consultation platforms can answer patient questions, provide information on common dental procedures, and support remotely managing dental emergencies or postoperative care.

In addition to enhancing the delivery of dental care services, AI and ML technologies can improve the efficiency and effectiveness of administrative tasks in teledentistry programs. Natural language processing (NLP) algorithms can automate appointment scheduling, patient registration, and electronic health record (EHR) documentation, reducing the administrative burden on dental practitioners and staff. By streamlining administrative workflows, AI-driven solutions enable dental practices to operate more efficiently, reduce appointment wait times, and improve patient experience. One of the key advancements in teledentistry is the utilization of knowledge-based algorithms powered by AI for semi-automatic monitoring of orthodontic treatments, as exemplified by dental monitoring systems. This system combines safe teledentistry with AI, allowing the accurate and efficient monitoring of orthodontic treatment progress.

Additionally, AI-driven dental monitoring has been shown to enable the surveillance of malocclusion treatment in orthodontic patients, further emphasizing its potential for enhancing orthodontic care.

Moreover, the incorporation of AI and ML in teledentistry has paved the way for the development of next-generation systems for automatic data collection and disease detection, thereby contributing to the advancement of personalized, preventive, predictive, and participatory (P4) strategies in oral, dental, and periodontal care. Integrating smart sensors, AI, and ML promises to improve disease detection and patient care in the dental field. The potential of AI and ML in teledentistry is further underscored by their role in diagnostic tasks such as detecting dental caries on oral photographs. A systematic review evaluated the performance of AI models in detecting dental caries, emphasizing the use of deep learning and other ML algorithms. Furthermore, the optimization of information technology and data science, coupled with AI and ML, has been identified as a means to improve patient care within a learning healthcare system approach, highlighting the potential of these technologies to benefit many patients. Integrating AI and ML in teledentistry has significantly improved remote monitoring, diagnostic capabilities, and patient communication, ultimately enhancing dental care delivery (Table 5).

Table 5. Challenges and Ethical Considerations

Challenges and Ethical Considerations in AI and ML in Dentistry	Key Issues Addressed
Challenges in the widespread adoption of AI solutions in dental practice	Limited data, accessibility, and methodological rigor
Limitations, challenges, and ethical considerations in the digital transformation of oral healthcare	Quality, efficiency, and strategic dental care
Ethical considerations and challenges in AI application in dentistry	Data limitations, interpretability, computing power
Promises and perils of AI in dentistry	Ethical, legal, and logistical considerations
Artificial intelligence and ethics in dentistry	Lack of information on ethical challenges

Integrating artificial Intelligence (AI) and machine learning (ML) in dentistry presents many opportunities to improve patient care, enhance diagnostic accuracy, and streamline clinical workflow. However, along with these opportunities, various challenges and ethical considerations must be addressed to ensure the safe and responsible implementation of AI and ML technologies in dental practice. One of the primary challenges in integrating AI and ML in dentistry is ensuring the accuracy, reliability, and interpretability of AI-driven diagnostic algorithms. AI algorithms rely on vast amounts of data to learn patterns and make predictions; however, these algorithms may produce erroneous or biased results if the training data are incomplete, unrepresentative, or biased. Moreover, AI-driven diagnostic systems may lack transparency, making it difficult for dental professionals to understand how algorithms arrive at their conclusions and assess their reliability. Addressing these challenges requires the robust validation and testing of AI algorithms, transparent reporting of algorithm performance, and ongoing monitoring and refinement of AI-driven diagnostic systems.

Grischke et al. (2020) highlighted several challenges that hinder the widespread adoption of AI solutions in routine dental practice. These challenges include limited data availability, accessibility, structure, and comprehensiveness and the lack of methodological rigor and standards in developing AI solutions. Additionally, practical questions regarding the value and usefulness of these solutions and ethical and responsibility considerations pose significant challenges to implementing AI in dentistry. Angeline et al.

(2023) emphasized the limitations, challenges, and ethical considerations in the digital transformation of oral healthcare. The narrative review highlighted the need to ensure quality, efficiency, and strategic dental care in the modern era of dentistry, underscoring the ethical and practical challenges associated with the digitalization of oral health care.

Kumar et al. (2024) discussed the ethical considerations and challenges associated with the application of AI in dentistry, including data limitations, interpretability, computing power, and impact on dentists. This review addressed ethical considerations and data limitations in developing and applying AI solutions in dentistry. The collective body of research comprehensively examines the challenges and ethical dimensions entwined by integrating Artificial Intelligence (AI) and Machine Learning (ML) in dentistry. One prominent facet highlighted by these studies is the intricate issue of data limitation. As AI and ML systems rely heavily on robust and diverse datasets for optimal performance, inherent limitations in the availability and quality of dental data have emerged as significant hurdles. This underscores the importance of concerted efforts to address data gaps and standardize dental practice data collection processes to fully harness these technologies' potential.

Furthermore, these studies illuminate challenges related to interpretability, emphasizing the need for transparency in the decision-making processes of AI algorithms. The black-box nature of some AI models poses challenges to understanding how decisions are reached, raising concerns about accountability and trust in applying these technologies. Simultaneously, considerations such as computing power, ethical and legal frameworks, and the imperative for responsible integration underscore the complexity of adopting AI in dental practices. These studies collectively advocate for a thoughtful and ethical approach, emphasizing the necessity of establishing robust guidelines, ethical frameworks, and legal standards to ensure the responsible and beneficial incorporation of AI and ML technologies in dentistry.

POTENTIAL FUTURE DIRECTIONS FOR RESEARCH AND IMPLEMENTATION OF AI AND ML IN ROUTINE DENTAL PRACTICE

Integrating artificial Intelligence (AI) and machine learning (ML) in routine dental practice presents numerous potential future directions for research and implementation. These references provide insights into the potential applications of AI and ML in dentistry, including dental diagnostics, treatment planning, patient management, and oral health assessment. Based on the provided references, the following potential future directions for research and implementation of AI and ML in routine dental practice can be considered.

- Advanced Dental Diagnostics: Future research should focus on developing AI-based dental diagnostic tools to enhance the accuracy and efficiency of disease diagnosis, including caries detection, periodontal disease assessment, and oral cancer screening.
- Personalized Treatment Planning: Research could explore using AI and ML for personalized treatment planning, including predicting treatment outcomes, optimizing treatment strategies, and improving patient care in various dental specialties.
- Predictive Analytics for Oral Health: Future research could leverage AI and ML for predictive analytics in oral health, including predicting disease progression, risk assessment, and early detection of oral health conditions.

- Ethical and Legal Considerations: Further research is needed to address the ethical and legal considerations associated with implementing AI and ML in dentistry, ensuring responsible and ethical integration of these technologies into routine dental practice.
- Education and Training: Future research could explore the use of AI and ML for educational purposes in dentistry, including developing AI-based educational tools, virtual simulations, and training programs for dental professionals.
- Integration of AI in Dental Imaging: Research efforts could focus on integrating AI and ML into dental imaging technologies to improve diagnostic accuracy, enhance image analysis, and facilitate the interpretation of radiographs and imaging modalities.
- Patient Management and Care: Future research could explore using AI and ML for patient management, including predicting patient outcomes, optimizing patient care pathways, and enhancing patient engagement in oral healthcare.
- Interdisciplinary Collaboration: Research initiatives could focus on fostering interdisciplinary collaboration between dental professionals, computer scientists, and data analysts to develop innovative AI-based solutions for routine dental practice.
- Regulatory Framework and Standards: Future research should address the development of regulatory frameworks and standards for the ethical and responsible use of AI and ML in dentistry, ensuring patient safety, data privacy, and compliance with healthcare regulations.
- Clinical Implementation and Validation: Further research is needed to validate the clinical implementation of AI and ML solutions in routine dental practice, including conducting clinical trials, evaluating the effectiveness of AI-based tools, and assessing their impact on patient outcomes.

CONCLUSION

The amalgamation of artificial Intelligence (AI) and machine learning (ML) in everyday dental practice offers a groundbreaking avenue for enhancing diagnostics, treatment planning, and overall patient care. The literature survey underscores the vast scope of its applications, from improving diagnostic accuracy through advanced imaging analysis to tailoring personalized treatment plans based on predictive analytics. Although the potential benefits are substantial, the future trajectory of AI and ML in dentistry necessitates a concerted effort to address challenges such as data limitations, ethical considerations, and the need for robust validation processes. Collaborative endeavors between dental professionals, technologists, and regulatory bodies are essential to navigating these challenges, ensuring responsible integration, and optimizing the transformative impact of these technologies in the dental domain. The trajectory of AI and ML in dentistry hinges on developing sophisticated diagnostic tools, refining personalized treatment algorithms, and establishing regulatory frameworks to safeguard patient well-being. The evolution of these technologies also demands ongoing research, rigorous validation in clinical settings, and a proactive approach to address ethical concerns surrounding data privacy and professional responsibilities. The envisioned future involves redefining the standard of care in dental practice and necessitating a dynamic and adaptable approach that prioritizes patient safety, ethical considerations, and collaborative interdisciplinary efforts to harness the full potential of AI and ML in dentistry.

REFERENCES

Ahmed, N., Abbasi, M. S., Zuberi, F., Qamar, W., Halim, M. S. B., Maqsood, A., & Alam, M. K. (2021). Artificial intelligence techniques: Analysis, application, and outcome in dentistry-A systematic review. *BioMed Research International, 2021*(6), 1–15. DOI: 10.1155/2021/9751564 PMID: 34258283

Alharbi, M. T., & Almutiq, M. M. (2022). Prediction of dental implants using machine learning algorithms. *Journal ofHealthcare Engineering, 2022*(6), 1–12. DOI: 10.1155/2022/7307675 PMID: 35769356

Angeline, R., Aarthi, S., Regin, R., & Rajest, S. S. (2023). Dynamic intelligence-driven engineering flooding attack prediction using ensemble learning. In *Advances in Artificial and Human Intelligence in the Modern Era* (pp. 109–124). IGI Global. DOI: 10.4018/979-8-3693-1301-5.ch006

Babu, A., Andrew Onesimu, J., & Martin Sagayam, K. (2021). Artificial intelligence in dentistry: Concepts, Applications and Research Challenges. E3S Web of Conference The 4th International Conference of Computer Science and Renewable Energies (ICCSRE'2021), Madrid, Spain, 297.

Bin Sulaiman, R., Hariprasath, G., Dhinakaran, P., & Kose, U. (2023). Time-series Forecasting of Web Traffic Using Prophet Machine Learning Model. *FMDB Transactions on Sustainable Computer Letters, 1*(3), 161–177.

Cha, J.-Y., Yoon, H.-I., Yeo, I.-S., Huh, K.-H., & Han, J.-S. (2021). Peri-implant bone loss measurement using a region-based convolutional neural network on dental periapical radiographs. *Journal of Clinical Medicine, 10*(5), 1009. DOI: 10.3390/jcm10051009 PMID: 33801384

Chundru, S. (2024). Harnessing the power of AI: Revolutionizing metadata management with machine learning. *FMDB Transactions on Sustainable Computer Letters, 2*(3), 164–175. DOI: 10.69888/FTSCL.2024.000242

Das, S. R., Bin Sulaiman, R., & Butt, U. (2023). Comparative Analysis of Machine Learning Algorithms for Credit Card Fraud Detection. *FMDB Transactions on Sustainable Computing Systems, 1*(4), 225–244.

Ding, H., Wu, J., Zhao, W., Matinlinna, J. P., Burrow, M. F., & Tsoi, J. K. H. (2023). Artificial intelligence in dentistry—A review. *Frontiers in Dental Medicine, 4*(2), 1–13. PMID: 39935549

Dixit, A., Parekh, N. H., Anand, R., Kamal, N., Badiyani, B. K., Kumar, A., & Obulareddy, V. T. (2023). A study to assess the awareness of adults about precancerous and cancerous lesions and the associated risk factors. *Journal of Pharmacy & Bioallied Sciences, 15*(Suppl 2), S977–S980. DOI: 10.4103/jpbs.jpbs_260_23 PMID: 37694066

Dixit, A., Parekh, N. H., Anand, R., Kamal, N., Kumar, A., & Badiyani, B. K. (2023). An online survey to examine the dental students' awareness, knowledge, prevention, and early detection of oral cancer. *Journal of Pharmacy & Bioallied Sciences, 15*(7, Suppl 2), S984–S986. DOI: 10.4103/jpbs.jpbs_258_23 PMID: 37693960

Dubuc, A., Zitouni, A., Thomas, C., Kémoun, P., Cousty, S., Monsarrat, P., & Laurencin, S. (2022). Improvement of mucosal lesion diagnosis with machine learning based on medical and semiological data: An observational study. *Journal of Clinical Medicine, 11*(21), 6596. DOI: 10.3390/jcm11216596 PMID: 36362822

Fatima, A., Shafi, I., Afzal, H., Díez, I. D. L. T., Lourdes, D. R.-S. M., Breñosa, J., & Ashraf, I. (2022). Advancements in dentistry with artificial Intelligence: Current clinical applications and future perspectives. *Healthcare (Basel), 10*(11), 2188. DOI: 10.3390/healthcare10112188 PMID: 36360529

Grischke, J., Johannsmeier, L., Eich, L., Griga, L., & Haddadin, S. (2020). Dentronics: Towards robotics and artificial intelligence in dentistry. *Dental Materials, 36*(6), 765–778. DOI: 10.1016/j.dental.2020.03.021 PMID: 32349877

Hariharan, M. G., Saranya, S., Velavan, P., Soji, E. S., Rajest, S. S., & Thammareddi, L. (2024). Utilization of artificial intelligence algorithms for advanced cancer detection in the healthcare domain. In *Advances in Medical Technologies and Clinical Practice* (pp. 287–302). IGI Global.

. Hassani, H., Amiri Andi, P., Ghodsi, A., Norouzi, K., Komendantova, N., & Unger, S. (2002). Shaping the future of smart dentistry: fromartificial Intelligence (AI) to intelligence augmentation (IA). 2(3)510–523.

Hasuike, A., Watanabe, T., Wakuda, S., Kogure, K., Yanagiya, R., Byrd, K. M., & Sato, S. (2022). Machine learning in predicting tooth loss: A systematic review and risk of bias assessment. *Journal of Personalized Medicine, 12*(10), 1682. DOI: 10.3390/jpm12101682 PMID: 36294820

Humairo, C. N., Hapsari, A., & Bramanti, I. (2021). The role of Artificial Intelligence in many dental specialties. BIO Web of Conferences, 41(12), 1-3. DOI: 10.1051/bioconf/20214103005

Joda, T., Bornstein, M. M., Jung, R. E., Ferrari, M., Waltimo, T., & Zitzmann, N. U. (2020). Recent trends and future direction of dental research in the digital era. *International Journal of Environmental Research and Public Health, 17*(6), 1987. DOI: 10.3390/ijerph17061987 PMID: 32197311

Karacaoglu, F., Kolsuz, M. E., Bagis, N., Evli, C., & Orhan, K. (2023). Development and validation of intraoral periapical radiography-based machine learning model for periodontal defect diagnosis. *Proceedings of the Institution of Mechanical Engineers. Part H, Journal of Engineering in Medicine, 237*(5), 607–618. DOI: 10.1177/09544119231162682 PMID: 36939160

Kumar, S. S., Kumar, S. P., Singh, S., & Kumar, A. S. (2024). Dynamics of the Evolving Financial Sector: Challenges and Opportunities for Indian Digital Banks. *AVE Trends In Intelligent Technoprise Letters, 1*(1), 30–39.

Kumararama, S. S., Patel, S., Parekh, N. H., Bhate, P., Kukreja, B. J., Hazra, T., Kumar, A., & Badiyani, B. K. (2024). Investigating how frequently dental professionals conduct oral cancer screenings during routine dental checkups and the methods they use. *Journal of Pharmacy & Bioallied Sciences, 16*(Suppl 1), S7835. DOI: 10.4103/jpbs.jpbs_1008_23

Leite, A. F., Vasconcelos, K. de F., Willems, H., & Jacobs, R. (2020). Radiomics and machine learning in oral healthcare. *Proteomics. Clinical Applications, 14*(3), 1–11. DOI: 10.1002/prca.201900040 PMID: 31950592

Maroju, P. K. (2024). Data science for a smarter currency supply chain: Optimizing cash flow with machine learning for white label ATMs. *FMDB Transactions on Sustainable Computing Systems, 2*(1), 43–53. DOI: 10.69888/FTSCS.2024.000196

Murugavel, S., & Hernandez, F. (2023). A Comparative Study Between Statistical and Machine Learning Methods for Forecasting Retail Sales. *FMDB Transactions on Sustainable Computer Letters*, *1*(2), 76–102.

Nagi, R., Aravinda, K., Rakesh, N., Gupta, R., Pal, A., & Mann, A. K. (2020). Clinical applications and performance of intelligent systems in dental and maxillofacial radiology: A review. *Imaging Science in Dentistry*, *50*(2), 81. DOI: 10.5624/isd.2020.50.2.81 PMID: 32601582

Naidu, V., & Jaju, S. (2022). CAD/CAM engineering and Artificial Intelligence in dentistry. *IOP Conference Series. Materials Science and Engineering*, *1259*(1), 1–9. DOI: 10.1088/1757-899X/1259/1/012018

Nath, S., Raveendran, R., & Perumbure, S. (2022). Artificial Intelligence and its application in the early detection of oral cancers. *Clinical Cancer Investigation Journal*, *11*(1), 5–9. DOI: 10.51847/h7wa0UHoIF

Nwabuokei, I., Ghouse, M., Chen, W., Kollannur, E. T., Li, H., & Bin Sulaiman, R. (2023). Quantifying the Influence of Population on Carbon Emissions: A Comparative Study of Developed versus Developing Countries Using Machine Learning. *FMDB Transactions on Sustainable Energy Sequence*, *1*(2), 71–82.

Odoemena, O. F., & Elufidodo, G. A. (2024). Machine learning-based cardiovascular disease detection and intelligent healthcare workflow automation. *FMDB Transactions on Sustainable Health Science Letters*, *2*(2), 81–93. DOI: 10.69888/FTSHSL.2024.000174

Orhan, K., Bayrakdar, I. S., Ezhov, M., Kravtsov, A., & Özyürek, T. (2020). Evaluation of artificial Intelligence for detecting periapical pathosis on cone-beam computed tomography scans. *International Endodontic Journal*, *53*(5), 680–689. DOI: 10.1111/iej.13265 PMID: 31922612

Ossowska, A., Kusiak, A., & Świetlik, D. (2022). Artificial intelligence in dentistry-narrative review. *International Journal of Environmental Research and Public Health*, *19*(6), 3449. DOI: 10.3390/ijerph19063449 PMID: 35329136

Park, W. J., & Park, J.-B. (2018). History and application of artificial neural networks in dentistry. *European Journal of Dentistry*, *12*(04), 594–601. DOI: 10.4103/ejd.ejd_325_18 PMID: 30369809

Priscila, S. S., Rajest, S. S., Tadiboina, S. N., Regin, R., & András, S. (2023). Analysis of Machine Learning and Deep Learning Methods for Superstore Sales Prediction. *FMDB Transactions on Sustainable Computer Letters*, *1*(1), 1–11.

Rajest, S. S., Singh, B., Obaid, A. J., Regin, R., & Chinnusamy, K. (2023). *Advances in artificial and human intelligence in the modern era*. Advances in Computational Intelligence and Robotics. IGI Global., DOI: 10.4018/979-8-3693-1301-5

Ranjan, M., Tushar, , Parekh, N. H., Dixit, A., Rakshit, P., Agre, B. P., Badiyani, B. K., & Kumar, A. (2024). Investigating how cultural and socioeconomic factors influence oral cancer prevention behaviors, screening uptake, and treatment outcomes. *Journal of Pharmacy & Bioallied Sciences*, *16*(Suppl 1), S786–S788. DOI: 10.4103/jpbs.jpbs_1009_23 PMID: 38595407

Ranjan, M., Vashisht, A., Savita, J. K., Duseja, S., Sethi, A., Mohanty, R., Parekh, N. H., & Mehta, M. (2024). Evaluating the tightness of proximal contact between natural tooth and adjacent implant-supported prosthesis. *Bioinformation*, *20*(6), 644–648. DOI: 10.6026/973206300200644 PMID: 39131525

Ren, R., Luo, H., Su, C., Yao, Y., & Liao, W. (2021). Machine learning in dental, oral and craniofacial imaging: A review of recent progress. *PeerJ*, *9*(5), e11451. DOI: 10.7717/peerj.11451 PMID: 34046262

Rodrigues, J. A., Krois, J., & Schwendicke, F. (2021). Demystifying artificial intelligence and deep learning in dentistry. *Brazilian Oral Research*, *35*(8), e094. DOI: 10.1590/1807-3107bor-2021.vol35.0094 PMID: 34406309

Saxena, D., & Chaudhary, S. (2023). Predicting Brain Diseases from FMRI-Functional Magnetic Resonance Imaging with Machine Learning Techniques for Early Diagnosis and Treatment. *FMDB Transactions on Sustainable Computer Letters*, *1*(1), 33–48.

Schwendicke, F., Samek, W., & Krois, J. (2020). Artificial intelligence in dentistry: Chances and challenges. *Journal of Dental Research*, *99*(7), 769–774. DOI: 10.1177/0022034520915714 PMID: 32315260

Shan, T., Tay, F. R., & Gu, L. (2021). Application of artificial Intelligence in dentistry. *Journal of Dental Research*, *100*(3), 232–244. DOI: 10.1177/0022034520969115 PMID: 33118431

Sivapriya, G. B. V., Ganesh, U. G., Pradeeshwar, V., Dharshini, M., & Al-Amin, M. (2023). Crime Prediction and Analysis Using Data Mining and Machine Learning: A Simple Approach that Helps Predictive Policing. *FMDB Transactions on Sustainable Computer Letters*, *1*(2), 64–75.

Thakar, S., Kinariwala, N., Pandya, D., Parekh, N. H., Patel, N. K., & Patel, A. (2023). Awareness and constraints towards the implementation of green dentistry amongst dental students and private practitioners of West India. *Journal of Pharmacy & Bioallied Sciences*, *15*(Suppl 2), S1287–S1290. DOI: 10.4103/jpbs.jpbs_116_23 PMID: 37694014

Vemula, V. R. (2024). Cognitive artificial intelligence systems for proactive threat hunting in AI-driven cloud applications. *AVE Trends in Intelligent Computing Systems*, *1*(3), 173–183.

Chapter 18
Transforming Mental Wellness via Developing Mindful Machines With an AI Therapist Guidance

S. Rubin Bose
https://orcid.org/0000-0001-5560-8580
SRM Institute of Science and Technology, Ramapuram, India

Panjagala Divya
SRM Institute of Science and Technology, Ramapuram, India

J. Yohaan Manu
SRM Institute of Science and Technology, Ramapuram, India

M. Deebiga
SRM Institute of Science and Technology, Ramapuram, India

M. B. Sudhan
SRM Institute of Science and Technology, Ramapuram, India

R. Regin
https://orcid.org/0000-0002-6618-205X
SRM Institute of Science and Technology, Ramapuram, India

M. Kandan
Dhaanish Ahmed College of Engineering, India

ABSTRACT

The chapter introduces an innovative platform merging technology and mental health support, incorporating advanced AI models such as LSTM (Long Short-Term Memory) to enhance its capabilities. This concept envisions an AI-driven system employing sophisticated algorithms, including LSTM and natural language processing, to offer personalized guidance, therapeutic interventions, and accessible resources for emotional well-being. By leveraging LSTM models, the platform can analyze user input, understand emotions, sentiments, and intentions, and provide tailored support and interventions. Emphasizing 24/7 availability and privacy safeguards, the platform aims to complement traditional mental health services by providing immediate, tailored support and tracking users' progress. Ethical considerations and potential human professional intervention are also addressed to create a comprehensive and accessible approach to enhancing mental wellness.

DOI: 10.4018/979-8-3693-9420-5.ch018

INTRODUCTION

The chapter is an innovative initiative to revolutionize mental health care by integrating Artificial Intelligence (AI) technology. The main goal is to create an AI-driven platform that provides personalized and easily accessible mental health support. Leveraging cutting-edge AI advancements, this platform delivers continuous counseling, therapeutic interventions, and various tailored resources, addressing the gap between the demand for mental health services and their availability. While AI technology is increasingly utilized in physical health care, its adoption in mental health has been slower. Mental health practitioners rely more on interpersonal skills and direct patient interactions, with clinical data often subjective and qualitative (Tak and Sundararajan, 2023).

Nevertheless, the mental health field stands to gain significant benefits from AI technology. Clinical data in mental health often comprises subjective patient statements and written notes, yet the field stands to gain significantly from AI technology. AI holds promise in reshaping our understanding and diagnosis of mental illnesses. While an individual's bio-psycho-social profile offers the most comprehensive insight into their mental health, our understanding of the interactions within these systems remains limited. Mental illnesses exhibit considerable heterogeneity in their pathophysiology, and identifying biomarkers may lead to more precise definitions. Utilizing AI techniques can facilitate the development of improved screening tools and risk models for identifying predispositions to mental illness. Achieving personalized mental healthcare as a long-term objective requires harnessing computational approaches suitable for big data analysis. By exploiting cutting-edge advancements in AI, this platform provides round-the-clock counsel, therapeutic interventions, and a wealth of resources customized to individual needs, thus bridging the gap between the demand for mental health services and their availability.

LITERATURE REVIEW

Mental health apps and websites assist by tracking moods and offering meditation guidance. Some facilitated connections to therapists via messaging or video calls. However, a comprehensive AI-powered system functioning as a genuine therapist, like "Enhancing Mental Health Support: A Chatbot Powered by Natural Language Processing," was lacking. Although AI was beginning to be utilized, it was not yet fully developed for mental health support (Silvia Priscila et al., 2023).

Galderisi et al. (2015) introduced Generative AI applications in the Health and well-being Domain in March 2024. The article offers a comprehensive overview of the anticipated growth of AI in the Healthcare market by 2028. Natural Language Processing holds the potential for providing psychological counseling for social and mental health issues. Virtual and embodied bots are increasingly involved in managing emotions, stress, and outcomes at the intersection of healthcare professionals and patients (Venkatasubramanian et al., 2023). However, in the current state of technology for both virtual and embodied socially assistive robots (SARs), users interact with an artificial system operating based on pre-trained databases, providing only a temporary illusion of relational interaction. SARs can only sustain brief engagements, posing significant challenges for broader user acceptance. These databases may also contain biases related to situational, cultural, gender, racial, and other factors (Chandratreya, 2024).

Zhang et al. (2023) introduced Deploying AI Methods for Mental Health in Singapore. Hopes arise for individuals coping with severe mental illnesses as machine learning is utilized to forecast clinical conditions. Another endeavor midline.sg emerges as a platform dedicated to mental well-being within the general populace. This initiative caters to the requirements of individuals grappling with severe mental illnesses, as classified by the US National Institute of Mental Health (NIMH) as conditions causing significant functional impairment and hindering major life activities (Kumar et al., 2024). Simultaneously, the team addresses the mental wellness needs of the community through mental health promotion. The Singapore Association for Mental Health defines mental wellness as a positive mental state extending beyond the absence of mental illness, enabling individuals to think, feel, and act in ways that positively influence their physical and social well-being.

Huang et al. (2022) introduced a Mind Talker that explains how AI helps early-stage Dementia patients engage socially. Individuals living with Dementia face a heightened risk of social isolation, and conversational AI agents have the potential to alleviate their loneliness. Eight individuals engaged with MindTalker for one month or longer, with data gathered through interviews. Our results highlighted that participants appreciated the novelty of AI but desired more consistent and deeper interactions. They preferred a personal touch from AI while emphasizing the irreplaceable value of human interactions. These findings underscore the intricacies of AI engagement dynamics, with participants commenting on the artificial nature of AI, offering crucial insights into the future design of conversational AI for this demographic.

Minerva and Giubilini (2023) introduced the Ethics of Digital Well-Being in 2020. The discussion has focused on the development of AI applications for predicting treatment outcomes in internet-delivered Cognitive Behavioral Therapy for depression and anxiety. It presents a human-centered approach integrating insights from Human-Computer Interaction (HCI), AI, and healthcare to tackle specific challenges in designing AI tools for mental health contexts. In the realm of mental health, both practical barriers (such as geographic location) and societal barriers prevent people from accessing treatment. Even among those who manage to overcome some of the most commonly cited barriers to care, there remains a shortage of providers compared to the demand for assistance. Therefore, there is an unmet need for a significant improvement in mental health services, which chatbots could potentially address. Despite extensive discussion of the negative possibilities, the paragraph underscores the importance of AI in mental health care (Obeta et al., 2024).

Graham et al. (2019) introduced Designing human-centered AI for mental health. The article outlines the hurdles in creating AI systems capable of delivering psychotherapy, emphasizing the importance of understanding the effectiveness of human-delivered therapy, the feasibility of forming therapeutic bonds with non-human agents, and the constraints of narrow AI in handling intricate therapeutic tasks. Despite these obstacles, the authors believe progress is achievable through a mindful approach to developing AI-based psychotherapy. They elaborate on how this analysis and the resulting design principles facilitated the integration of prediction models into a production interface. Addressing the identified risks of excessive reliance on AI outputs, the necessity for balanced information assessment, and a focus on personalized care, the authors discuss and contemplate what constitutes a responsible, human-centered approach to AI design within this healthcare domain (Hariharan et al., 2024).

Margam (2023) introduced an article in 2023, Role of AI and Machine Learning in Mental Healthcare is pivotal, with numerous brain illnesses effectively diagnosed through AI technologies. This study aims to consolidate findings from previous research on the effectiveness of AI models in identifying mental health issues. Specifically, it examines AI chatbots delivered via Smartphone Applications and their potential societal implications. Moreover, it adds to the expanding literature on how AI can bolster mental health support. The literature review delves into AI's utilization in healthcare and explores its applications in mental health. However, societal acceptance is essential for AI chatbots and SMHApps to be genuinely impactful, and appropriate regulatory measures must be implemented to mitigate potential risks (Paramasivan et al., 2024). The paper also explores target demographics and emphasizes the importance of machine learning algorithms in crafting effective models, alongside recommendations for future research avenues.

Lavrentyeva (2022) introduced an article in 2023, Beyond the Asylum Walls, that explores the evolution of mental health therapies from traditional to modern methods, emphasizing human rights and cultural sensitivity. The paragraph explores the diverse and evidence-based nature of contemporary approaches, which include advancements like virtual environments. Cultural competency remains crucial, and the future promises further innovation through telepsychiatry and artificial intelligence (Sengupta et al., 2023). The ultimate aim is to cultivate a society that prioritizes, celebrates, and values mental health. Amidst the escalating refugee movements and the resulting tragedies at borders, European nations opt to construct more barriers instead of providing refuge. Instead of proposing a new theoretical or conceptual framework, this article aims to critically analyze these border practices and their underlying material and discursive foundations, drawing upon the frameworks provided by critical border studies.

Van Cuylenburg et al. (2021) introduced Deploying AI Methods for Mental Health in Singapore; the paragraph describes three digital health initiatives in Singapore leveraging machine learning and AI for mental health. Project HOPES, which began as an observational study on the digital characteristics of schizophrenia patients, now assists in early patient prioritization and predicting clinical status. Mindline.sg provides mental wellness resources, including self-assessments and an AI chatbot, accessed by 10 to 20% of the national population by 2023. Let's Talk, an online peer-support mental health network, supports over 80,000 users with trained moderators and therapists, employing generative models to assist therapists in offering pertinent resources.

Huang et al. (2022) introduced an article in 2024; the chapter discusses the growing demand for AI in healthcare due to population aging, presenting various opportunities for generative AI in research, clinical, operational, and behavioral applications. The paragraph delves into the obstacles faced in behavioral applications, specifically in examining extensive datasets for client behavior trends to enhance engagement and welfare. Natural language processing is underscored for its capability to offer psychological counseling and aid. Nevertheless, existing technological constraints in virtual and physically embodied socially assistive robots (SARs) lead to short interactions and potential biases in pre-established databases. The forthcoming progress hinges on specialized language models (NLMs), necessitating cooperation among involved parties for successful deployment. Furthermore, assistive technologies ought to be incorporated into healthcare professional training.

Oh (2016) introduced an article in 2020; the paper introduces the concept of Personalized Mental Health Navigation (MHN), a therapist-in-the-loop cybernetic system aimed at providing personalized mental health treatment (Chitra et al., 2024). MHN employs wearable and mobile technology to assess, estimate, and direct individuals toward mental well-being. It stresses the significance of capturing an individual's comprehensive mental health model over time, incorporating various layers of knowledge such as emotion, biology, sociology, behavior, and cognition. A preliminary case study illustrates the viability of MHN in reducing stress and managing depression among college students, showcasing proactive interventions customized to each person's requirements. MHN seeks to revolutionize mental healthcare from a reactive, sporadic approach to a continuous, individualized paradigm.

Oh (2017) published AI in Mental Health: Predictive Analytics and Intervention Strategies. The article underscores the growing utilization of artificial intelligence (AI) in medical domains such as oncology and radiology while acknowledging its restricted implementation in mental healthcare and neurobiological studies. It stresses the pressing requirement for AI to assist in identifying individuals at high risk and delivering interventions for psychiatric conditions, given the scarcity of mental health professionals. Despite limited exploration in neuropsychiatry, the potential for AI to transform diagnosis, prediction, and intervention approaches in mental health is encouraging, as outlined in the paper addressing predictive analytics and intervention strategies (Kler et al., 2024).

Cho et al. (2014) introduced Ethics of Digital Well-Being: A Multidisciplinary Approach, 207-219, 2020. Approach, 207-219, 2020 The article discusses the creation of AI applications for forecasting treatment outcomes in internet-delivered Cognitive Behavioral Therapy (CBT) for depression and anxiety. It presents a human-centered strategy incorporating insights from Human-Computer Interaction (HCI), AI, and healthcare to tackle specific challenges in crafting AI tools for mental health settings. Through interviews and design workshops with iCBT advocates, the research underscores the influence of design decisions on AI predictions, advocate motivation, and sense of control. The results underscore the significance of a responsible, human-centered approach to AI design in mental healthcare.

Kothuru (2023) introduced Artificial Intelligence for Mental Health Care in 2021, and the use of AI in mental health care and neurobiological research has been modest. Given the significant morbidity and mortality rates among individuals with psychiatric disorders, alongside a worsening shortage of mental health care providers, there is an urgent necessity for AI to assist in identifying high-risk individuals and providing interventions to prevent and treat mental illnesses (Bala Kuta and Bin Sulaiman, 2023). Although published research on AI in neuropsychiatry is relatively scarce, there is a growing number of successful instances where AI has been utilized with brain imaging, sensor-based monitoring systems, and social media platforms to predict, classify, or subgroup mental illnesses, as well as issues such as suicidality. Despite these advancements, AI must address concerns regarding bias, privacy, transparency, and other ethical considerations while potentially reshaping the understanding of mental illnesses, identifying them early, personalizing treatments, and empowering patients in their care. These objectives align with human wisdom, pivotal in individual and societal well-being.

Santhosh et al. (2023) introduced Minding the AI in 2022. Health tools utilizing AI present particular challenges for regulation, both in terms of the technical aspects and because many of the applications may be used outside of healthcare settings and thus are outside of the traditional frameworks for regulating health issues. AI presents opportunities to tackle existing inequalities in mental health care. Safeguarding patients and other users of mental health AI tools from potential misuse of their health information and adverse consequences of data sharing is another vital area of concern.

Tak and Sundararajan (2023).introduced the idea of a phone being your therapist. There has been an explosion of digital interventions that aim to supplement or replace face-to-face mental health services. More recently, various automated conversational agents have become available, interacting with users in real-life conversations. From the perspective of young individuals, we discuss the strengths and limitations of using chatbots in mental health support. Additionally, we delineate what we view as the minimum ethical standards for these platforms, covering issues related to privacy and confidentiality, effectiveness, and safety. We assess three existing platforms based on our proposed framework (Woebot, Joy, and Wysa). Our aim is for this article to spark ethical discussions among app developers, professionals, young people, and other stakeholders, encouraging ethically responsible practices in digital mental health.

In the context of the evolving mental health care landscape, a growing disparity emerges between the increasing demand for mental wellness support and the limited accessibility of traditional therapeutic services (Vashishtha and Dhawan, 2023). This disparity necessitates innovative solutions. The "Mindful Machine," an AI Therapist, aims to tackle this issue by utilizing artificial intelligence to offer scalable, personalized, and accessible mental health support. Nonetheless, developing and implementing such a system presents challenges related to ethics, privacy, user trust, and the necessity for a comprehensive understanding of mental health nuances. Insufficient additional information provided in existing apps exacerbates this issue. This problem statement seeks to delineate and address these challenges, laying the groundwork for effective solutions in AI-driven mental wellness support.

METHODOLOGY

Accurately gathering and analyzing data from various sources is essential for constructing a dataset for the model. Precision in data collection facilitates informed business decisions, ensures quality assurance, and maintains research integrity. Furthermore, data can be categorized into qualitative and quantitative types. Qualitative data encompasses descriptions such as color, size, quality, and appearance, while quantitative data involves numbers such as statistics, poll numbers, percentages, etc. Although the concept of data collection is not new, the landscape has evolved significantly. Today, a wealth of data is available in previously unimaginable forms, necessitating adaptation and growth in data collection to keep pace with technological advancements. Various data collection tools, such as Word Association, Sentence Completion, Role Playing, In-Person Surveys, Mobile Surveys, and Observation, contribute to this evolving landscape (Figure 1).

Figure 1. Functional Block diagram of Mindful Machines using LSTM Model

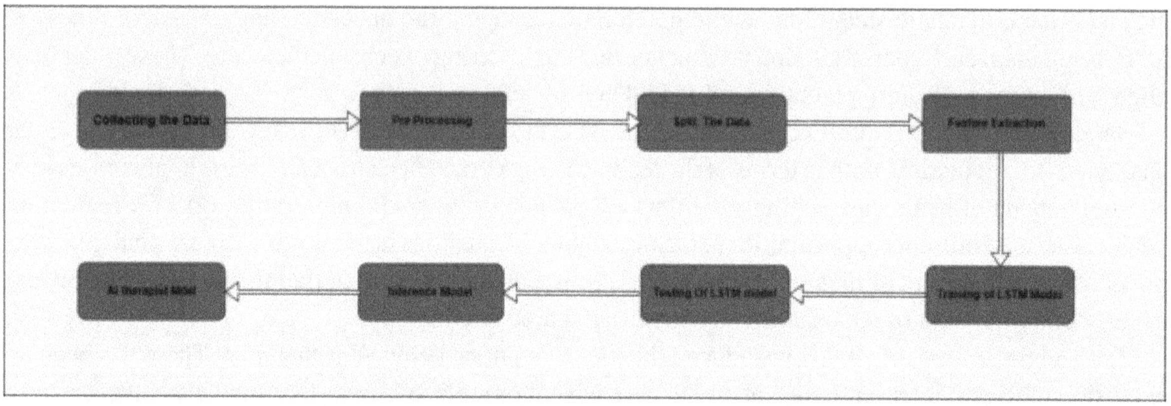

The collected raw data undergoes preprocessing to prepare for Long Short Term Memory (LSTM). This involves cleaning, transforming, and integrating the data to ready it for analysis. Data preprocessing aims to enhance data quality and suitability for specific data mining tasks. The preprocessing pipeline utilized can significantly impact the outcomes of subsequent analyses, highlighting the importance of data representation and quality before analysis. Data preprocessing is a crucial phase in machine learning projects, particularly in computational biology. High levels of irrelevant or redundant information and noisy or unreliable data can complicate knowledge discovery during training. Consequently, data preparation and filtering steps may require substantial processing time.

Data splitting is a crucial aspect of this model, especially for constructing data-based models. It involves dividing the data into two subsets: one for testing and the other for training. Additionally, the data may be split into more than two subsets. The testing dataset is utilized post-training to assess the model's performance. In machine learning, data is commonly divided into three or more sets, with the additional set, often referred to as the dev set, used for adjusting learning process parameters. Data splitting prevents overfitting, where a model fits the training data excessively and struggles to generalize to new data. Typically, the original data in a machine-learning model is divided into three or four sets.

Feature extraction, accomplished through Machine Learning and Data Analysis, involves identifying pertinent features from raw data. These features are subsequently utilized to enhance dataset informativeness for tasks such as Classification and Prediction. The initial raw data set is partitioned and condensed into more manageable subsets, facilitating easier processing. Notably, large datasets often entail numerous variables, demanding substantial computing resources. Feature extraction addresses this challenge by selecting and combining variables into features, effectively reducing data volume. This technique proves beneficial when dealing with extensive datasets, aiming to minimize resource usage without compromising essential information. Moreover, feature extraction aids in reducing redundant data, streamlining model-building efforts, and accelerating learning and generalization processes in machine learning. Reducing the data helps build the model with less machine effort and increases the speed of learning and generalization steps in the machine learning process.

Training the LSTM Model includes memory consumption, which can be mitigated by employing Mini Batches. These batches, subsets of the training data, are fed to the model during each iteration, enabling parallelized computation and more frequent model parameter updates. Selecting the appropriate size for mini-batches is crucial, as excessively small or large batches can impact convergence and model accuracy. To prevent overfitting, dropout can be utilized wherein the model learns noise or specific training data patterns rather than general features. Additionally, Bidirectional LSTMs, comprising two LSTMs processing input sequences in both forward and backward directions, can capture more contextual information and dependencies, accessing past and future states.

Expanding the number of timesteps or lagging features to forecast the label can be effective, but only to a certain extent. Increasing epochs can prolong computation unnecessarily if the approach is flawed. Reducing the number of epochs may be beneficial if your algorithm is correctly configured. With the right algorithm, optimal loss values can typically be achieved within 20–25 epochs. To refine your algorithm for improved accuracy and precision, utilize early stopping to monitor a specific loss metric, preferably Root Mean Squared Error (RMSE) for LSTMs. Incorporating Batch Normalization has demonstrated enhanced algorithm performance. The Inference Application Model is employed to generate results. Model inference, or deploying the model into a production environment, marks the phase where the model executes its designated task in the live business environment. Deploying the model involves transitioning it to a live environment where it processes new and unseen data, distinct from the model training phase typically conducted locally or offline. LSTM model inference is typically overseen by a separate team from the one that trained the model.

The AI Therapist Model utilizes automated, text-based conversations to deliver mental health assistance. For individuals who prefer to avoid direct human interaction, AI is a non-intrusive and non-judgmental platform for seeking support. Virtual assistants and chatbots offer an alternative avenue for expressing emotions and discussing mental health concerns. AI-driven algorithms analyze patient data to prioritize high-risk cases and distribute resources efficiently, thereby reducing inefficiencies in the mental health system and ensuring timely, targeted support for those in need. While therapy chatbots may provide accessible tools for managing mental health, concerns persist regarding their effectiveness and ethical implications in addressing the complex emotional needs of individuals.

LSTM

The model comprises interconnected layers aimed at efficiently processing and understanding sequential speech input. At its core lies the LSTM layer, composed of stacked LSTM cells. These cells specialized recurrent neural network units, retain information across extended sequences crucial for detecting temporal relationships in speech signals. Each LSTM cell maintains hidden states, enabling the model to learn and recall patterns over multiple time steps. After the LSTM layer, fully connected (FC) layers extract additional high-level features and representations from the sequential data. ReLU activation functions follow each FC layer to introduce nonlinearity and facilitate the model's learning of intricate mappings between input characteristics and emotional states. The final output layer, incorporating a softmax activation function, produces the model's predictions by modeling the probability distribution across various emotion classes. This architecture empowers the model to effectively learn and discern emotional cues in voice signals, offering valuable insights into speakers' underlying emotional states. In natural language processing (NLP) and sequence modeling tasks, such as language translation, text generation, and sentiment analysis, conventional RNNs often encounter difficulty retaining information over lengthy sequences due to the vanishing gradient problem. This issue arises as gradients propagated through numerous time steps during backpropagation can diminish significantly, leading to the model forgetting earlier information (Figure 2).

Figure 2. Architectural Block Diagram of LSTM mode

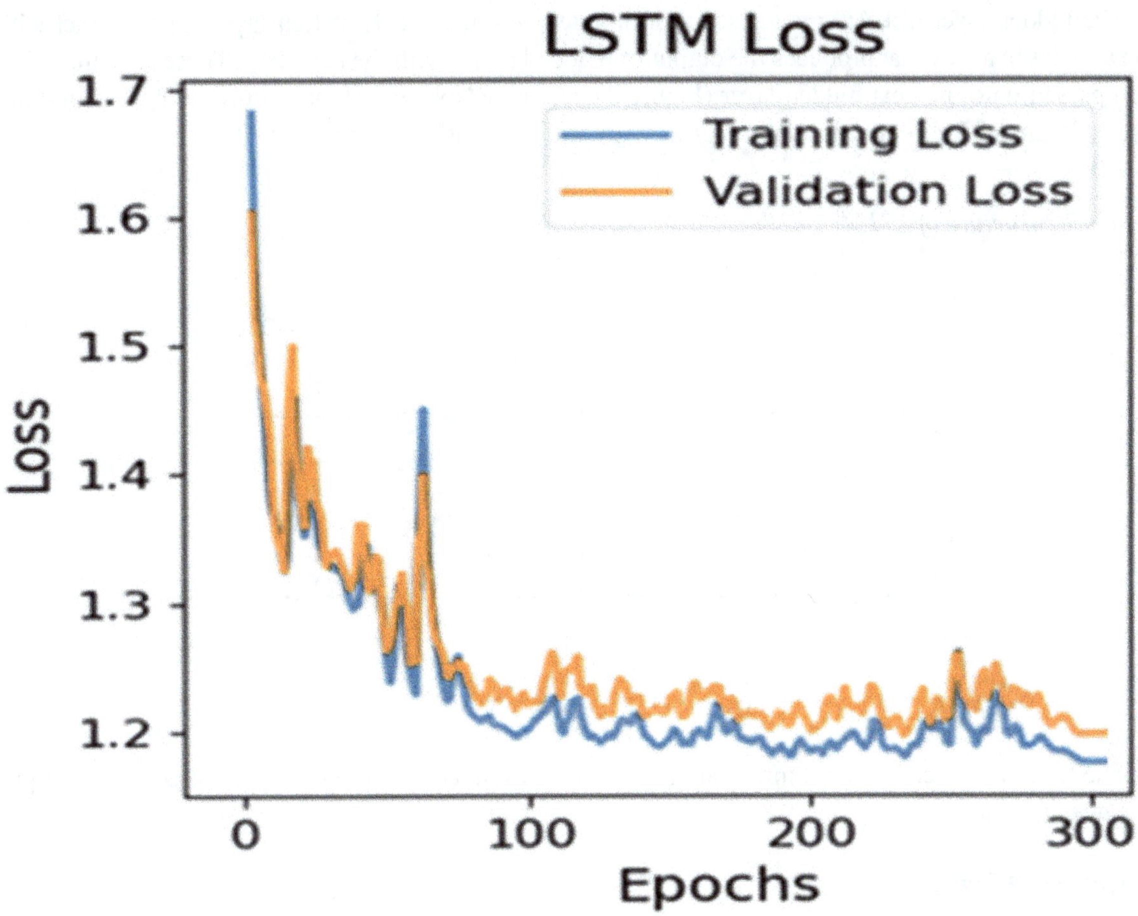

Preprocessing: In this stage, our system conducts word segmentation, part-of-speech tagging, named entity recognition, dependency parsing, and semantic role label parsing. As the subsequent sections detail, this data is crucial for simplifying sentences and generating questions.

Sentence Simplification: Our method utilizes transformation processes to simplify the original sentence. This involves eliminating parentheses, which serve as explanatory or qualifying remarks within a sentence and lack clear dependent relations with other sentence elements. Additionally, adverbial modifiers located between commas and certain types of phrases, such as sentence-level modifying phrases (e.g., manner adverb), are removed. However, there are instances where we retain specific adverbial modifiers, particularly if they contain information about a person's name, place, number, or time, as this information can be utilized to generate potential questions.

Experimental Setup

The hidden layer of LSTM is a gated unit or gated cell. It consists of four layers that interact with one another in a way that produces the output of that cell along with the cell state. These two things are then passed onto the next hidden layer (Figure 3). Unlike RNNs, which have only a single neural net layer of tanh, LSTMs comprise three logistic sigmoid gates and one tanh layer.

Figure 3. Structure of LSTM

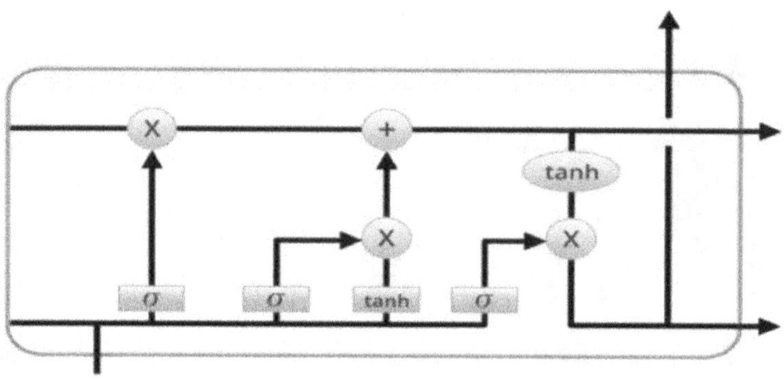

The task of extracting useful information from the current cell state will be presented as the output gate does output.

Training of Data

Data Collection: Collect a sizable dataset of conversational text. This may involve chat logs, transcripts, or any other dialogue appropriate for your chatbot's purpose. Prepare the data for training by tokenizing it into individual words or sub-words, removing punctuation, converting text to lowercase, and possibly performing other text-cleaning operations. Additionally, encoding the text into numerical vectors may be necessary. Arrange the data into fixed-length sequences depicting a series of words or tokens. These sequences will serve as input to the LSTM model. Additionally, prepare target sequences that are shifted by a one-time step to train the model in predicting the next word/token in a sequence. Convert the integer-encoded words/tokens into dense vectors (embeddings) utilizing an embedding layer. This process aids the model in understanding the connections between words within a continuous vector space.

Validation of the data

Throughout training, regularly assess the performance of the LSTM model on the validation set, such as after each epoch. If no further improvement or performance declines, it could suggest potential overfitting or convergence problems. Utilize the validation set to adjust hyperparameters like learning rate, batch size, LSTM layer size, dropout rate, etc. Explore various values for these hyperparameters and select the ones that produce optimal performance on the validation set. Besides quantitative metrics, qualitative assessment is performed by manually examining model-generated responses from the validation set. Assess whether the responses are relevant, coherent, and contextually appropriate. Consider using ensemble methods to combine multiple LSTM models or other architectures to improve performance. Ensemble methods often result in more robust and reliable models. Consider employing ensemble methods to merge multiple LSTM models or alternative architectures to enhance performance. Ensemble methods frequently lead to more resilient and dependable models. If the dataset is restricted, think about utilizing methods such as k-fold cross-validation for a more dependable evaluation of the model's performance. This process entails dividing the dataset into k subsets and training/testing the model k times, with each iteration using a different subset for testing and the remainder for training/validation.

RESULT AND DISCUSSION

It's crucial to summarize the methodology's results, assess the developed system's performance, and contemplate the broader impacts. The objective is to raise awareness and comprehension regarding artificial intelligence's transformative influence on mental health care. By exploring AI's potential, readers will acquire insights into its ability to tackle significant challenges, provide personalized interventions, facilitate early detection, and offer remote support. The article also underscores prevailing trends and the significance of ethical considerations and data privacy in advancing responsible AI adoption, ultimately nurturing trust and contributing to a future where mental well-being support is accessible, efficacious, and compassionate for all individuals (Table 1).

Table 1. Performance metrics of an AI therapist model using LSTM for mental well-being

Epochs	Training				Validation			
	Accuracy (%)	Precision (%)	Recall (%)	F1-Score (%)	Accuracy (%)	Precision (%)	Recall (%)	F1-Score (%)
300	99.59	99.59	99.59	99.59	96.96	97.01	96.96	96.96
200	89.08	89.13	89.08	89.06	84.89	85.60	84.89	84.06
150	84.89	85.60	84.89	84.06	71.88	70.95	71.88	71.11
100	83.42	83.69	83.42	83.31	70.83	69.78	70.83	69.89
50	82.86	82.95	82.86	82.80	67.71	60.1	67.71	62.39

Assessing the LSTM model's performance across varying numbers of training epochs uncovers insightful trends. The model consistently attains high accuracy, precision, recall, and F1-score on the training set, with accuracy ranging from 82.86% to 99.59%. This suggests the model effectively learns from the training data and makes accurate predictions. However, on the validation set, there's a noticeable decline in performance, with accuracy ranging from 67.71% to 96.96%. This indicates potential overfitting to the training data, resulting in a lack of generalization to unseen data. Despite the decrease in performance, the model maintains relatively high precision, recall, and F1-score on the validation set, suggesting it still performs reasonably well, albeit not as robustly as on the training set. Various strategies can be utilized to mitigate the observed overfitting, including regularization techniques, dropout, or early stopping. These approaches prevent the model from memorizing the training data and encourage it to learn more generalized patterns. Such techniques can significantly enhance the model's capacity to generalize to unseen data, improving overall performance.

Additionally, fine-tuning hyperparameters and optimizing the model architecture could also contribute to bolstering its generalization capabilities. Although the LSTM model exhibits strong performance on the training dataset, there is a potential enhancement to ensure its resilience and dependability in real-world scenarios. Artificial intelligence holds the potential to transform mental health care (Figure 4(a) and (b)). By providing personalized treatment strategies, detecting symptoms early, and offering continuous virtual support, AI-driven interventions bring significant advantages to mental well-being. Nonetheless, it's vital to prioritize ethical concerns, guaranteeing data privacy, transparency, and a balanced approach that integrates human care. Through the thoughtful adoption of AI, we can envision a future where mental health assistance is accessible, compassionate, and inclusive, nurturing an environment where everyone can flourish on their mental health path (Figure 4(c) and (d)).

Figure 4. a: Training and Validation Loss

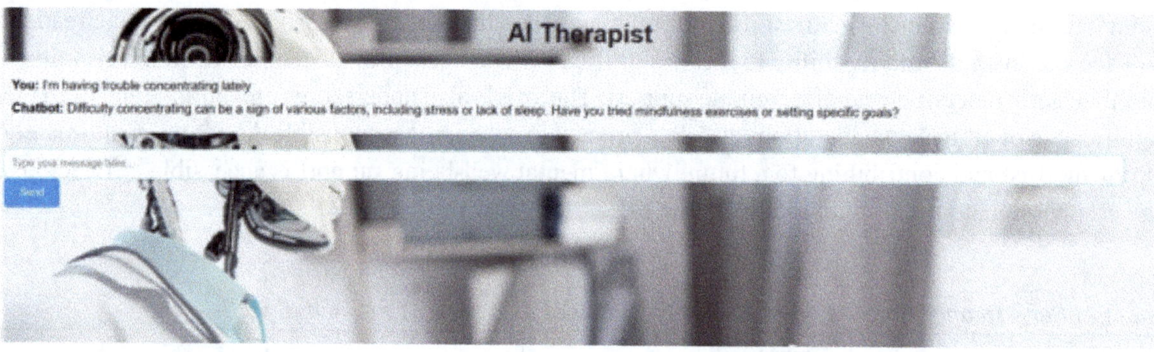

Figure 5. b: Training and Validation Accuracy

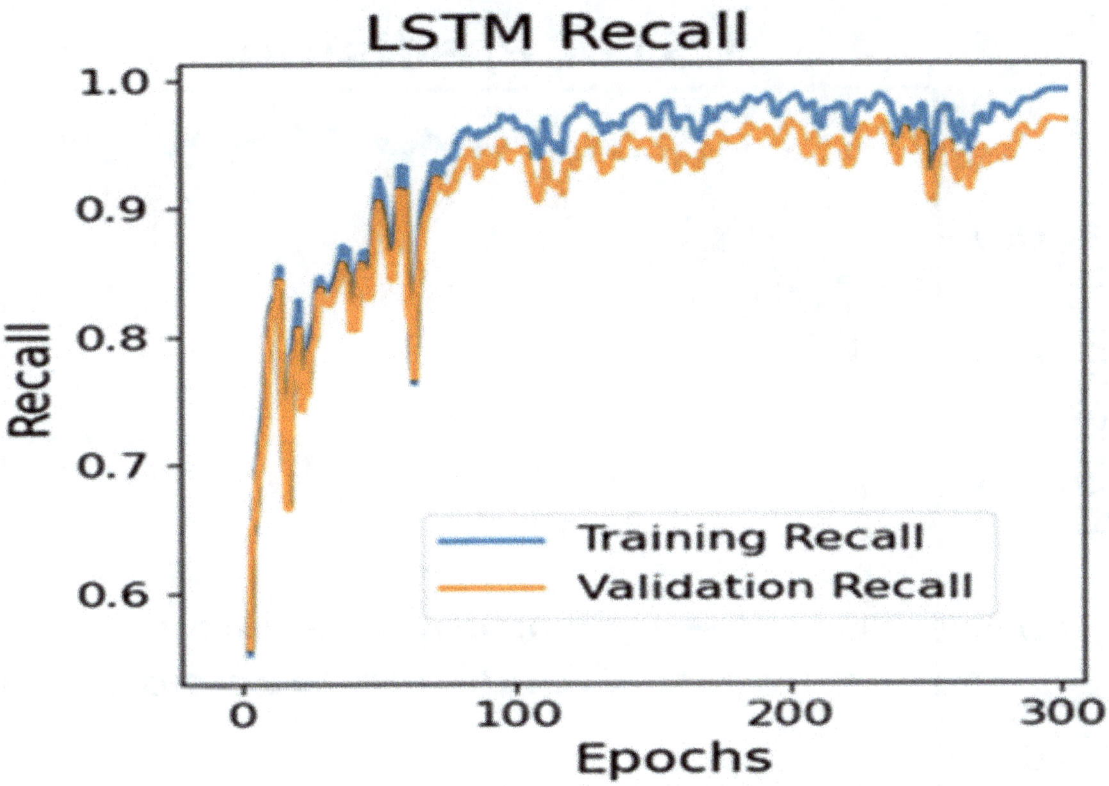

Figure 6. c: Training and Validation Precision

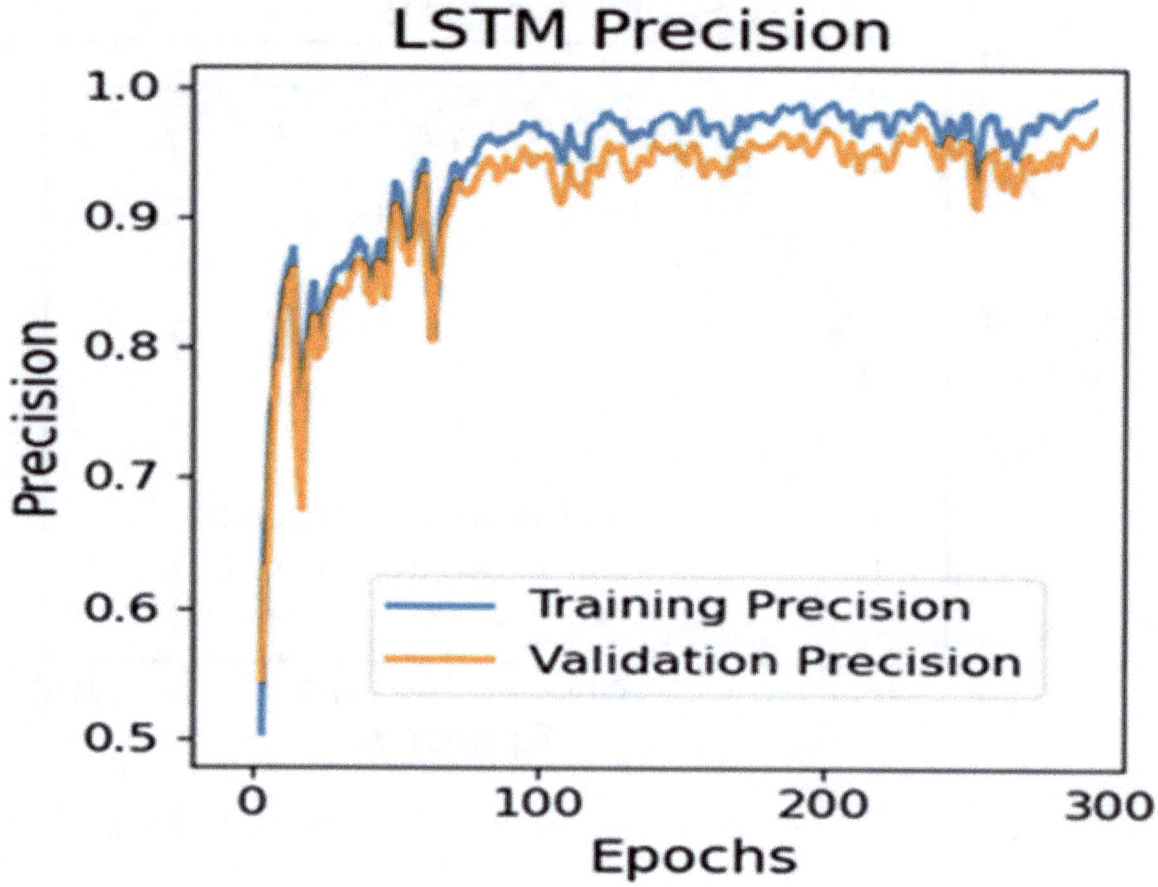

Figure 7. d: Training and Validation Recall of LSTM model.

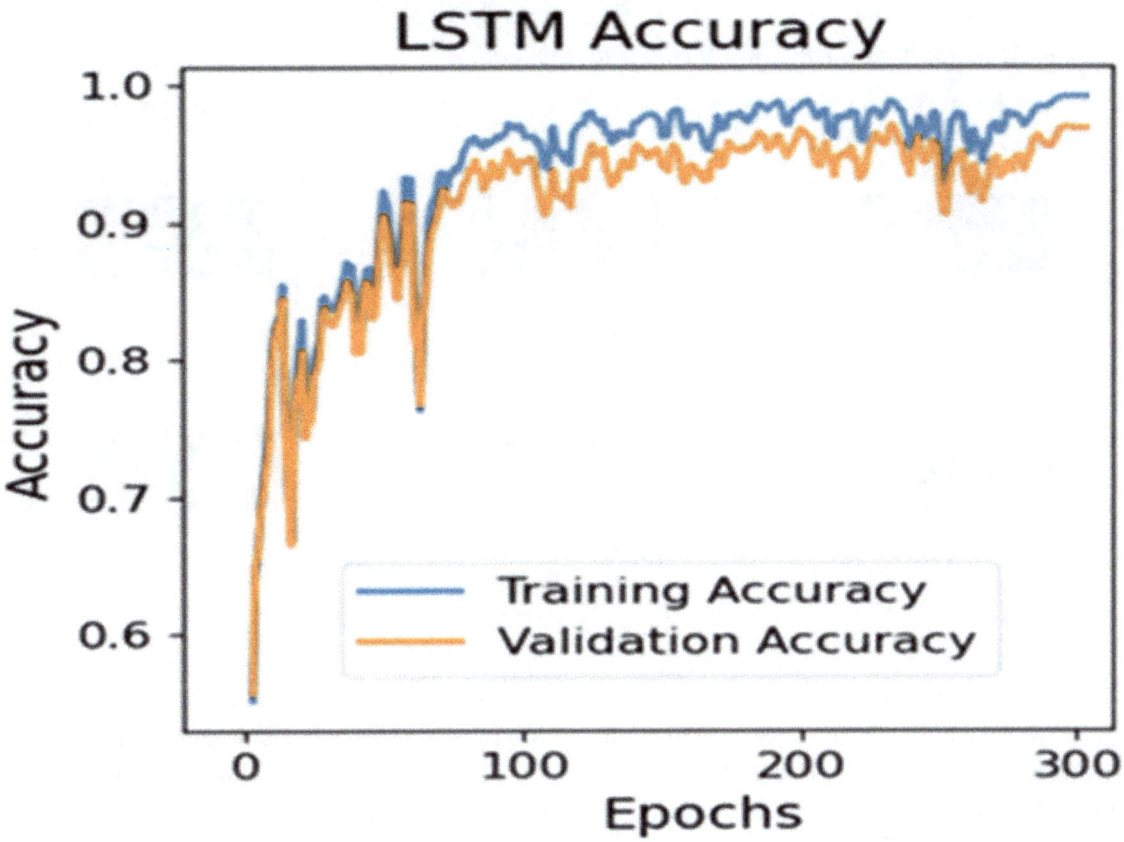

When evaluating the performance of our LSTM model, we examined several important metrics such as accuracy, loss, precision-recall curves, and other evaluation criteria. Firstly, we computed the model's accuracy on the training, validation, and test datasets. The training accuracy gauges the proportion of correctly predicted labels on the training dataset, whereas the validation accuracy assesses the model's performance on data it hasn't encountered during training. Ultimately, the test accuracy evaluates the model's performance on unseen data. Secondly, we calculated the loss metrics for our LSTM model. The training loss reflects the mean loss computed during the training phase on the training dataset, while the validation loss quantifies the mean loss on the validation dataset. Likewise, the test loss signifies the mean loss on the test dataset. Additionally, precision-recall curves were generated to depict the balance between precision and recall across various threshold values. Precision-recall curves evaluate the model's capability to make pertinent predictions while mitigating false positives.

Finally, we reported other evaluation metrics such as precision, recall, F1-Score, and ROC-AUC. Precision represents the fraction of relevant instances among the retrieved instances, while recall measures the fraction of relevant instances retrieved over the total amount of relevant instances. The F1-Score is the harmonic mean of precision and recall, providing a balanced assessment of the model's performance. ROC-AUC (Receiver Operating Characteristic - Area Under the Curve) is another important metric that evaluates the model's ability to distinguish between classes. These metrics collectively offer a comprehensive evaluation of the LSTM model's performance.

Figure 8. AI therapist for mental well-being web Application

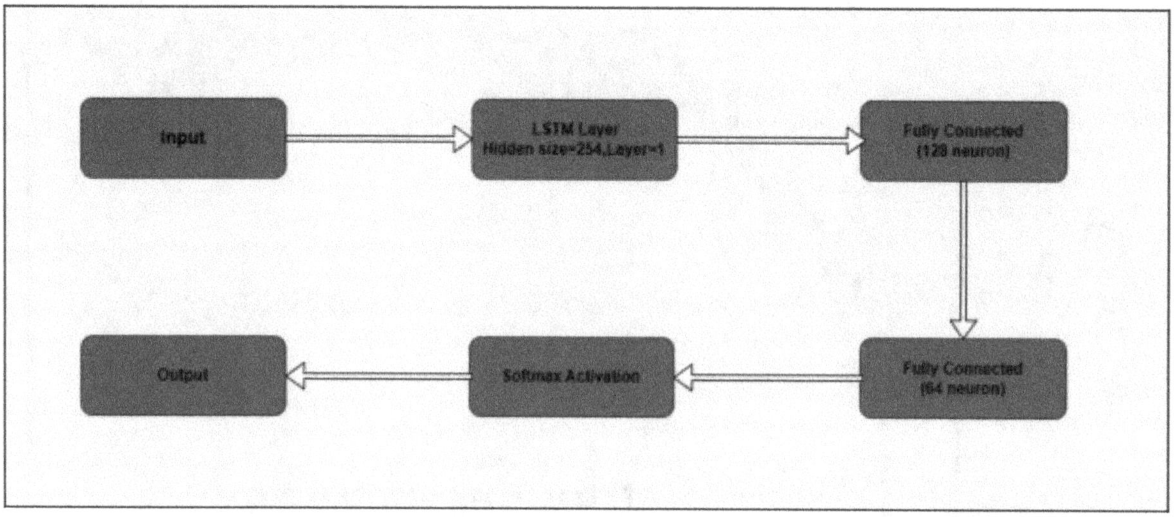

Figure 5 illustrates the AI therapist for mental well-being web Application. An AI therapist for mental well-being leverages advanced technologies such as long-term memory (LSTM) and machine learning to provide personalized support and guidance to individuals struggling with mental health issues. These digital platforms offer a safe and non-judgmental space for users to express their thoughts, feelings, and concerns through natural language conversations. By analyzing user input, AI therapists can understand emotions, sentiments, and intentions, allowing them to offer relevant insights, coping strategies, and resources tailored to the individual's needs. One of the significant advantages of AI therapists is their round-the-clock availability, ensuring that users can access support whenever they need it, without the constraints of scheduling appointments or travel time. Additionally, AI therapists provide anonymity and privacy, enabling users to discuss sensitive issues without the fear of stigma or privacy breaches.

While AI therapists are not meant to substitute human therapists, they enhance traditional therapy by providing supplementary support and guidance between therapy sessions. These platforms widen access to mental health assistance for individuals who may encounter obstacles such as cost, location, or the stigma associated with traditional therapy. AI therapists continuously learn and refine their responses based on user interactions and feedback, ensuring that the assistance provided remains accurate and beneficial over time. By offering evidence-based therapeutic techniques and principles, AI therapists equip users with valuable tools and resources to manage their mental health effectively. With their scalability, accessibility, and personalized approach, AI therapists have the potential to transform the delivery of mental health support, fostering overall well-being on a larger scale.

CONCLUSION

The chapter signifies a significant advancement in merging technology and mental health support. By integrating sophisticated AI models like LSTM (Long Short-Term Memory), the platform delivers tailored guidance, therapeutic interventions, and readily available resources for emotional well-being. Utilizing LSTM models enables the analysis of user input, comprehension of emotions, sentiments, and intentions, and the delivery of personalized support and interventions. Prioritizing daily accessibility, privacy protections, and user progress tracking, the platform seeks to supplement traditional mental health services effectively. By addressing ethical concerns and allowing for potential human professional involvement, this innovative approach offers a comprehensive and accessible solution to enhance mental wellness. As technology progresses, incorporating LSTM models in mental health support signifies a promising path for delivering timely, effective, personalized assistance to those in need. The model delivers support responsibly and inclusively by prioritizing ethical considerations, bias mitigation, and user privacy. As technology advances, the AI therapist model is a valuable tool for promoting mental well-being and enhancing individuals worldwide' access to mental health resources.

REFERENCES

Bala Kuta, Z., & Bin Sulaiman, R. (2023). Analysing Healthcare Disparities in Breast Cancer: Strategies for Equitable Prevention, Diagnosis, and Treatment among Minority Women. *FMDB Transactions on Sustainable Health Science Letters*, *1*(3), 130–143.

Chandratreya, A. (2024). Psychological impacts of climate change and environmental degradation on mental well-being. *FMDB Transactions on Sustainable Techno Learning*, *2*(2), 75–87. DOI: 10.69888/FTSTL.2024.000208

Chitra, A., Rajpriya, R., Karras, D. A., & Sridharlakshmi, N. R. B. (2024). An Exhaustive Study of Parasitic Organisms and Pathological Effects on Human Health. *AVE Trends In Intelligent Health Letters*, *1*(1), 10–18.

Cho, K., van Merrienboer, B., Gulcehre, C., Bahdanau, D., Bougares, F., Schwenk, H., & Bengio, Y. (2014). Learning phrase representations using RNN encoder–decoder for statistical machine translation. *Proceedings of the 2014 Conference on Empirical Methods in Natural Language Processing (EMNLP)*, Doha, Qatar. DOI: 10.3115/v1/D14-1179

Galderisi, S., Heinz, A., Kastrup, M., Beezhold, J., & Sartorius, N. (2015). Toward a new definition of mental health. *World Psychiatry; Official Journal of the World Psychiatric Association (WPA)*, *14*(2), 231–233. DOI: 10.1002/wps.20231 PMID: 26043341

Graham, S., Depp, C., Lee, E. E., Nebeker, C., Tu, X., Kim, H.-C., & Jeste, D. V. (2019). Artificial intelligence for mental health and mental illnesses: An overview. *Current Psychiatry Reports*, *21*(11), 116. DOI: 10.1007/s11920-019-1094-0 PMID: 31701320

Hariharan, M. G., Saranya, S., Velavan, P., Soji, E. S., Rajest, S. S., & Thammareddi, L. (2024). Utilization of artificial intelligence algorithms for advanced cancer detection in the healthcare domain. In *Advances in Medical Technologies and Clinical Practice* (pp. 287–302). IGI Global.

Huang, J. A., Hartanti, I. R., Colin, M. N., & Pitaloka, D. A. (2022). Telemedicine and artificial intelligence to support self-isolation of COVID-19 patients: Recent updates and challenges. *Digital Health*, *8*(4), 1–10. DOI: 10.1177/20552076221100634 PMID: 35603328

Kler, R., Jamoliddinov, J., Nematjonov, J., Kadirov, I., & Muzaffarov, M. (2024). Locating contribution of health and education in regional growth in Uzbekistan. *AVE Trends In Intelligent Techno Learning*, *1*(1), 11–22.

Kothuru, S. K. (2023). Emerging Technologies for Health and Wellness Monitoring at Home. *FMDB Transactions on Sustainable Health Science Letters*, *1*(4), 208–218.

Kumar, M. P. N. V., Chitra, A., Rajpriya, R., Gayathri, B., Roberts, C., & Rajest, S. S. (2024). Brain-optimized U-Net model for intraretinal cystoid fluid segmentation in optical coherence tomography. *AVE Trends in Intelligent Health Letters*, *1*(1), 38–50.

Lavrentyeva, Y. (2022). The big promise AI holds for mental health. *Emerging Tech Analyst*, *10*(1), 1–7.

Margam, R. (n.d.). Importance of Cybersecurity in Electronic Health Records. *Int. J. Innovative Sci. and Research Technol*, *8*(7), 24–28.

. Minerva, F., & Giubilini, A. (2023). Is AI the future of mental healthcare? Topoi: An International Review of Philosophy, 1–9.

Obeta, U. M., Mantu, E. C., Orshio, D. A., Obeta, N. L., & Sara, S. B. V. J. (2024). Social theories for diagnosis and management of HIV in Nigerian healthcare. *AVE Trends in Intelligent Health Letters*, *1*(2), 82–91.

Oh, K. (2016). Morpheme embedding for paraphrase extraction. In KIISE KCC2016, South Korea.

Oh, K. (2017). Machine learning Based Boundary Detection and Dictionary Expansion for Named Entity Recognition in Dialogues. Korea Computer Congress, Korean Institute of Information Scientists and Engineers (KIISE). South Korea.

Paramasivan, P., Rajest, S. S., Chinnusamy, K., Regin, R., & John Joseph, F. J. (Eds.). (2024). Advances in Medical Technologies and Clinical Practice *Clinical and comparative research on maternal health.* IGI Global., DOI: 10.4018/979-8-3693-5941-9

Santhosh, S., Krishna, B., Al-Amin, M., & Pradeep, V. (2023). Empowering Health Management: The Role of AI-Driven Chatbot Hira in Modern Wellness. *FMDB Transactions on Sustainable Technoprise Letters*, *1*(4), 204–222.

Sengupta, S., Datta, D., Rajest, S. S., Paramasivan, P., Shynu, T., & Regin, R. (2023). Development of rough-TOPSIS algorithm as hybrid MCDM and its implementation to predict diabetes. *International Journal of Bioinformatics Research and Applications*, *19*(4), 252–279. DOI: 10.1504/IJBRA.2023.135363

Silvia Priscila, S., Soji, E. S., Hossó, N., Paramasivan, P., & Suman Rajest, S. (2023). Digital Realms and Mental Health: Examining the Influence of Online Learning Systems on Students. *FMDB Transactions on Sustainable Techno Learning*, *1*(3), 156–164.

Tak, A., & Sundararajan, V. (2023). Pervasive Technologies and Social Inclusion in Modern Healthcare: Bridging the Digital Divide. *FMDB Transactions on Sustainable Health Science Letters*, *1*(3), 118–129.

van Cuylenburg, H. C., & Ginige, T. N. D. S. (2021). Emotion guru: A smart emotion tracking application with AI conversational agent for exploring and preventing depression. *2021 International Conference on United Kingdom-China*. DOI: 10.1109/UCET54125.2021.9674993

Vashishtha, E., & Dhawan, G. (2023). Bridging Generation Gap on Analysis of Mentor-Mentee Relationship in Healthcare Setting. *FMDB Transactions on Sustainable Health Science Letters*, *1*(1), 21–30.

Venkatasubramanian, S., Sakthikeerthika, T., & Saltanat Yerbolovna, K. (2023). Examine the Relationship Between Online Learning Students' Screen Time, Digital Fatigue, and Mental Health Issues. *FMDB Transactions on Sustainable Techno Learning*, *1*(4), 179–188.

Wali, G. (2024). Evaluating centralized and decentralized maintenance strategies for improved operational efficiency. *AVE Trends in Intelligent Technoprise Letters*, *1*(2), 91–99.

Zhang, W., Yang, C., Cao, Z., Li, Z., Zhuo, L., Tan, Y., He, Y., Yao, L., Zhou, Q., Gong, Q., Sweeney, J. A., Shi, F., & Lui, S. (2023). Detecting individuals with severe mental illness using artificial intelligence applied to magnetic resonance imaging. *EBioMedicine*, *90*(4), 104541. DOI: 10.1016/j.ebiom.2023.104541 PMID: 36996601

Chapter 19

Sentinal.AI on Emergency Call Operator Using Artificial Intelligence and Blockchain

M. S. Minu
https://orcid.org/0000-0001-6532-4530
SRM Institute of Science and Technology, Ramapuram, India

S. S. Subashka Ramesh
https://orcid.org/0000-0002-7163-6335
SRM Institute of Science and Technology, Ramapuram, India

Prayasu Satapathy
SRM Institute of Science and Technology, Ramapuram, India

M. B. Sudhan
SRM Institute of Science and Technology, Ramapuram, India

Ishaan Dwivedi
SRM Institute of Science and Technology, Ramapuram, India

G. Agalya
Dhaanish Ahmed College of Engineering, India

ABSTRACT

Emergency call centers in India face critical challenges that can significantly impact response times and, ultimately, the lives of needy individuals. Factors such as call center overload and understaffing can lead to delays in attending to emergency calls, resulting in severe consequences. The Importance of Prompt Response in Life-Threatening Situations Prompt response is crucial in life-threatening situations, as it can significantly save lives and minimize property damage. However, overloaded or understaffed emergency call centers can hinder the promptness of response. One such innovative solution that addresses these challenges is Sentinel.AI, which leverages the power of artificial intelligence to prioritize emergency calls and efficiently relay vital information to emergency handlers. Sentinel.AI is an innovative solution designed specifically for emergency call centers in India to address these critical challenges.

DOI: 10.4018/979-8-3693-9420-5.ch019

INTRODUCTION

In today's technologically advanced society, implementing AI-powered emergency call management systems has revolutionized the handling of emergency calls. These systems, such as Sentinel.AI, utilize natural language processing and machine learning algorithms to quickly analyze and assess the urgency of each call, ensuring that the most urgent situations are prioritized and addressed promptly. The use of AI in emergency call management has significantly improved the efficiency and effectiveness of emergency response systems. By rapidly classifying information from a vast number of calls, AI can identify the urgent needs of victims and share this information with relevant emergency services. This has led to quicker response times and a more coordinated and targeted emergency approach. One of the key features of AI-powered emergency call management systems is the ability to grade calls based on context. This means that the system can analyze the content of the caller's description and determine the level of urgency based on the context and phrases used. This enables the system to quickly identify and transfer urgent calls to emergency handlers, ensuring that critical situations receive immediate attention. Location tracking is another crucial feature of AI-powered emergency call management systems. By recording each caller's location, Sentinel.AI can provide this information to emergency handlers, allowing them to locate the caller and respond accurately.

Furthermore, AI-powered systems like Sentinel.AI provide a transcript of each call to the emergency handler. This transcript includes a record of the conversation between the caller and the AI system, which aids in quickly and accurately assessing the situation. Automated responses are also a valuable feature of AI-powered emergency call management systems. They can provide automated guidance and instructions to callers until an emergency handler is available. These automated responses help ensure callers receive immediate support and guidance, even if there is a delay in connecting them with an emergency handler. Integrating AI-based tools into emergency call management systems has improved emergency response efficiency and effectiveness. With AI-powered call management systems, emergencies can be accurately classified and prioritized, leading to prompt attention and response. This saves valuable time and ensures that resources are allocated most effectively and efficiently. Appropriate resource management is a top priority for emergency professionals, and AI-powered call management systems address this concern by efficiently classifying and prioritizing emergency calls based on their urgency.

LITERATURE SURVEY

This survey paper delves into the prominent security challenges content management systems (CMS) face (Tas and Tanriover, 2019). It proposes an efficient proposal for constructing a decentralized application (DApp) for CMS using the Ethereum platform. Content Management Systems are fundamental tools for website management but are often susceptible to various security vulnerabilities (Minu et al., 2023). This paper comprehensively looks at the primary security concerns plaguing CMS. These issues encompass a variety of threats, including SQL injection, cross-site scripting (XSS), and authentication vulnerabilities, highlighting the pressing need for heightened security measures in this domain (Swetha et al., 2020). In response to these challenges, the paper introduces a novel approach—developing a CMS DApp on the Ethereum blockchain platform. Ethereum's unique features, such as its smart contract capabilities, decentralized nature, and immutability, offer an appealing solution to the security predicaments commonly encountered in traditional CMS setups (Sasikala et al., 2022).

By leveraging Ethereum's blockchain infrastructure, developers can create an inherently secure CMS resistant to tampering, ushering in a new content management system security (Bhargavi et al., 2020). This survey paper sheds light on the critical security issues affecting CMS. It advocates for a transformative solution by implementing a decentralized application on the Ethereum platform, aiming to bolster the security and resilience of content management systems in an ever-evolving digital landscape (Wang et al., 2023). This article provides valuable insights into the firsthand experience of developing a decentralized application (DApp) utilizing the Ethereum blockchain platform. It serves as a practical exploration of the Ethereum ecosystem, offering a glimpse into its advantages for creating decentralized applications (Sureshbhai et al., 2020).

Throughout the article, the advantages of Ethereum for crafting DApps are thoughtfully emphasized (Bagadia et al., 2020). Ethereum's prominent features, including its robust smart contract capabilities, decentralized architecture, and immutability, are discussed in detail. These attributes contribute to the platform's appeal and make it an ideal choice for DApp development (Kyriacou et al., 2020). By sharing their experiences and highlighting these advantages, the article not only showcases the potential of Ethereum as a powerful DApp development platform but also serves as a valuable resource for developers and enthusiasts looking to harness the benefits of blockchain technology in their projects (Thamarai Kannan et al., 2023). It underscores the transformative impact Ethereum can have on creating decentralized applications fostering innovation and security in the blockchain space (Minu et al., 2020).

This article embarks on a comprehensive exploration of the integration of blockchain technology within healthcare systems, with a primary focus on bolstering the security of patient information and enabling decentralized control over data access (Deschamps-Berger et al., 2021). A notable highlight of this exploration is the prominent role assigned to the Hyperledger framework in ensuring robust data access control (Shi-Jim Yen and Kavak, 2021). The safeguarding of patient information is of paramount importance within the healthcare sector, given its sensitivity. Blockchain technology is showcased as a potent solution to enhance the security of this data (Zhao et al., 2022).

Utilizing Blockchain's immutable and tamper-resistant ledger can securely store and access patient records, reducing the risk of data breaches and unauthorized alterations. The article underscores the significance of Hyperledger, a permissioned blockchain platform, in this context (Gupta et al., 2020). Hyperledger's tailored features for data access control and its permissioned nature make it a strategic choice for healthcare applications (Minu and Canessane, 2021). It empowers healthcare institutions with the capability to determine and regulate who can access patient data, further strengthening privacy and security measures (Pervez et al., 2018). In summary, this article sheds light on the promising fusion of blockchain technology and healthcare systems, emphasizing the pivotal role of Hyperledger in achieving decentralized data access control and heightened patient data security (Joshi et al., 2023). It paves the way for transformative advancements in healthcare data management, fostering trust and integrity within the industry (Kathirvelu et al., 2022). This article zeroes in on the practical application of blockchain technology within data storage management systems.

A key area of focus is the encryption of metering assets and the myriad benefits of leveraging Blockchain for data validation and storage. In data storage management, security and integrity are paramount concerns (Kler et al., 2024). The article delves into how blockchain technology is a robust solution for addressing these challenges. Data can be securely stored and verified by employing Blockchain's inherent attributes of immutability and transparency (Nagaraj, 2023). This is especially pertinent in the case of metering assets, where accurate and tamper-proof records are crucial (Frank et al., 2023).

Furthermore, the article underscores the advantages of Blockchain in data validation and storage (Angeline et al., 2023). It highlights how Blockchain's decentralized nature eliminates the need for a central authority, reducing the risk of data manipulation and unauthorized access (Maroju, 2024). This not only enhances data security but also streamlines data management processes. This article illuminates the practical benefits of integrating blockchain technology into data storage management systems, emphasizing its role in securing metering assets and improving data validation and storage procedures. It heralds a paradigm shift in data management practices, driven by the transparency and security offered by blockchain solutions (Mudunuri, 2024).

This research paper introduces an innovative decentralized framework, KaRuNa, to assess risks associated with fraudulent cryptocurrency schemes. KaRuNa leverages the combined power of blockchain technology and sentiment analysis to achieve an impressive 98.99% accuracy in detecting fraudulent activities within the cryptocurrency space (Hullurappa, 2024). Cryptocurrency markets have become increasingly susceptible to various fraudulent schemes, posing a substantial challenge for investors and regulatory authorities. KaRuNa represents a pioneering effort to mitigate these risks effectively.

The framework employs blockchain technology to enhance transparency and traceability within cryptocurrency transactions, enabling the identification of suspicious patterns or activities. Additionally, sentiment analysis is harnessed to gauge public sentiment and reactions to specific cryptocurrencies or projects. This multifaceted approach significantly improves the accuracy of fraud detection. In conclusion, KaRuNa stands as a groundbreaking solution in cryptocurrency security. By merging Blockchain's transparency and immutability with sentiment analysis, it offers an exceptionally accurate means of identifying and mitigating risks associated with fraudulent cryptocurrency schemes, contributing to the overall integrity and trustworthiness of the cryptocurrency ecosystem.

This research report delves into a comprehensive analysis of Ethereum's transaction space to better understand the behavioral patterns inherent in transactional activities. This analysis applies supervised and unsupervised characteristic analysis techniques to infer these behavioral traits. Within the Ethereum network, transactions form a vital part of its functionality, and their patterns can reveal valuable insights into user behavior, network dynamics, and potential anomalies. The report adopts a dual-pronged approach: supervised analysis, where predefined traits are examined using labeled data, and unsupervised analysis, which involves identifying and categorizing traits without prior labeling. This research holds significant implications for Ethereum and blockchain networks at large. Discerning behavioral traits within transactional activities can facilitate improved network monitoring, anomaly detection, and security enhancements (Hariharan et al., 2024).

Moreover, it contributes to a deeper comprehension of user dynamics within the Ethereum ecosystem, aiding in developing more robust and efficient blockchain applications (Usman and Ullah, 2024). This research report analyses the performance of a decentralized Ethereum blockchain system for crowdfunding. It evaluates the scalability and efficiency of the system (Sayedelahl and Farouk, 2024). This paper outlines the conceptualization, design, and implementation of an electronic system known as the emergency system. The primary objective of this system is to provide comprehensive support for the management of emergency calls and the efficient dispatch of ambulance services. The emergency system encompasses a range of critical features, including the coordination and management of ambulance fleets, assistance in evaluating emergency calls, facilitating the triage process, and enhancing communication channels between the emergency call center and ambulance vehicles.

This system revolutionizes the emergency response process by introducing automation and advanced tools to streamline the workflow (Vemula, 2024). It ensures that emergency calls are promptly assessed and routed to the appropriate resources, optimizing the allocation of ambulance services and potentially saving lives. Additionally, by fostering improved communication between the call center and ambulance units, the emergency system aims to enhance the coordination and effectiveness of emergency responses, ultimately contributing to the overall efficiency and reliability of emergency services.

This paper uses semantic analysis and machine learning techniques for real-time sentiment analysis of online content, specifically focusing on Twitter data, particularly during emergencies (Vignesh Raja et al., 2023). The primary objective is to equip emergency responders with valuable insights into online networks' evolving sentiment and dynamics, thereby minimizing the delay between a disaster event and initiating a timely and effective disaster response (Mittal et al., 2024). By harnessing semantic analysis and machine learning algorithms, this research strives to keep pace with the rapid dissemination of information on social media platforms, such as Twitter, during emergencies (Vashishtha and Kapoor, 2023).

The aim is to swiftly gauge public sentiment and identify critical patterns or trends that could inform emergency response strategies (Farhan and Bin Sulaiman, 2023). This paper addresses a crucial aspect of modern disaster management—leveraging cutting-edge technology to process and interpret real-time online sentiment data (Panyaram, 2024). By reducing response time lags and enhancing the understanding of public sentiment, this approach holds significant promise in improving the efficiency and efficacy of disaster response efforts (Sharma et al., 2020).

EXISTING SYSTEM

Emergency call operator systems, an indispensable cornerstone of public safety infrastructure, operate with meticulous precision and a sophisticated array of components. They commence with the reception of distress calls, primarily dialed through telephone or mobile devices, directed to specialized call centers known as Public Safety Answering Points (PSAPs). Simultaneously, the system undertakes the intricate task of pinpointing the caller's location, utilizing known landline data or advanced techniques such as GPS or cell tower triangulation in mobile scenarios. Upon receipt of the call at the PSAP, highly trained call operators assume the triage role, meticulously assessing the nature and gravity of the emergency. This assessment is the linchpin for dispatching the most appropriate emergency services, whether police, fire, or medical responders. The operator's astute judgment directs the response, determining the allocation of resources and their destination.

A pivotal facet of the system is the comprehensive recording of data. Call operators diligently record pertinent information, encompassing the caller's identity, location, a detailed description of the emergency, and any additional critical details. This meticulous data is channeled into a sophisticated Computer-Aided Dispatch (CAD) system, orchestrating the management and real-time tracking of the responding emergency units. Communication between call operators and the dispatched responders is facilitated via radio systems, where critical information and updates are exchanged, ensuring that responders are well-informed as they approach the scene. The CAD system further optimizes the allocation of resources, continually monitoring the availability and proximity of emergency units to minimize response times and maximize efficiency.

Call operators maintain vigilant oversight throughout this intricate process, offering guidance and support to callers and responding units. They may dispense pre-arrival instructions for medical emergencies or furnish safety directives for other incidents, underscoring their role as the lynchpin in the emergency response chain. Detailed records of every emergency call, response, and subsequent outcome are meticulously maintained for legal, statistical, and analytical purposes. These records are instrumental in ensuring accountability and refining and enhancing emergency response procedures.

Data Analysis

The technological underpinnings of the system have evolved significantly, encompassing advanced technologies such as Geographic Information Systems (GIS) mapping, which aids in the precise geolocation of callers. Enhanced 911 (E911) systems, a hallmark of modernization, automate the transmission of caller location data to PSAPs, further augmenting response accuracy. Complementing the technical sophistication is a robust framework of training and protocols. Emergency call operators undergo exhaustive training to navigate various situations, from medical emergencies to fires and criminal incidents. They adhere to established protocols and guidelines, ensuring the consistency and effectiveness of responses.

In summation, the extant emergency call operator system is a testament to meticulous planning and technological prowess, bridging the critical gap between individuals in distress and the swift arrival of emergency services. Its operational success hinges on efficient call handling, precise location determination, astute response coordination, and a perpetual commitment to refinement and enhancement, all within rigorous training and protocols. It remains an indomitable bulwark of public safety infrastructure, a beacon of hope during society's most vulnerable moments. Emergency call operator systems, an indispensable cornerstone of public safety infrastructure, operate with meticulous precision and a sophisticated array of components. They commence with the reception of distress calls, primarily dialed through telephone or mobile devices, directed to specialized call centers known as Public Safety Answering Points (PSAPs). Simultaneously, the system undertakes the intricate task of pinpointing the caller's location, utilizing known landline data or advanced techniques such as GPS or cell tower triangulation in mobile scenarios.

Upon receipt of the call at the PSAP, highly trained call operators assume the triage role, meticulously assessing the nature and gravity of the emergency. This assessment is the linchpin for dispatching the most appropriate emergency services, whether police, fire, or medical responders. The operator's astute judgment directs the response, determining the allocation of resources and their destination. A pivotal facet of the system is the comprehensive recording of data. Call operators diligently record pertinent information, encompassing the caller's identity, location, a detailed description of the emergency, and any additional critical details. This meticulous data is channeled into a sophisticated Computer-Aided Dispatch (CAD) system, orchestrating the management and real-time tracking of the responding emergency units.

Communication between call operators and the dispatched responders is facilitated via radio systems, where critical information and updates are exchanged, ensuring that responders are well-informed as they approach the scene. The CAD system further optimizes the allocation of resources, continually monitoring the availability and proximity of emergency units to minimize response times and maximize efficiency. Call operators maintain vigilant oversight throughout this intricate process, offering guidance and support to callers and responding units. They may dispense pre-arrival instructions for medical emergencies or furnish safety directives for other incidents, underscoring their role as the lynchpin in the emergency response chain. Detailed records of every emergency call, response, and subsequent outcome are meticulously maintained for legal, statistical, and analytical purposes. These records are instrumental in ensuring accountability and refining and enhancing emergency response procedures.

The technological underpinnings of the system have evolved significantly, encompassing advanced technologies such as Geographic Information Systems (GIS) mapping, which aids in the precise geolocation of callers. Enhanced 911 (E911) systems, a hallmark of modernization, automate the transmission of caller location data to PSAPs, further augmenting response accuracy.

Complementing the technical sophistication is a robust framework of training and protocols. Emergency call operators undergo exhaustive training to navigate various situations, from medical emergencies to fires and criminal incidents. They adhere to established protocols and guidelines, ensuring the consistency and effectiveness of responses. In summation, the extant emergency call operator system is a testament to meticulous planning and technological prowess, bridging the critical gap between individuals in distress and the swift arrival of emergency services. Its operational success hinges on efficient call handling, precise location determination, astute response coordination, and a perpetual commitment to refinement and enhancement, all within rigorous training and protocols. It remains an indomitable bulwark of public safety infrastructure, a beacon of hope during society's most vulnerable moments.

PROPOSED SYSTEM

The Emergency Call Operator System represents a meticulously architected confluence of sophisticated technologies and services meticulously engineered to optimize the efficacy of emergency response procedures. At its core, this system boasts a meticulously designed frontend interface, serving as the primary conduit through which end-users initiate emergency calls. The backbone of this operational marvel is fortified by the robust Twilio communication platform, orchestrating the intricate symphony of inbound and outbound emergency calls. At the same time, the Python Flask backend takes the helm in orchestrating the intricate interplay of these calls, user data, and a multifaceted array of interconnected services.

At the crux of this intricate machinery, Assembly AI emerges as a pivotal player, harnessing advanced voice-to-text transcription capabilities to deliver seamless real-time conversion of voice calls into textual data. In parallel, GPT, an advanced Natural Language Processing (NLP) model, is pivotal in processing this transcribed data, showcasing unparalleled acumen in discerning critical keywords, thus expediting swift and precise response strategies. The system adorns itself with the venerable Ethereum blockchain technology in data fidelity, serving as an impervious citadel for secure data storage. Data is enshrined in an immutable ledger format, with meticulously timestamped records and crucial minutiae about each emergency call. This architectural marvel coalesces harmoniously with a traditional database framework, accommodating the storage of user profiles and ancillary non-blockchain data with seamless grace, ensuring the comprehensive integration of data within the system's expansive architecture.

For the virtuosos manning the operational helm, the Operator Dashboard emerges as an indispensable sanctum, endowing them with real-time insights into the intricacies of incoming emergencies bolstered by an arsenal of indispensable tools designed to facilitate precise management of these difficult situations. Operators remain ceaselessly vigilant by implementing a real-time alert system, which consistently beckons their attention to incoming emergency calls, heralding the situation's urgency. Furthermore, the system employs stringent user authentication protocols and security fortifications, standing as unwavering sentinels, zealously safeguarding the sanctity of sensitive information, and fortifying the system against potential breaches.

The sagacity with which this system approaches scalability and redundancy engenders it with formidable resilience, allowing it to gracefully accommodate surges in call volume and navigate unforeseen operational challenges. The continuum of model refinement is realized through a rigorous regime of exhaustive testing and iterative training, elevating the system's proficiency and efficacy to unprecedented heights. The bedrock of this entire endeavor is the unswerving commitment to regulatory compliance, diligently navigating the labyrinthine nexus of legal obligations, thus ensuring the system's unwavering adherence to the tapestry of pertinent laws and regulations.

The collaborative ethos inherent to this system extends its reach to local emergency services, forging a seamless nexus of coordination for the prompt dispatch of first responders in difficult circumstances. An overarching vigilance, fortified by meticulous monitoring and proactive maintenance protocols, stands as the vanguard of system health and operational performance. Comprehensive documentation and training resources proffer consummate guidance to users and administrators alike, facilitating the adept and proficient operation of the system. A user-centric feedback loop forms the sine qua non of this system, iteratively assimilating end-user insights into its ongoing calibration and enhancement, perpetually finessing its functional repertoire. Its robust approach to the labyrinthine domain of legal considerations bespeaks a mastery over intricacies related to liability and data privacy, thereby ensuring the sanctity of the system's operational framework.

In summation, this system stands as a testament to the zenith of technical sophistication, poised to reimagine the contours of emergency response paradigms through an exquisite fusion of cutting-edge technology and meticulous planning, ultimately advancing public safety and, in the process, preserving lives. As it evolves, its potential for expansion lies in integrating AI-driven decision support tools and assimilating emerging technologies within the ever-evolving emergency response domain. The Emergency Call Operator System, a meticulously designed and executed masterpiece of technological innovation and operational excellence, represents a critical nexus within the framework of public safety infrastructure. This system is meticulously architected to orchestrate and optimize the complex and time-sensitive emergency response process. Its core features a meticulously designed frontend interface, the user's first point of contact when initiating an emergency call. Behind this user-friendly façade lies a sophisticated infrastructure powered by a meticulously integrated and orchestrated constellation of technologies.

The Twilio communication platform is the muscular workhorse that underpins the system, facilitating the reception and dispatch of emergency calls. It seamlessly manages the intricate flow of inbound and outbound calls, ensuring that critical communications are efficiently routed and promptly addressed. The Python Flask backend, a robust and versatile system component, takes center stage in coordinating the multifaceted interactions between these calls, user data, and a network of interconnected services. This backend acts as the operational nerve center, orchestrating exchanging information and commands to ensure a swift and effective response to each emergency.

Assembly AI emerges as a pivotal player within this intricate web of technology. Leveraging advanced voice-to-text transcription capabilities, Assembly AI converts real-time voice calls into textual data. This transformation is a linchpin in the system's ability to process and analyze the information provided by callers effectively. The textual data, now in a format that can be readily analyzed, is passed on to another essential component: GPT, an advanced Natural Language Processing (NLP) model. GPT plays a pivotal role in processing the transcribed data, displaying unparalleled acumen in discerning critical keywords and patterns. Its capabilities expedite the swift and precise formulation of response strategies, ensuring that the appropriate emergency services are dispatched efficiently.

In the realm of data fidelity and security, the system showcases a robust architectural design. At its core, the venerable Ethereum blockchain technology is revered for its immutability and security attributes. Within this Blockchain, data is enshrined in an immutable ledger format, meticulously timestamped to provide an indisputable record of each emergency call. Blockchain's robust security measures ensure that sensitive information remains protected and that the integrity of the data is preserved. To accommodate the storage of user profiles and ancillary non-blockchain data seamlessly, the system

ADVANTAGES OF THE PROPOSED SYSTEM OVER THE EXISTING SYSTEM

The proposed emergency call operator system significantly advances emergency response infrastructure. In contrast to the existing system, which relies on dated technologies and methodologies, the proposed system incorporates a cutting-edge arsenal of components, including AI-driven transcription and blockchain data storage. These innovations collectively provide a substantial accuracy, efficiency, and data security advantage. One of the pivotal enhancements offered by the proposed system is its real-time voice-to-text transcription capabilities, a feature conspicuously absent in the existing system. The proposed system further elevates location accuracy to unprecedented levels, primarily through implementing advanced Geographic Information Systems (GIS) mapping and Enhanced 911 (E911) capabilities. These technologies ensure that responders are precisely guided to the emergency coordinates, leaving no room for ambiguity or error. The paramount importance of such precision becomes evident in scenarios where every passing second carries profound implications for the safety and well-being of those in distress.

In data security and integrity, the proposed system leverages blockchain technology, specifically Ethereum, to erect an impervious bulwark against data breaches and tampering. Utilizing blockchain technology is an unassailable citadel of data integrity and transparency in emergency call processing. Each data fragment associated with an emergency call is securely enshrined within an immutable ledger format. These records are meticulously timestamped, with critical details meticulously preserved. This stringent approach guarantees data integrity and effectively thwarts tampering or unauthorized access attempts. Additionally, this architectural innovation seamlessly harmonizes with a conventional database framework, accommodating the storage of user-profiles and ancillary non-blockchain data within the comprehensive architecture of the system.

To address the inherent limitations of the existing system, the proposed model is meticulously engineered to withstand surges in call volumes and unforeseen technical difficulties. It is architected to ensure uninterrupted service and the seamless coordination of emergency response efforts, even in the face of the most challenging scenarios. This capacity for scalability and redundancy is indispensable, as it guarantees that the system remains fully operational during high-stress situations, such as natural disasters or large-scale emergencies. The proposed system is built to adapt dynamically, ensuring its continued relevance and effectiveness in meeting the evolving demands of emergency response.

RESULT AND DISCUSSION

The proposed system does not merely equip call operators with advanced tools; it empowers them with a comprehensive suite of capabilities designed to enhance their proficiency in managing emergencies efficiently and effectively. At the core of this empowerment is the Operator Dashboard, a central hub that provides real-time insights into the intricacies of incoming emergencies. The dashboard is fortified with various indispensable tools and features to facilitate precise emergency management. Operators are the recipients of a real-time alert system that consistently draws their attention to incoming emergency calls, underscoring the urgency of each situation. These alerts guarantee that no call goes unnoticed and that each emergency is addressed promptly and urgently.

Furthermore, the proposed system emphasizes security, incorporating stringent user authentication protocols and robust security measures to safeguard the sanctity of sensitive information. The system functions as a steadfast guardian, unflinchingly defending against potential breaches and ensuring that all sensitive data is handled carefully and diligently. Additionally, robust privacy safeguards are deeply embedded within the system's architecture to protect user data and uphold stringent privacy standards. The proposed system exhibits a commendable prowess in navigating the intricate landscape of regulatory compliance and legal considerations. It adeptly traverses the labyrinthine nexus of legal obligations, assuring that the system operates diligently within the confines of applicable laws and regulations. This meticulous approach effectively mitigates legal risks, ensuring the system conducts its operations consistent with legal and ethical standards. The system's commitment to delivering exceptional emergency response extends to its dedication to operating within a legally compliant framework.

Furthermore, the collaborative ethos that defines the proposed system extends its reach to local emergency services, forging a seamless nexus of coordination for the prompt dispatch of first responders in difficult circumstances. The system actively fosters a culture of cooperation and coordination, ensuring that local emergency services are seamlessly integrated into the emergency response process. This collaborative approach optimizes response times and enhances the overall efficiency of emergency services, underscoring the system's commitment to delivering swift and effective aid in times of crisis. The proposed system is marked by a relentless commitment to proactive monitoring and maintenance, constituting an overarching vigilance that serves as the vanguard of system health and operational performance. The system boasts robust monitoring capabilities that enable real-time system performance assessment. This proactive approach facilitates the rapid identification and resolution of any issues or anomalies, guaranteeing that the system remains operational.

The proposed model addresses the existing system's limitations in scalability and redundancy with precision. Designed to weather surges in call volumes and technical difficulties, it guarantees uninterrupted service and seamless response coordination during challenging scenarios. The proposed system doesn't merely endow call operators with advanced tools; it empowers them with real-time alerts and AI-driven decision support, enhancing their ability to manage emergencies efficiently and effectively. The intricate maze of regulatory compliance and legal considerations is navigated with dexterity, mitigating legal risks through robust data management and privacy safeguards.

Moreover, the proposed system fosters a culture of continuous improvement driven by a user-centric feedback loop. This iterative approach ensures adaptability to evolving needs and harnesses emerging technologies to further augment its capabilities. The proposed emergency call operator system is a testament to technological prowess and meticulous planning, poised to redefine the emergency response landscape, enhance public safety, and preserve lives. The proposed emergency call operator system represents a quantum leap in the evolution of emergency response infrastructure, outshining the existing system across multiple dimensions. While the existing system is functional, its reliance on dated technologies and methodologies parallels the proposed system's technologically advanced arsenal (Figure 1).

Figure 1. Architecture Diagram of E.C.O. (Emergency Call Operator)

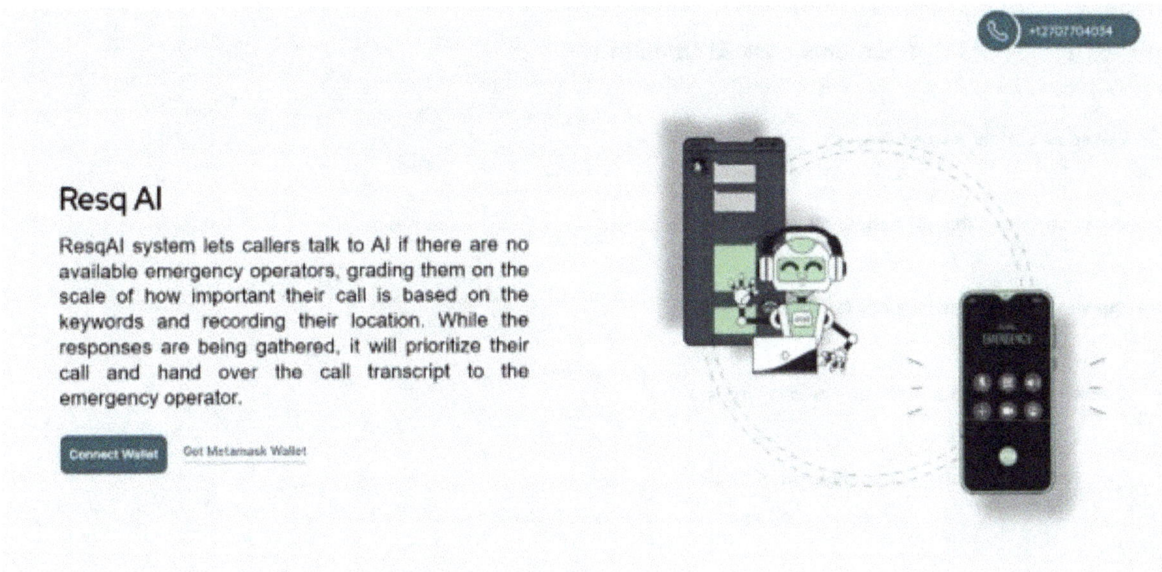

The latter incorporates state-of-the-art components, including AI-driven transcription and blockchain data storage, bestowing it superior accuracy, efficiency, and data security. These innovations collectively provide a substantial accuracy, efficiency, and data security advantage. One of the pivotal enhancements offered by the proposed system is its real-time voice-to-text transcription capabilities, a feature conspicuously absent in the existing system. This capability represents a foundational pillar of the proposed system's efficiency. Assembly AI and GPT, two formidable AI tools, synergistically expedite the extraction of vital information from incoming emergency calls. This acceleration reduces response times and mitigates the risk of human error in the call processing pipeline. The seamless transformation of voice calls into textual data empowers operators with a wealth of information, enabling them to make rapid and well-informed decisions (Figure 2).

Figure 2. A Map of the area the WebApp covers

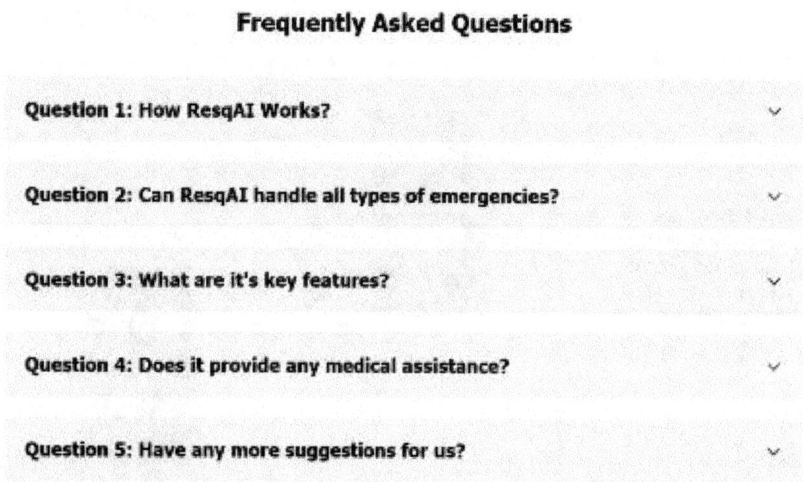

In data security and integrity, the proposed system leverages blockchain technology, specifically Ethereum, to erect an impervious bulwark against data breaches and tampering. Utilizing blockchain technology is an unassailable citadel of data integrity and transparency in emergency call processing. Each data fragment associated with an emergency call is securely enshrined within an immutable ledger format. These records are timestamped, with critical details meticulously preserved (Figure 3).

Figure 3.An alert is generated at the Receiver's end

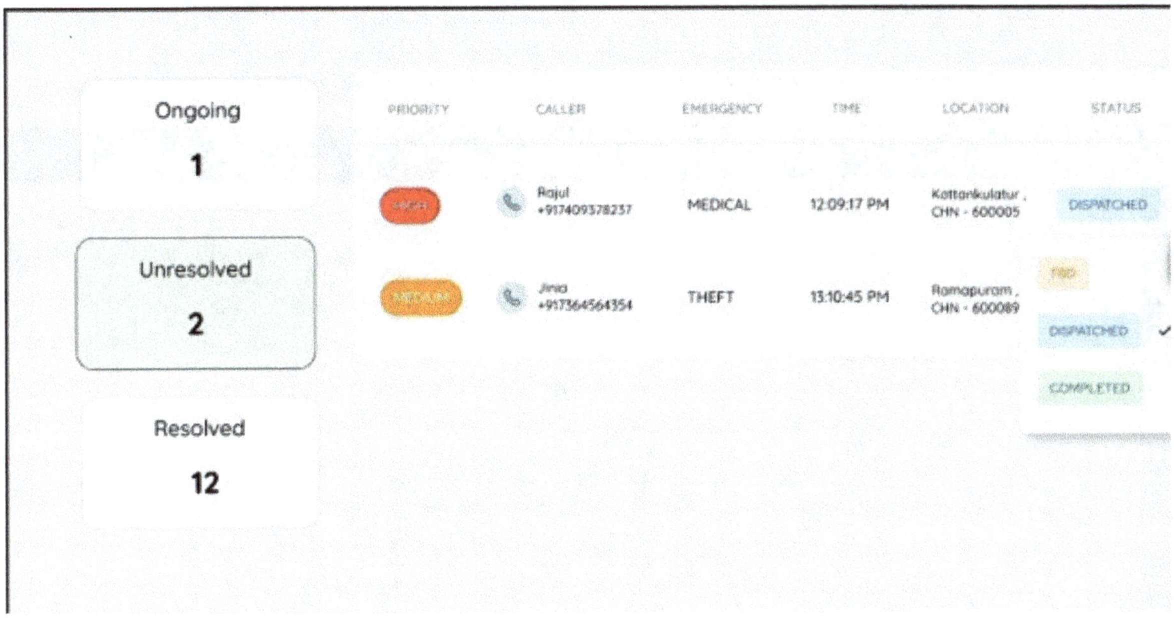

This stringent approach guarantees data integrity and effectively thwarts tampering or unauthorized access attempts. Furthermore, this architectural innovation seamlessly harmonizes with a conventional database framework, accommodating the storage of user-profiles and ancillary non-blockchain data within the comprehensive architecture of the system (Figure 4).

Figure 4. All the unresolved cases

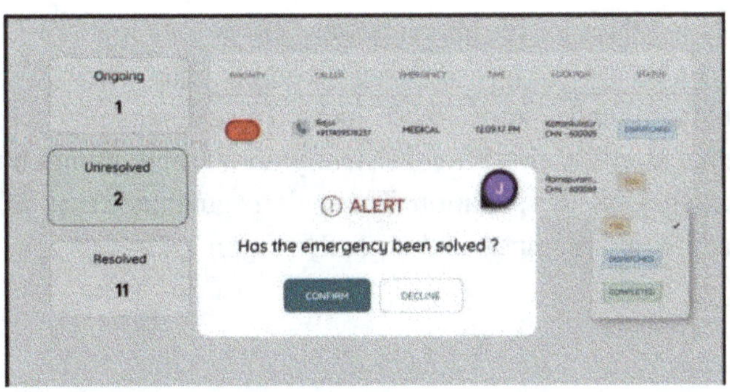

To address the inherent limitations of the existing system, the proposed model is meticulously engineered to withstand surges in call volumes and unforeseen technical difficulties. It is architected to ensure uninterrupted service and the seamless coordination of emergency response efforts, even in the face of the most challenging scenarios. This capacity for scalability and redundancy is indispensable, as it guarantees that the system remains fully operational during high-stress situations, such as natural disasters or large-scale emergencies. The proposed system is built to adapt dynamically, ensuring its continued relevance and effectiveness in meeting the evolving demands of emergency response (Figure 5).

Figure 5. FAQs to help the users understand what it is WebApp about and how it is used

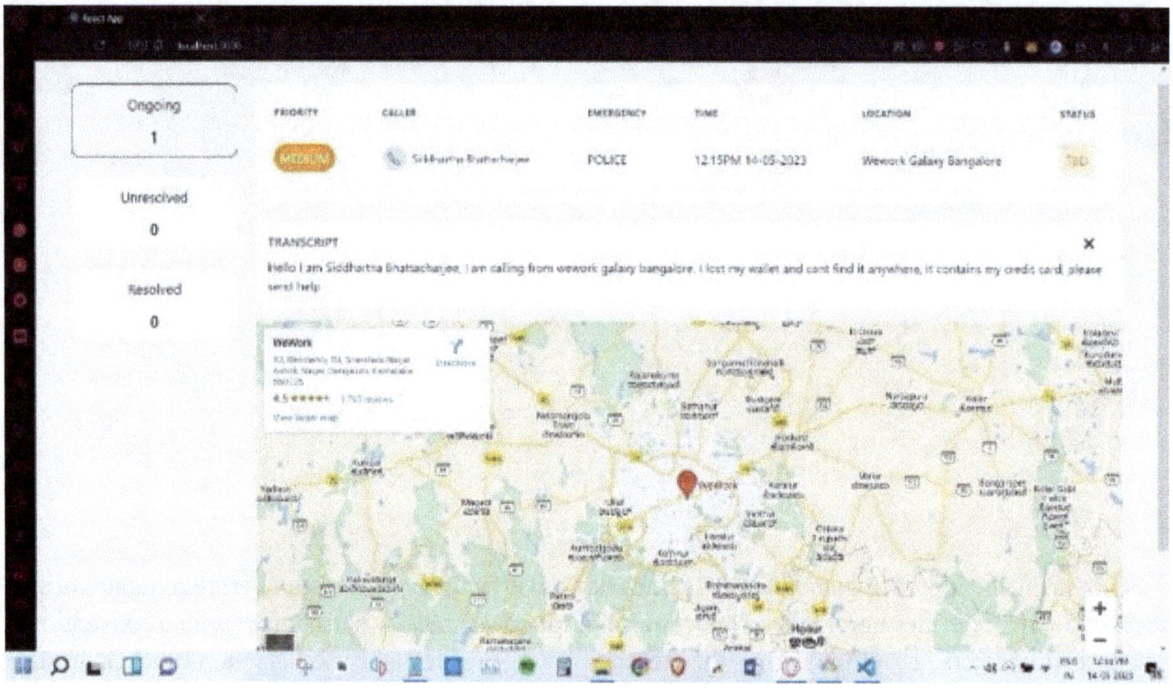

The proposed system does not merely equip call operators with advanced tools; it empowers them with a comprehensive suite of capabilities designed to enhance their proficiency in managing emergencies efficiently and effectively. At the core of this empowerment is the Operator Dashboard, a central hub that provides real-time insights into the intricacies of incoming emergencies. The dashboard is fortified with various indispensable tools and features to facilitate precise emergency management. Operators are the recipients of a real-time alert system that consistently draws their attention to incoming emergency calls, underscoring the urgency of each situation. These alerts guarantee that no call goes unnoticed and that each emergency is addressed promptly and urgently (Figure 6).

Figure 6. The Welcome Page

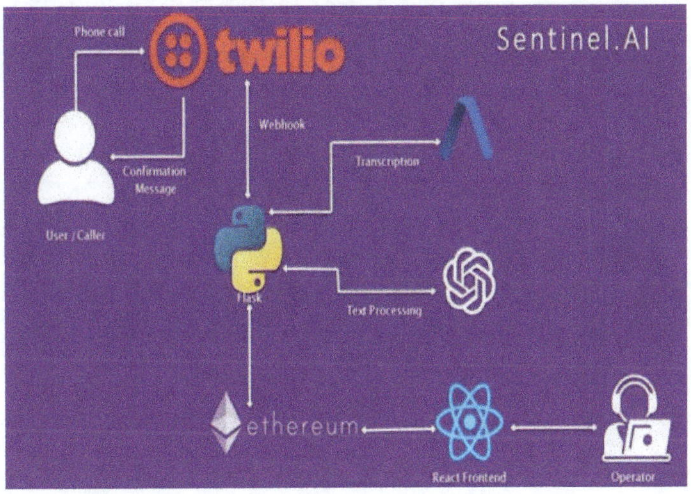

Furthermore, the proposed system emphasizes security, incorporating stringent user authentication protocols and robust security measures to safeguard the sanctity of sensitive information. The system. Functions as a steadfast guardian, unflinchingly defending against potential breaches and ensuring that all sensitive data is handled carefully and diligently. Additionally, robust privacy safeguards are deeply embedded within the system's architecture to protect user data and uphold stringent privacy standards. The proposed system exhibits a commendable prowess in navigating the intricate landscape of regulatory compliance and legal considerations. It adeptly traverses the labyrinthine nexus of legal obligations, assuring that the system operates diligently within the confines of applicable laws and regulations. This meticulous approach effectively mitigates legal risks, ensuring the system conducts its operations consistent with legal and ethical standards. The system's commitment to delivering exceptional emergency response extends to its dedication to operating within a legally compliant framework. Furthermore, the collaborative ethos that defines the proposed system extends its reach to local emergency services, forging a seamless nexus of coordination for the prompt dispatch of first responders in difficult circumstances.

CONCLUSION

In today's technologically evolved culture, AI-powered emergency call management systems have altered the processing of emergency calls. These systems, such as Sentinel.AI, use natural language processing and machine learning to quickly assess call urgency, ensuring that essential situations are prioritized. The contextual analysis of caller descriptions performed by AI allows for rapidly detecting critical calls and their routing to emergency handlers. By pinpointing callers' places, location monitoring assists in proper resource allocation. Providing phone transcripts to handlers expedites scenario evaluation. Automated answers improve caller help by providing rapid guidance until human handlers are available. Artificial intelligence-based techniques improve emergency response efficiency and coordination while optimizing resource allocation. These methods save time and money, allowing for a more targeted and timely reaction to catastrophes. This technology enhances public safety, but human monitoring is still required, especially in complicated and dynamic circumstances. AI augments emergency responders, increasing the efficacy of emergency call handling while providing quick reactions to urgent occurrences.

REFERENCES

Angeline, R., Aarthi, S., Regin, R., & Rajest, S. S. (2023). Dynamic intelligence-driven engineering flooding attack prediction using ensemble learning. In *Advances in Artificial and Human Intelligence in the Modern Era* (pp. 109–124). IGI Global. DOI: 10.4018/979-8-3693-1301-5.ch006

Bagadia, U., Bodkurwar, J., Bhat, J., & Halbe, A. (2020). Performance Analysis of Decentralized Ethereum Blockchain System. *2020 International Conference on Inventive Computation Technologies (ICICT)*. IEEE, Coimbatore, India. DOI: 10.1109/ICICT48043.2020.9112550

Bhargavi, M. S., Katti, S. M., Shilpa, M., Kulkarni, V. P., & Prasad, S. (2020). Transactional Data Analytics for Inferring Behavioural Traits in Ethereum Blockchain Network. 2020 IEEE 16th International Conference on Intelligent Computer Communication and Processing (ICCP), Cluj-Napoca, Romania.

Deschamps-Berger, T., Lamel, L., & Devillers, L. (2021). End-to-End Speech Emotion Recognition: Challenges of Real-Life Emergency Call Centers Data Recordings". In 2021, 9th International Conference on Affective Computing and Intelligent Interaction, Nara, Japan.

Farhan, M., & Bin Sulaiman, R. (2023). Developing Blockchain Technology to Identify Counterfeit Items Enhances the Supply Chain's Effectiveness. *FMDB Transactions on Sustainable Technoprise Letters*, *1*(3), 123–134.

Frank, M. S., Angel, M. S., & Shajahan, M. A. (2023). The Role of Artificial Intelligence on Enhancing Customer Experience. *FMDB Transactions on Sustainable Technoprise Letters*, *1*(4), 223–230.

Gupta, V., Zhu, G., Yu, A., & Brown, D. E. (2020). A Comparative Study of the Performance of Unsupervised Text Segmentation Techniques on Dialogue Transcripts". *2020 Systems and Information Engineering Design Symposium (SIEDS)*, Charlottesville, VA, United States of America. DOI: 10.1109/SIEDS49339.2020.9106639

Hariharan, M. G., Saranya, S., Velavan, P., Soji, E. S., Rajest, S. S., & Thammareddi, L. (2024). Utilization of artificial intelligence algorithms for advanced cancer detection in the healthcare domain. In *Advances in Medical Technologies and Clinical Practice* (pp. 287–302). IGI Global.

Hullurappa, M. (2024). Uniting quantum computing and artificial intelligence: Exploring new frontiers. *FMDB Transactions on Sustainable Computer Letters*, *2*(2), 120–130. DOI: 10.69888/FTSCL.2024.000186

Joshi, M., Shen, Z., & Kausar, S. (2023). Enhancing Inclusive Education on Leveraging Artificial Intelligence Technologies for Personalized Support and Accessibility in Special Education for Students with Diverse Learning Needs. *FMDB Transactions on Sustainable Techno Learning*, *1*(3), 125–142.

Kathirvelu, M., Janaranjani, A., Pranav, N., & Pradeep, A. T. (2022). Voice Recognition Chat bot for Consumer Product Applications". In *2022 IEEE International Conference on Data Science and Information System (ICDSIS)*, Hassan, India. DOI: 10.1109/ICDSIS55133.2022.9915884

Kler, R., Jamoliddinov, J., Nematjonov, J., Kadirov, I., & Muzaffarov, M. (2024). Locating contribution of health and education in regional growth in Uzbekistan. *AVE Trends In Intelligent Techno Learning*, *1*(1), 11–22.

Kyriacou, E., Constantinou, R., Kronis, C., Hadjichristofi, G., & Pattichis, C. (2020). eEmergency System to Support Emergency call Evaluation and Ambulance dispatch Procedures. 2020 IEEE 20th Mediterranean Electrotechnical Conference (MELECON), Palermo, Italy.

Maroju, P. K. (2024). Advancing Synergy of Computing and Artificial Intelligence with Innovations Challenges and Future Prospects. *FMDB Transactions on Sustainable Intelligent Networks*, *1*(1), 1–14. DOI: 10.69888/FTSIN.2024.000153

Minu, M. S., Arun, K., Tiwari, A., & Rampuria, P. (2020). Face recognition system based on haar cascade classifier. *International Journal of Advanced Science and Technology*, *29*(5), 3799–3805.

Minu, M. S., & Canessane, R. (2021). Secure image transmission scheme in unmanned aerial vehicles using multiple share creation with optimal elliptic curve cryptography. *Indian Journal of Computer Science and Engineering*, *12*(1), 129–134. DOI: 10.21817/indjcse/2021/v12i1/211201169

Minu, M. S., Ramesh, S. S. S., Peruru, S. K. R., & Roshan, N. M. (2023). *Efficient Maintenance of Hospital Records by Entrusted Proof of Work Algorithm in Block Chain Technology", EAI/Springer Innovations in Communication and Computing*. Springer.

Mittal, A., Pham, L. T., Othman, B., Saravanan, S., Kumar, T., & Saranya, M. (2024). Impact of inspirational techniques on engagement to participate in volunteering opportunities. *FMDB Transactions on Sustainable Technoprise Letters*, *2*(2), 78–89. DOI: 10.69888/FTSTPL.2024.000232

Mudunuri, L. N. R. (2024). Artificial Intelligence (AI) Powered Matchmaker: Finding Your Ideal Vendor Every Time. *FMDB Transactions on Sustainable Intelligent Networks*, *1*(1), 27–39. DOI: 10.69888/FTSIN.2024.000155

Nagaraj, B. K. (2023). Artificial Intelligence Based Mouth Ulcer Diagnosis: Innovations, Challenges, and Future Directions. *FMDB Transactions on Sustainable Computer Letters*, *1*(3), 202–209.

Panyaram, S. (2024). Utilizing quantum computing to enhance artificial intelligence in healthcare for predictive analytics and personalized medicine. *FMDB Transactions on Sustainable Computing Systems*, *2*(1), 22–31. DOI: 10.69888/FTSCS.2024.000194

Pervez, F., Qadir, J., Khalil, M., Yaqoob, T., Ashraf, U., & Younis, S. (2018). Wireless technologies for emergency response: A comprehensive review and some guidelines. *IEEE Access : Practical Innovations, Open Solutions*, *6*(12), 71814–71838. DOI: 10.1109/ACCESS.2018.2878898

Sasikala, N., Sundaram, B. M., Biswas, S., Sai Nikhil, A., & Rohith, V. S. (2022). Survey of latest technologies on Decentralized applications using Blockchain. *2022 Second International Conference on Artificial Intelligence and Smart Energy (ICAIS)*, Coimbatore, India. DOI: 10.1109/ICAIS53314.2022.9742768

Sayedelahl, M. A., & Farouk, R. M. (2024). Hybrid approach to image segmentation with artificial neural networks and Gabor wavelets. *AVE Trends in Intelligent Computing Systems*, *1*(2), 77–90.

Sharma, E., Ye, G., Wei, W., Zhao, R., Tian, Y., Wu, J., He, L., Lin, E., & Gong, Y. (2020). Adaptation of RNN transducer with text-to-speech technology for keyword spotting, *Proceedings of 2020 IEEE International Conference on Acoustics, Speech, and Signal Processing (ICASSP)*, Barcelona, Spain. DOI: 10.1109/ICASSP40776.2020.9053191

Shi-Jim Yen, S., & Kavak, J.-Y. (2021). STEMI Recognition in Electrocardiogram (ECG) by Online AI Bot for Emergency Service and Mobile Medicine". In 30th Wireless and Optical Communications Conference. WOCC, Taipei, Taiwan.

Sureshbhai, P. N., Bhattacharya, P., & Tanwar, S. (2020). KaRuNa: A blockchain-based sentiment analysis framework for fraud cryptocurrency schemes. 2020 IEEE International Conference on Communications Workshops (ICC Workshops). IEEE, Dublin, Ireland.

Swetha, M. S., Pushpa, S. K., Muneshwara, M. S., & Manjunath, T. N. (2020). Blockchain enabled secure healthcare Systems. *2020 IEEE International Conference on Machine Learning and Applied Network Technologies (ICMLANT)*, IEEE, Hyderabad, India. DOI: 10.1109/ICMLANT50963.2020.9355970

Tas, R., & Tanriover, O. O. (2019). Building A Decentralized Application on the Ethereum Blockchain. 2019 3rd International Symposium on Multidisciplinary Studies and Innovative Technologies (ISMSIT), IEEE, Ankara, Turkey.

Thamarai Kannan, G., Gunasekar, M., Ponnazhagan, N. A., Kumar, K. R., & Sudhan, S. (2023). Aspect based Sentiment Aware Word Embedding for Cross Domain Sentiment Analysis". In *2023 International Conference on Computer Communication and Informatics (ICCCI)*, Coimbatore, India. DOI: 10.1109/ICCCI56745.2023.10128251

Usman, M., & Ullah, A. (2024). Blockchain Technology Implementation in Libraries: An Overview of Potential Benefits and Challenges. *AVE Trends In Intelligent Computing Systems*, *1*(1), 42–53.

Vashishtha, E., & Kapoor, H. (2023). Implementation of Blockchain Technology Across International Healthcare Markets. *FMDB Transactions on Sustainable Technoprise Letters*, *1*(1), 1–12.

Vemula, V. R. (2024). Cognitive artificial intelligence systems for proactive threat hunting in AI-driven cloud applications. *AVE Trends in Intelligent Computing Systems*, *1*(3), 173–183.

Vignesh Raja, A. S., Jasper, K. D., Aljaafreh, R., Yogeshwarran, S. K., & Saleem, M. (2023). A Comprehensive Exploration of Blockchain-Based Decentralized Applications and Federated Learning in Reshaping Data Management. *FMDB Transactions on Sustainable Computer Letters*, *1*(4), 228–240.

Wang, X., Jia, J., Cao, Y., Du, J., Hu, A., Liu, Y., & Wang, Z. (2023). Application of data storage management system in blockchain-based technology. 2023 IEEE 2nd International Conference on Electrical Engineering, Big Data and Algorithms (EEBDA). IEEE, Changchun, China.

Zhao, Q., Zhang, H., & Shang, J. (2022). Interpretable sentiment analysis based on sentient words' syntax information". In *2022 International Conference on Industrial Automation*, Chengdu, China.

Compilation of References

Abbad Ur Rehman, H., Lin, C.-Y., & Mushtaq, Z. (2021). Effective K-nearest neighbor algorithms performance analysis of thyroid disease. *Zhongguo Gongcheng Xuekan*, *44*(10), 1–11. DOI: 10.1080/02533839.2020.1831967

Abdulkareem, N. M., & Abdulazeez, A. M. (2021). Machine learning classification based on random forest algorithm: A review. *International Journal of Science and Business*, *5*(2), 128–142.

Abràmoff, M. D., Lou, Y., Erginay, A., Clarida, W., Amelon, R., Folk, J. C., & Niemeijer, M. (2016). Improved automated detection of Diabetic Retinopathy on a publicly available dataset through integration of deep learning. *Investigative Ophthalmology & Visual Science*, *57*(13), 5200–5206. DOI: 10.1167/iovs.16-19964 PMID: 27701631

Aditya Komperla, R. C. (2023). Revolutionizing Patient Care with Connected Healthcare Solutions. *FMDB Transactions on Sustainable Health Science Letters*, *1*(3), 144–154.

Ahmed, H. M., & Taha, M. A. (2021). A brief survey on modern iris feature extraction methods. *Engineering and Technology Journal*, *39*(1), 123–129. DOI: 10.30684/etj.v39i1A.1680

Ahmed, N., Abbasi, M. S., Zuberi, F., Qamar, W., Halim, M. S. B., Maqsood, A., & Alam, M. K. (2021). Artificial intelligence techniques: Analysis, application, and outcome in dentistry-A systematic review. *BioMed Research International*, *2021*(6), 1–15. DOI: 10.1155/2021/9751564 PMID: 34258283

Ajitha, Y., Talukder, M. S. H., & Shuvo, S. A. (2024). Advanced radar range prediction and performance analysis in aircraft adhoc networks (AANET). *FMDB Transactions on Sustainable Computer Letters*, *2*(1), 1–13. DOI: 10.69888/FTSCL.2024.000177

Akhtar, T., Gilani, S. O., Mushtaq, Z., Arif, S., Jamil, M., Ayaz, Y., Butt, S. I., & Waris, A. (2021). Effective voting ensemble of homogenous ensembling with multiple attribute-selection approaches for improved identification of thyroid disorder. *Electronics (Basel)*, *10*(23), 3026. DOI: 10.3390/electronics10233026

Ak, T. A., & Steluta, A. (2021). An iris recognition system using a new method of iris local-ization. *International Journal of Open Information Technologies*, *9*(7), 67–76.

Alharbi, M. T., & Almutiq, M. M. (2022). Prediction of dental implants using machine learning algorithms. *Journal of Healthcare Engineering*, *2022*(6), 1–12. DOI: 10.1155/2022/7307675 PMID: 35769356

Ali, S., Shah, M. H., & Naqvi, K. J. (2023). A CNN-based obesity prediction model for adults using electronic health records. *Journal of King Saud University. Computer and Information Sciences*, *35*(3), 422–431.

Almomani, W., El-Shafai, A., AlKhayer, A., Alsumayt, S., Aljameel, K., & Alissa, K. (2023). Computational materials and continuum mechanics. *Computers, Materials & Continua*, *74*(2), 3515–3537. DOI: 10.32604/cmc.2023.033765

Alqarni, R. S., Alqahtani, F. A., & Almutairi, B. (2021). Predictive analysis of adult obesity using deep learning models with real-time data from IoT devices. *Applied Sciences (Basel, Switzerland)*, *11*(22), 10672.

Al-Tawalbeh, J., ... (2022). Classification of lung cancer by using machine learning algorithms. In IICETA 2022 - 5th International Conference on Engineering Technology Its Applications, Al-Najaf, Iraq DOI: 10.1109/IICETA54559.2022.9888332

Alzubaidi, L., Zhang, J., Humaidi, A. J., Al-Dujaili, A., Duan, Y., Al-Shamma, O., Santama-Ría, J., Fadhel, M. A., Al-Amidie, M., & Farhan, L. (2021). Review of deep learning: Con-cepts, CNN architec-tures, challenges, applications, future directions. *Journal of Big Data*, *8*(1), 1–74. DOI: 10.1186/s40537-021-00444-8 PMID: 33425651

Anand, P. P., Sulthan, N., Jayanth, P., & Deepika, A. A. (2023). A Creating Musical Compositions Through Recurrent Neural Networks: An Approach for Generating Melodic Creations. *FMDB Transactions on Sustainable Computing Systems*, *1*(2), 54–64.

Angeline, R., Aarthi, S., Regin, R., & Rajest, S. S. (2023). Dynamic intelligence-driven engineering flooding attack prediction using ensemble learning. In *Advances in Artificial and Human Intelligence in the Modern Era* (pp. 109–124). IGI Global. DOI: 10.4018/979-8-3693-1301-5.ch006

Anitha, K., Nagaraj, B. K., Paramasivan, P., & Shynu, T. (2023). Enhancing Clustering Performance with the Rough Set C-Means Algorithm. *FMDB Transactions on Sustainable Computing Systems*, *1*(4), 190–203.

Anushya, A., Begum, S., Shiwani, S., & Shrivastava, A. (2024). Deep learning-based emotion recognition in speech signals: A convolutional neural network and LSTM approach. *AVE Trends in Intelligent Computing Systems*, *1*(4), 198–208.

Arabahmadi, M., Farahbakhsh, R., & Rezazadeh, J. (2022). Deep learning for smart healthcare-A survey on brain tumor detection from medical imaging. *Sensors (Basel)*, *22*(5), 1960. DOI: 10.3390/s22051960 PMID: 35271115

Arjunan, P., & Ramesh, R. (2020). Deep learning methods for accurate obesity prediction using biomedical datasets. *Journal of Medical Systems*, *44*(189), 1–9.

Asiri, A. A., Shaf, A., Ali, T., Shakeel, U., Irfan, M., Mehdar, K. M., Halawani, H. T., Alghamdi, A. H., Alshamrani, A. F. A., & Alqhtani, S. M. (2023). Exploring the power of deep learning: Fine-tuned vision transformer for accurate and efficient brain tumor detection in MRI scans. *Diagnostics (Basel)*, *13*(12), 2094. DOI: 10.3390/diagnostics13122094 PMID: 37370989

Aversano, L., Bernardi, M. L., Cimitile, M., Iammarino, M., Macchia, P. E., Nettore, I. C., & Verdone, C. (2021). Thyroid Disease Treatment prediction with machine learning approaches. *Procedia Computer Science*, *192*(1), 1031–1040. DOI: 10.1016/j.procs.2021.08.106

Babu, A., Andrew Onesimu, J., & Martin Sagayam, K. (2021). Artificial intelligence in dentistry: Concepts, Applications and Research Challenges. E3S Web of Conference The 4th International Conference of Computer Science and Renewable Energies (ICCSRE'2021), Madrid, Spain, 297.

Bagadia, U., Bodkurwar, J., Bhat, J., & Halbe, A. (2020). Performance Analysis of Decentralized Ethereum Blockchain System. *2020 International Conference on Inventive Computation Technologies (ICICT)*. IEEE, Coimbatore, India. DOI: 10.1109/ICICT48043.2020.9112550

Bala Kuta, Z., & Bin Sulaiman, R. (2023). Analysing Healthcare Disparities in Breast Cancer: Strategies for Equitable Prevention, Diagnosis, and Treatment among Minority Women. *FMDB Transactions on Sustainable Health Science Letters*, *1*(3), 130–143.

Bala Kuta, Z., & Bin Sulaiman, R. (2023). Analyzing Healthcare Disparities in Breast Cancer: Strategies for Equitable Prevention, Diagnosis, and Treatment among Minority Women. *FMDB Transactions on Sustainable Health Science Letters*, *1*(3), 130–143.

Bhargavi, M. S., Katti, S. M., Shilpa, M., Kulkarni, V. P., & Prasad, S. (2020). Transactional Data Analytics for Inferring Behavioural Traits in Ethereum Blockchain Network. 2020 IEEE 16th International Conference on Intelligent Computer Communication and Processing (ICCP), Cluj-Napoca, Romania.

Bhaskaranand, M., Ramachandra, C., Bhat, S., Cuadros, J., Nittala, M. G., Sadda, S., & Solanki, K. (2016). Automated diabetic retinopathy screening and monitoring using retinal fundus image analysis. *Journal of Diabetes Science and Technology*, *10*(2), 254–261. DOI: 10.1177/1932296816628546 PMID: 26888972

Bhatia, S., Sinha, Y., & Goel, L. (2019). Lung cancer detection: A deep learning approach. In Soft Computing for Problem Solving, Springer Nature, Singapore. DOI: 10.1007/978-981-13-1595-4_55

Bin Sulaiman, R., Hariprasath, G., Dhinakaran, P., & Kose, U. (2023). Time-series Forecasting of Web Traffic Using Prophet Machine Learning Model. *FMDB Transactions on Sustainable Computer Letters*, *1*(3), 161–177.

Bose, S. R., Jeba, J. A., Kishore, V. K., Gnanaguru, G., & Shynu, T. (2024). Deep learning-driven acute lymphoblastic leukemia detection using CT scan imaging. *AVE Trends in Intelligent Health Letters*, *1*(2), 110–124.

Bose, S. R., Jeba, J. A., Regin, R., Tarunraj, S., Soji, E. S., & Rajest, S. S. (2024). Enhanced deep learning models for early detection of renal failure from CT imaging. *FMDB Transactions on Sustainable Health Science Letters*, *2*(3), 152–163. DOI: 10.69888/FTSHSL.2024.000251

Bose, S. R., Sirajudheen, M. A. S., Kirupanandan, G., Arunagiri, S., Regin, R., & Rajest, S. S. (2023). Fine-grained independent approach for workout classification using integrated metric transfer learning. In *Advanced Applications of Generative AI and Natural Language Processing Models* (pp. 358–372). IGI Global. DOI: 10.4018/979-8-3693-0502-7.ch017

Browning, D. J. (2010). Diabetic retinopathy: Evidence-based management. *The American Orthoptic Journal*, *60*(1), 108–108. DOI: 10.3368/aoj.60.1.108

Buia, S., Popescu, D., & Ichim, L. (2021). Blood vessel segmentation in retinal images using neural networks. In 2021 12th International Symposium on Advanced Topics in Electrical Engineering (ATEE) (pp. 1–6). Bucharest, Romania. DOI: 10.1109/ATEE52255.2021.9425035

Cha, J.-Y., Yoon, H.-I., Yeo, I.-S., Huh, K.-H., & Han, J.-S. (2021). Peri-implant bone loss measurement using a region-based convolutional neural network on dental periapical radiographs. *Journal of Clinical Medicine*, *10*(5), 1009. DOI: 10.3390/jcm10051009 PMID: 33801384

Chakravarthi, B., Ng, S.-C., Ezilarasan, M. R., & Leung, M.-F. (2022). EEG-based emotion recognition using hybrid CNN and LSTM classification. *Frontiers in Computational Neuroscience*, *16*(10), 1019776. DOI: 10.3389/fncom.2022.1019776 PMID: 36277613

Chandel, K., Kunwar, V., Sabitha, S., Choudhury, T., & Mukherjee, S. (2016). A comparative study on thyroid disease detection using K-nearest neighbor and Naive Bayes classification techniques. *CSI Transactions on ICT*, *4*(1), 313–319. DOI: 10.1007/s40012-016-0100-5

Chandratreya, A. (2024). Psychological impacts of climate change and environmental degradation on mental well-being. *FMDB Transactions on Sustainable Techno Learning*, *2*(2), 75–87. DOI: 10.69888/FTSTL.2024.000208

Chang, Y., Zheng, Z., Sun, Y., Zhao, M., Lu, Y., & Zhang, Y. (2023). DPAFNet: A residual dual-path attention-fusion convolutional neural network for multimodal brain tumor segmentation. *Biomedical Signal Processing and Control*, *79*(1), 104037. DOI: 10.1016/j.bspc.2022.104037

Chatterjee, S., Kumar, V., & Roy, S. (2021). Predictive Modelling for Obesity Using Deep Learning Frameworks and Demographic Data. *IEEE Transactions on Neural Networks and Learning Systems*, *32*(10), 4200–4212.

Chaudhari, P., Agarwal, H., & Bhateja, V. (2019). Data augmentation for cancer classification in oncogenomics: An improved KNN-based approach. *Evolutionary Intelligence*, *14*(4), 1–10.

Chen, D., Hu, J., Zhu, M., Tang, N., Yang, Y., & Feng, Y. (2020). Diagnosis of thyroid nodules for ultrasonographic characteristics indicative of malignancy using random forest. *BioData Mining*, *13*(1), 1–21. DOI: 10.1186/s13040-020-00223-w PMID: 32905307

Chen, X., Wu, S., & Tang, X. (2022). Predictive analysis of adult obesity using machine learning and deep neural networks on electronic health record data. *Electronics (Basel)*, *11*(9), 1534.

Chitra, A., Rajpriya, R., Karras, D. A., & Sridharlakshmi, N. R. B. (2024). An Exhaustive Study of Parasitic Organisms and Pathological Effects on Human Health. *AVE Trends In Intelligent Health Letters*, *1*(1), 10–18.

Cho, K., van Merrienboer, B., Gulcehre, C., Bahdanau, D., Bougares, F., Schwenk, H., & Bengio, Y. (2014). Learning phrase representations using RNN encoder–decoder for statistical machine translation. *Proceedings of the 2014 Conference on Empirical Methods in Natural Language Processing (EMNLP)*, Doha, Qatar. DOI: 10.3115/v1/D14-1179

Chundru, S. (2024). Harnessing the power of AI: Revolutionizing metadata management with machine learning. *FMDB Transactions on Sustainable Computer Letters*, *2*(3), 164–175. DOI: 10.69888/FTS-CL.2024.000242

Chunduri, V., Hannan, S. A., Devi, G. M., Nomula, V. K., Tripathi, V., & Rajest, S. S. (2024). Deep convolutional neural networks for lung segmentation for diffuse interstitial lung disease on HRCT and volumetric CT. In *Advances in Computational Intelligence and Robotics* (pp. 335–350). IGI Global.

Chunduri, V., Rajest, S. S., Allugunti, V. R., Verma, D., Aarthi, R., & Sharma, D. K. (2024). Deep neural network for brain tumour segmentation using guaranteed time slots (GTS) algorithm. In *Advances in Computer and Electrical Engineering* (pp. 371–390). IGI Global.

Dargan, S., & Kumar, M. (2020). A comprehensive survey on the biometric recognition sys-tems based on physiological and behavioral modalities. *Expert Systems with Applications*, *143*(4), 113114. DOI: 10.1016/j.eswa.2019.113114

Das, S. R., Bin Sulaiman, R., & Butt, U. (2023). Comparative Analysis of Machine Learning Algorithms for Credit Card Fraud Detection. *FMDB Transactions on Sustainable Computing Systems*, *1*(4), 225–244.

Das, S., Kruti, A., Devkota, R., & Bin Sulaiman, R. (2023). Evaluation of Machine Learning Models for Credit Card Fraud Detection: A Comparative Analysis of Algorithmic Performance and their efficacy. *FMDB Transactions on Sustainable Technoprise Letters*, *1*(2), 70–81.

Daugman, J. (2007). New methods in iris recognition. IEEE Transactions on Systems, Man, and Cybernetics. Part B, Cybernetics: A Publication of the IEEE Systems. *IEEE Transactions on Systems, Man, and Cybernetics. Part B, Cybernetics*, *37*(5), 1167–1175. DOI: 10.1109/TSMCB.2007.903540

De Marsico, M., Petrosino, A., & Ricciardi, S. (2016). Iris recognition through machine learning techniques: A survey. *Pattern Recognition Letters*, *82*(10), 106–115. DOI: 10.1016/j.patrec.2016.02.001

Debiasi, L., & Uhl, A. (2015). Techniques for a forensic analysis of the CASIA-IRIS V4 database. *3rd International Workshop on Biometrics and Forensics (IWBF 2015)*, Gjovik, Norway. DOI: 10.1109/IWBF.2015.7110236

Decencière, E., Zhang, X., Cazuguel, G., Lay, B., Cochener, B., Trone, C., Gain, P., Ordonez, R., Massin, P., Erginay, A., Charton, B., & Klein, J.-C. (2014). Feedback on a publicly distributed image database: The Messidor database. *Image Analysis & Stereology*, *33*(3), 231–234. DOI: 10.5566/ias.1155

Deschamps-Berger, T., Lamel, L., & Devillers, L. (2021). End-to-End Speech Emotion Recognition: Challenges of Real-Life Emergency Call Centers Data Recordings". In 2021, 9th International Conference on Affective Computing and Intelligent Interaction, Nara, Japan.

Devasia, J., Goswami, H., Lakshminarayanan, S., Rajaram, M., & Adithan, S. (2023). Deep learning classification of active tuberculosis lung zones wise manifestations using chest X-rays: A multi-label approach. *Scientific Reports*, *13*(1), 1–15. DOI: 10.1038/s41598-023-28079-0 PMID: 36650270

Ding, H., Wu, J., Zhao, W., Matinlinna, J. P., Burrow, M. F., & Tsoi, J. K. H. (2023). Artificial intelligence in dentistry—A review. *Frontiers in Dental Medicine*, *4*(2), 1–13. PMID: 39935549

Dixit, A., Parekh, N. H., Anand, R., Kamal, N., Badiyani, B. K., Kumar, A., & Obulareddy, V. T. (2023). A study to assess the awareness of adults about precancerous and cancerous lesions and the associated risk factors. *Journal of Pharmacy & Bioallied Sciences*, *15*(Suppl 2), S977–S980. DOI: 10.4103/jpbs.jpbs_260_23 PMID: 37694066

Dixit, A., Parekh, N. H., Anand, R., Kamal, N., Kumar, A., & Badiyani, B. K. (2023). An online survey to examine the dental students' awareness, knowledge, prevention, and early detection of oral cancer. *Journal of Pharmacy & Bioallied Sciences*, *15*(7, Suppl 2), S984–S986. DOI: 10.4103/jpbs.jpbs_258_23 PMID: 37693960

Doe, J., Sharma, R., & Singh, N. (2020). Prediction of Adult Obesity Using Deep Learning Techniques and Genetic Information. *International Journal of Environmental Research and Public Health*, *244*(8), 77–92.

Dubuc, A., Zitouni, A., Thomas, C., Kémoun, P., Cousty, S., Monsarrat, P., & Laurencin, S. (2022). Improvement of mucosal lesion diagnosis with machine learning based on medical and semiological data: An observational study. *Journal of Clinical Medicine*, *11*(21), 6596. DOI: 10.3390/jcm11216596 PMID: 36362822

Elaiyaraja, P., Sudha, G., & Shvets, Y. Y. (2023). Spectral Analysis of Breast Cancer is Conducted Using Human Hair Fibers Through ATR-FTIR. *FMDB Transactions on Sustainable Health Science Letters*, *1*(2), 70–81.

El-Sayed, M. A., & Abdel-Latif, M. A. (2022). Iris recognition approach for identity verification with DWT and multiclass SVM. *PeerJ. Computer Science*, *8*(6), e919. DOI: 10.7717/peerj-cs.919 PMID: 35494865

Farhan, A. M. Q., & Yang, S. (2023). Automatic lung disease classification from the chest X-ray images using hybrid deep learning algorithm. *Multimedia Tools and Applications*, *82*(25), 38561–38587. DOI: 10.1007/s11042-023-15047-z PMID: 37362647

Farhan, M., & Bin Sulaiman, R. (2023). Developing Blockchain Technology to Identify Counterfeit Items Enhances the Supply Chain's Effectiveness. *FMDB Transactions on Sustainable Technoprise Letters*, *1*(3), 123–134.

Fatima, A., Shafi, I., Afzal, H., Díez, I. D. L. T., Lourdes, D. R.-S. M., Breñosa, J., & Ashraf, I. (2022). Advancements in dentistry with artificial Intelligence: Current clinical applications and future perspectives. *Healthcare (Basel)*, *10*(11), 2188. DOI: 10.3390/healthcare10112188 PMID: 36360529

Folorunsho Ajayi, A., Tayo Adebayo, E., Oluwadunsi Adebayo, I., Simeon Oyekunle, O., Oluwaseyi Amos, V., Emmanuel Bamidele, S., & Olusayo Olatinwo, G. (2022). Application of data science approaches to investigate autoimmune thyroid disease in precision medicine. In *Hypothyroidism - New Aspects of an Old Disease*. Intech Open. DOI: 10.5772/intechopen.101220

Frank, M. S., Angel, M. S., & Shajahan, M. A. (2023). The Role of Artificial Intelligence on Enhancing Customer Experience. *FMDB Transactions on Sustainable Technoprise Letters*, *1*(4), 223–230.

Gab Allah, A. M., Sarhan, A. M., & Elshennawy, N. M. (2021). Classification of brain MRI tumor images based on deep learning PGGAN augmentation. *Diagnostics (Basel)*, *11*(12), 2343. DOI: 10.3390/diagnostics11122343 PMID: 34943580

Galderisi, S., Heinz, A., Kastrup, M., Beezhold, J., & Sartorius, N. (2015). Toward a new definition of mental health. *World Psychiatry; Official Journal of the World Psychiatric Association (WPA)*, *14*(2), 231–233. DOI: 10.1002/wps.20231 PMID: 26043341

Galdran, A., Anjos, A., Dolz, J., Chakor, H., Lombaert, H., & Ayed, I. B. (2022). State-of-the-art retinal vessel segmentation with minimalistic models. *Scientific Reports*, *12*(1), 6174. DOI: 10.1038/s41598-022-09675-y PMID: 35418576

Gandhi, M., & Dhanasekaran, R. (2013). Diagnosis of diabetic retinopathy using morphological process and SVM classifier. In *2013 International Conference on Communication and Signal Processing* (pp. 23–28). IEEE. Melmaruvathur, India. DOI: 10.1109/iccsp.2013.6577181

Gandhi, M., Satheesh, C., Soji, E. S., Saranya, M., Rajest, S. S., & Kothuru, S. K. (2024). Image recognition and extraction on computerized vision for sign language decoding. In *Explainable AI Applications for Human Behavior Analysis* (pp. 157–173). IGI Global. DOI: 10.4018/979-8-3693-1355-8.ch010

Ghazi, P., Ibrahim, S., & Mohanty, K. (2021). A comparative evaluation of machine learning techniques for obesity prediction. *IEEE Journal of Translational Engineering in Health and Medicine*, *9*(12), 1–10.

Gnanadurai, G. J., Raaza, A., Velayutham, R., Palani, S. K., & Bramwell, E. A. (2023). Detection of cardiac amyloidosis on electrocardiogram images using machine learning and deep learning techniques. *Computational Intelligence*, *39*(4), 554–576. DOI: 10.1111/coin.12505

Gnanaguru, G., Priscila, S. S., Sakthivanitha, M., Radhakrishnan, S., Rajest, S. S., & Singh, S. (2024). Thorough analysis of deep learning methods for diagnosis of COVID-19 CT images. In *Advances in Medical Technologies and Clinical Practice* (pp. 46–65). IGI Global.

Gonzalez-Amador, E., Arines, J., Charlón, P., Garcia-Porta, N., Abraldes, M. J., & Acosta, E. (2022). Improvement of retinal images affected by cataracts. *Photonics*, *9*(4), 251. DOI: 10.3390/photonics9040251

Gonzalez, R. C., & Woods, R. E. (2018). *Digital image processing. Pearson, N.J.* Prentice Hall.

Gore, D. V., & Deshpande, V. (2020). Comparative study of various techniques using Deep Learning for Brain Tumor Detection. 2020 International Conference for Emerging Technology (INCET). IEEE, Belgaum, India. DOI: 10.1109/INCET49848.2020.9154030

Goyal, N., Dehghani, A., & Maji, S. (2020). Accurate diabetic retinopathy classification through eligible region proposals. In *International Conference on Medical Image Computing and Computer-Assisted Intervention*, Graz, Austria.

Graham, S., Depp, C., Lee, E. E., Nebeker, C., Tu, X., Kim, H.-C., & Jeste, D. V. (2019). Artificial intelligence for mental health and mental illnesses: An overview. *Current Psychiatry Reports*, *21*(11), 116. DOI: 10.1007/s11920-019-1094-0 PMID: 31701320

Grischke, J., Johannsmeier, L., Eich, L., Griga, L., & Haddadin, S. (2020). Dentronics: Towards robotics and artificial intelligence in dentistry. *Dental Materials*, *36*(6), 765–778. DOI: 10.1016/j.dental.2020.03.021 PMID: 32349877

Gruenwald, J. T., Nistor, J., & Tusar, J. (2022). Powering our nuclear fleet with artificial intelligence. *Nucl. News*, *65*(2), 50–58.

Gupta, V., Zhu, G., Yu, A., & Brown, D. E. (2020). A Comparative Study of the Performance of Unsupervised Text Segmentation Techniques on Dialogue Transcripts". *2020 Systems and Information Engineering Design Symposium (SIEDS)*, Charlottesville, VA, United States of America. DOI: 10.1109/SIEDS49339.2020.9106639

Hafner, A., Peer, P., Emersic, Z., & Vitek, M. (2021). Deep iris feature extraction. In *2021 International Conference on Artificial Intelligence in Information and Communication*, Jeju Island, South Korea.

Hakim, A. (2022). Thesis Proposal: Implementation of Android-Based Artificial Intelligence in Early Detection of Thyroid Disorders and Mental Disorders, 229(3), 57-64.

Hakim, A., Titin, R., & Prihantinisetyowisnu, G. (2021). Expert System Framework Design for Diagnosis of Thyroid Disorders. In Conference: the 1st Science and Technology Student Conference (ISTECH), Klaster Mahasiswa, Indonesia.

Hariprasath, G., Dhinakaran, P., & Kumar, V. H. (2024). Exploring the efficacy of LightGBM, AdaBoost, and CatBoost in Alzheimer's disease classification. *FMDB Transactions on Sustainable Health Science Letters*, *2*(1), 41–55. DOI: 10.69888/FTSHSL.2024.000171

Haris, U. (2024). 'Warm water' politics in the Russia-Ukraine conflict. *FMDB Transactions on Sustainable Social Sciences Letters*, *2*(1), 11–18. DOI: 10.69888/FTSSSL.2024.000216

Harshavardhan, A., Cheerla, S., Parkavi, A., Latha Mary, S. A., Qureshi, K., & Mhaske, H. R. (2023). Deep learning modified neural networks with chicken swarm optimization-based lung disease detection and severity classification. *Journal of Electronic Imaging*, *32*(6), 062603. DOI: 10.1117/1.JEI.32.6.062603

Hasan Talukder, M. S., Sarkar, A., Akter, S., Nuhi-Alamin, M., & Bin Sulaiman, R. (2023). An Improved Model for Diabetic Retinopathy Detection by Using Transfer Learning and Ensemble Learning. *FMDB Transactions on Sustainable Health Science Letters*, *1*(2), 92–106.

Hassoun, N., Kateeb, R., & Thallaj, N. (2024). Effect of Ginger and Garlic Extracts on In-vitro Thrombolysis. *AVE Trends In Intelligent Health Letters*, *1*(1), 19–27.

Hasuike, A., Watanabe, T., Wakuda, S., Kogure, K., Yanagiya, R., Byrd, K. M., & Sato, S. (2022). Machine learning in predicting tooth loss: A systematic review and risk of bias assessment. *Journal of Personalized Medicine*, *12*(10), 1682. DOI: 10.3390/jpm12101682 PMID: 36294820

Hernandez, P., Fuentes, L., & Morales, F. (2022). Deep neural networks for adult obesity prediction based on physical health features. *IEEE Transactions on Biomedical Engineering*, *69*(8), 2367–2375.

He, Y., Deng, L., & Chen, S. (2021). Predictive analytics for obesity detection using convolutional neural networks and deep learning models. *Journal of Healthcare Engineering*, *10*(1), 1–11.

Hogarty, D. T., Mackey, D. A., & Hewitt, A. W. (2019). Current state and future prospects of artificial in-telligence in ophthalmology: A review. *Clinical & Experimental Ophthalmology*, *47*(1), 128–139. DOI: 10.1111/ceo.13381 PMID: 30155978

Huang, J. A., Hartanti, I. R., Colin, M. N., & Pitaloka, D. A. (2022). Telemedicine and artificial intelligence to support self-isolation of COVID-19 patients: Recent updates and challenges. *Digital Health*, *8*(4), 1–10. DOI: 10.1177/20552076221100634 PMID: 35603328

Huang, Z., Tang, C., Xu, M., & Lei, Z. (2020). Joint Retinex-based variational model and CLAHE-in-CIELUV for enhancement of low-quality color retinal images. *Applied Optics*, *59*(28), 8628–8637. DOI: 10.1364/AO.401792 PMID: 33104544

Hugar, P., Pranaygoud, G., Vishnuvardhan, K., & Faizuddin, M. (2020). Thyroid problem detection using Naive Bayesian classification. *International Journal of Creative Research Thoughts*, *8*(2), 1340–1343.

Hullurappa, M. (2024). Uniting quantum computing and artificial intelligence: Exploring new frontiers. *FMDB Transactions on Sustainable Computer Letters*, *2*(2), 120–130. DOI: 10.69888/FTSCL.2024.000186

Hu, M., Asami, C., Iwakura, H., Nakajima, Y., Sema, R., Kikuchi, T., Miyata, T., Sakamaki, K., Kudo, T., Yamada, M., Akamizu, T., & Sakakibara, Y. (2022). development and preliminary validation of a machine learning system for thyroid dysfunction diagnosis based on routine laboratory tests. *Communications Medicine*, *2*(1), 1–8. DOI: 10.1038/s43856-022-00071-1 PMID: 35603277

Humairo, C. N., Hapsari, A., & Bramanti, I. (2021). The role of Artificial Intelligence in many dental specialties. BIO Web of Conferences, 41(12), 1-3. DOI: 10.1051/bioconf/20214103005

Hu, Y., Ren, J., Yang, J., Bai, R., & Liu, J. (2021). Noise reduction by adaptive-SIN filtering for retinal OCT images. *Scientific Reports*, *11*(1), 19498. DOI: 10.1038/s41598-021-98832-w PMID: 34593894

Islam, S. S., Haque, M. S., Miah, M. S. U., Sarwar, T. B., & Nugraha, R. (2022). Application of machine learning algorithms to predict the thyroid disease risk: An experimental comparative study. *PeerJ. Computer Science*, *8*(10), 1–35. DOI: 10.7717/peerj-cs.898 PMID: 35494828

Izdiharbozkus, Z. (2016). MLTDD: Use of Machine Learning Techniques for Diagnosis of Thyroid Gland Disorder. *Computer Science and Information Technology*, *6*(4), 67–73.

Jalilian, E., Hofbauer, H., & Uhl, A. (2022). Iris image compression using deep convolutional neural networks. *Sensors (Basel)*, *22*(7), 2698. DOI: 10.3390/s22072698 PMID: 35408311

Jani, P., Nanban, D., Selvan, J., Richardson, N., Sivakani, R., & Subhashni, R. (2024). Studying Price Dynamics of Bus Services Using Machine Learning Algorithms. *AVE Trends In Intelligent Computing Systems*, *1*(1), 54–65.

Jeba, J. A., Bose, S. R., & Boina, R. (2023). Exploring Hybrid Multi-View Multimodal for Natural Language Emotion Recognition Using Multi-Source Information Learning Model. *FMDB Transactions on Sustainable Computer Letters*, *1*(1), 12–24.

Jeganathan, J., Vashist, S., Nirmala, G., & Deep, R. (2023). A Cross Sectional Study on Anxiety and Depression Among Patients with Alcohol Withdrawal Syndrome. *FMDB Transactions on Sustainable Health Science Letters*, *1*(1), 31–40.

Jha, R., Bhattacharjee, V., & Mustafi, A. (2022). Increasing the prediction accuracy for thyroid disease: A step towards better health for society. *Wireless Personal Communications*, *122*(2), 1921–1938. DOI: 10.1007/s11277-021-08974-3

Jiang, C., Chen, X., Yan, S., Kamijo, S., & Nomura, M. (2021). Multi-task attention network for retinal vessel and exudate segmentation. *Computers in Biology and Medicine*, *134*(2), 104335.

Jin, . (2019). A multi-task learning network with CRF for joint retinal vessel segmentation and optic disc localization. *IEEE Transactions on Medical Imaging*, *38*(11), 2647–2658.

Joda, T., Bornstein, M. M., Jung, R. E., Ferrari, M., Waltimo, T., & Zitzmann, N. U. (2020). Recent trends and future direction of dental research in the digital era. *International Journal of Environmental Research and Public Health*, *17*(6), 1987. DOI: 10.3390/ijerph17061987 PMID: 32197311

Johnson, K., Gupta, M., & Yadav, S. (2022). A Machine Learning Approach for Predicting Obesity Using Behavioural and Genetic Data. *Expert Systems with Applications*, *8*(1), 196–208.

Joshi, M., Shen, Z., & Kausar, S. (2023). Enhancing Inclusive Education on Leveraging Artificial Intelligence Technologies for Personalized Support and Accessibility in Special Education for Students with Diverse Learning Needs. *FMDB Transactions on Sustainable Techno Learning*, *1*(3), 125–142.

Jovanovic, A. S., & Popovic, P. M. (2022). An ensemble of deep learning methods for obesity prediction in adults using health records. *Biology and Medicine (Aligarh)*, *3*(3), 32.

Jung, Y., Kim, D., Son, B., & Kim, J. (2017). An eye detection method robust to eyeglasses for mobile iris recognition. *Expert Systems with Applications*, *67*(1), 178–188. DOI: 10.1016/j.eswa.2016.09.036

Kaewlek, T., Tanyong, K., Chakkaeo, J., Kladpree, S., Chusin, T., Yabsantia, S., & Udee, N. (2023). Classification of pneumonia, tuberculosis, and COVID-19 on computed tomography images using deep learning. *Trends in Sciences*, *20*(11), 6974. DOI: 10.48048/tis.2023.6974

Kagawade, V. C., & Angadi, S. A. (2022). A new scheme of polar Fast Fourier Transform Code for iris recognition through symbolic modelling approach. *Expert Systems with Applications*, *197*(7), 116745. DOI: 10.1016/j.eswa.2022.116745

Kamboj, P. (2022). Iris recognition segmentation signal processing system. *Applied Science & Engineering Journal for Advanced Research*, *1*(2), 2583–2468.

Karacaoglu, F., Kolsuz, M. E., Bagis, N., Evli, C., & Orhan, K. (2023). Development and validation of intraoral periapical radiography-based machine learning model for periodontal defect diagnosis. *Proceedings of the Institution of Mechanical Engineers. Part H, Journal of Engineering in Medicine*, *237*(5), 607–618. DOI: 10.1177/09544119231162682 PMID: 36939160

Karthikeyan, B., Devi, R. A., & Munshi, M. (2024). Utilizing Deep Learning for the Classification of Brain Tumours Using MRI. *AVE Trends In Intelligent Health Letters*, *1*(1), 1–9.

Karthik, S., Bhaggiaraj, S., Soji, E. S., Deve, L. S., Priscila, S. S., & Rajest, S. S. (2024). Real-time hand gesture recognition for stroke rehabilitation using deep learning approach. *AVE Trends in Intelligent Computing Systems*, *1*(3), 157–172.

Karthik, S., Soji, E. S., Priscila, S. S., Deve, L. S., Paramasivan, P., & Kumar, A. S. (2024a). Enhanced performance evaluation of vector images using SVA for tumor detection and sizing in brain MRI scans. *AVE Trends in Intelligent Health Letters*, *1*(2), 51–68.

Karthik, S., Soji, E. S., Priscila, S. S., Sakthivanitha, M., Rajest, S. S., & Kumar, A. S. (2024b). Enhancing tumour localization in brain MRI images using a scalable systematic vector algorithm for result-oriented accuracy. *FMDB Transactions on Sustainable Health Science Letters*, *2*(2), 110–127. DOI: 10.69888/FTSHSL.2024.000176

Kathirvelu, M., Janaranjani, A., Pranav, N., & Pradeep, A. T. (2022). Voice Recognition Chat bot for Consumer Product Applications". In *2022 IEEE International Conference on Data Science and Information System (ICDSIS)*, Hassan, India. DOI: 10.1109/ICDSIS55133.2022.9915884

Kayadibi, I., Güraksın, G. E., Ergün, U., & Özmen Süzme, N. (2022). An eye state recognition system using transfer learning: AlexNet-based deep convolutional neural network. *International Journal of Computational Intelligence Systems*, *15*(7), 1–19. DOI: 10.1007/s44196-022-00108-2

Khade, S., Gite, S., & Pradhan, B. (2022). Iris liveness detection using multiple deep convolution networks. *Big Data and Cognitive Computing*, *6*(2), 67. DOI: 10.3390/bdcc6020067

Kharayat, A., Rawat, D., & Panwar, N. (2024). A Study on the Efficiency of Structured Instruction on Dengue Fever Prevention and Control among People. *AVE Trends In Intelligent Social Letters*, *1*(1), 25–40.

Khoje, S., & Shinde, S. (2023). Evaluation of ripplet transform as a texture characterization for iris recognition. Journal of Thc Institution of Engineers (India) Series B, 104(2), 369–380.

Kler, R., Jamoliddinov, J., Nematjonov, J., Kadirov, I., & Muzaffarov, M. (2024). Locating contribution of health and education in regional growth in Uzbekistan. *AVE Trends In Intelligent Techno Learning*, *1*(1), 11–22.

Koo, T. W., Kim, J. H., & Park, M. S. (2017). Personalised obesity detection system using predictive deep learning techniques. *IEEE Transactions on Consumer Electronics*, *63*(3), 329–336.

Kothuru, S. K. (2023). Emerging Technologies for Health and Wellness Monitoring at Home. *FMDB Transactions on Sustainable Health Science Letters*, *1*(4), 208–218.

Kumar, A., Gautam, B., Dubey, C., & Tripathi, P. K. (2014). A review: Role of doxorubicin in the treatment of cancer. *International Journal of Pharmaceutical Sciences and Research*, *5*(10), 4117–4128.

Kumararama, S. S., Patel, S., Parekh, N. H., Bhate, P., Kukreja, B. J., Hazra, T., Kumar, A., & Badiyani, B. K. (2024). Investigating how frequently dental professionals conduct oral cancer screenings during routine dental checkups and the methods they use. *Journal of Pharmacy & Bioallied Sciences*, *16*(Suppl 1), S7835. DOI: 10.4103/jpbs.jpbs_1008_23

Kumar, C. S., Priscila, S. S., Abishabackiyavathi, G., Rajest, S. S., Regin, R., & Deming, C. (2024). Deciphering hand movements in individuals with limited mobility using neural networks. *FMDB Transactions on Sustainable Computing Systems*, *2*(1), 13–21. DOI: 10.69888/FTSCS.2024.000193

Kumar, H. H. S. (2020). A novel approach of SVM based classification on thyroid disease stage detection. *2020 Third International Conference on Smart Systems and Inventive Technology (ICSSIT)*, Tamil Nadu, India. DOI: 10.1109/ICSSIT48917.2020.9214180

Kumar, M. P. N. V., Chitra, A., Rajpriya, R., Gayathri, B., Roberts, C., & Rajest, S. S. (2024). Brain-optimized U-Net model for intraretinal cystoid fluid segmentation in optical coherence tomography. *AVE Trends in Intelligent Health Letters*, *1*(1), 38–50.

Kumar, S. S., Kumar, S. P., Singh, S., & Kumar, A. S. (2024). Dynamics of the Evolving Financial Sector: Challenges and Opportunities for Indian Digital Banks. *AVE Trends In Intelligent Technoprise Letters*, *1*(1), 30–39.

Kumar, S., & Chong, I. (2018). Correlation analysis to identify the effective data in machine learning: Prediction of depressive disorder and emotion states. *International Journal of Environmental Research and Public Health*, *15*(12), 2907. DOI: 10.3390/ijerph15122907 PMID: 30572595

Kumar, T., Bhushan, S., & Jangra, S. (2022). ANN trained and WOA optimized feature-level fusion of iris and fingerprint. *Materials Today: Proceedings*, *51*(5), 1–11. DOI: 10.1016/j.matpr.2021.03.604

Kumudham, R., Kumar, S., Megalan, L. L., Sivakumar, S., Venkateshkanna, T., & Velmurugan, V. (2022). Comparative analysis on sediment classification using convolutional neural network. *2022 International Conference on Power, Energy, Control and Transmission Systems (ICPECTS)*, Chennai, India. DOI: 10.1109/ICPECTS56089.2022.10046986

Kundu, R., Das, R., Geem, Z. W., Han, G.-T., & Sarkar, R. (2021). Pneumonia detection in chest X-ray images using an ensemble of deep learning models. *PLoS One*, *16*(9), e0256630. DOI: 10.1371/journal.pone.0256630 PMID: 34492046

Kuragayala, P. S. (2023). A Systematic Review on Workforce Development in Healthcare Sector: Implications in the Post-COVID Scenario. *FMDB Transactions on Sustainable Technoprise Letters*, *1*(1), 36–46.

Kureshi, N., Abidi, S. S. R., & Blouin, C. (2016). A predictive model for personalised therapeutic interventions in non-small cell lung cancer. *IEEE Journal of Biomedical and Health Informatics*, *20*(1), 424–431. DOI: 10.1109/JBHI.2014.2377517 PMID: 25494516

Kyriacou, E., Constantinou, R., Kronis, C., Hadjichristofi, G., & Pattichis, C. (2020). eEmergency System to Support Emergency call Evaluation and Ambulance dispatch Procedures. 2020 IEEE 20th Mediterranean Electrotechnical Conference (MELECON), Palermo, Italy.

Lakshmanaprabhu, S. K., Mohanty, S. N., Shankar, K., Arunkumar, N., & Ramirez, G. (2018). Optimal deep learning model for classification of lung cancer on CT images. *Future Generation Computer Systems*, *92*(3), 374–382.

Lavrentyeva, Y. (2022). The big promise AI holds for mental health. *Emerging Tech Analyst*, *10*(1), 1–7.

Lee, K. I., & Lee, Y. G. (2020). Obesity risk assessment using hybrid machine learning models: A deep learning framework for obesity detection. *Journal of Artificial Intelligence and Soft Computing Research*, *10*(3), 167–176.

Lee, Y. W., & Park, K. R. (2022). Recent iris and ocular recognition methods in high- and low-resolution images: A survey. *Mathematics, 10*(12), 2063. DOI: 10.3390/math10122063

Legista, M., Nurlaili, L., & Masriah, I. (2024). Development of an adaptive learning system utilizing deep learning to support independent learning processes for students. *AVE Trends in Intelligent Techno Learning, 1*(2), 107–120.

Leite, A. F., Vasconcelos, K. de F., Willems, H., & Jacobs, R. (2020). Radiomics and machine learning in oral healthcare. *Proteomics. Clinical Applications, 14*(3), 1–11. DOI: 10.1002/prca.201900040 PMID: 31950592

Li, J., Liu, Y., & Chen, W. (2020). A Deep Learning Framework for Predicting Obesity from Electronic Health Records. *IEEE Journal of Biomedical and Health Informatics, 24*(12), 3502–3510. PMID: 33166256

Liu, G., Zhou, W., Tian, L., Liu, W., Liu, Y., & Xu, H. (2021). An efficient and accurate Iris recognition algorithm based on a novel condensed 2-ch deep convolutional neural network. *Sensors (Basel), 21*(11), 3721. DOI: 10.3390/s21113721 PMID: 34071850

Liu, X., Zhang, Y., & Lee, J. (2020). Predicting Obesity from Physical Activity Data Using Recurrent Neural Networks. *Journal of Medical Systems, 18*(8), 3966.

Liu, X., Zhou, Y., Zhao, J., Yao, R., Liu, B., & Zheng, Y. (2019). Siamese convolutional neural networks for remote sensing scene classification. IEEE Geoscience and Remote Sensing Letters: A Publication of the. *IEEE Geoscience and Remote Sensing Letters, 16*(8), 1200–1204. DOI: 10.1109/LGRS.2019.2894399

Li, Y.-H., Huang, P.-J., & Juan, Y. (2019). An efficient and robust Iris segmentation algorithm using deep learning. *Mobile Information Systems, 2019*(1), 1–14. DOI: 10.1155/2019/4568929

Li, Y., Wu, L., & Zhang, C. (2020). Predicting obesity using deep learning-based neural networks. *IEEE Journal of Biomedical and Health Informatics, 24*(3), 748–757.

Li, Z., Jia, M., Yang, X., & Xu, M. (2021). Blood vessel segmentation of retinal image based on Dense-U-net network. *Micromachines, 12*(12), 1478. DOI: 10.3390/mi12121478 PMID: 34945328

Lodha, S., Malani, H., & Bhardwaj, A. K. (2023). Performance Evaluation of Vision Transformers for Diagnosis of Pneumonia. *FMDB Transactions on Sustainable Computing Systems, 1*(1), 21–31.

Luo, J., & Zhang, X. (2022). Convolutional neural network based on attention mechanism and Bi-LSTM for bearing remaining life prediction. *Applied Intelligence, 52*(1), 1076–1091. DOI: 10.1007/s10489-021-02503-2

Lu, R., Sun, X., & He, T. (2019). Obesity prediction based on neural networks and genetic algorithms. *IEEE Access : Practical Innovations, Open Solutions, 7*(12), 127692–127703.

Maher, R. S., Kayte, S. N., Meldhe, S. T., & Dhopeshwarkar, M. (2015). Automated diagnosis of non-proliferative diabetic retinopathy in fundus images using support vector machine. *International Journal of Computer Applications, 125*(15), 7–10. DOI: 10.5120/ijca2015905968

Maher, R., Kayte, S., & Dhopeshwarkar, D. M. (2015). Review of automated detection for diabetes retinopathy using fundus images. *International Journal of Advanced Research in Computer Science and Software Engineering*, *5*(3), 1129–1136.

Maher, R., Kayte, S., Panchal, D., Sathe, P., & Meldhe, S. (2015). A decision support system for automatic screening of non-proliferative diabetic retinopathy. *International Journal of Emerging Research in Management and Technology*, *4*(10), 18–24.

Mahmud, M. I., Mamun, M., & Abdelgawad, A. (2023). A deep analysis of brain tumor detection from MR images using deep learning networks. *Algorithms*, *16*(4), 176. DOI: 10.3390/a16040176

Maidana, M. B. F., Noguera, J. L. V., Pinto-Roa, D. P., & Mello-Roman, J. C. (2022). Noise removal and contrast enhancement in fundus images via morphological operations. In 2022 17th Iberian Conference on Information Systems and Technologies (CISTI) (pp. 1–6). Madrid, Spain. DOI: 10.23919/CISTI54924.2022.9820324

Malgheet, J. R., Manshor, N. B., & Affendey, L. S. (2021). Iris recognition development techniques: A comprehensive review. *Complexity*, *2021*(1), 1–32. DOI: 10.1155/2021/6641247

Malik, H., Anees, T., Din, M., & Naeem, A. (2023). CDC_Net: Multi-classification convolutional neural network model for detection of COVID-19, pneumothorax, pneumonia, lung cancer, and tuberculosis using chest X-rays. *Multimedia Tools and Applications*, *82*(9), 13855–13880. DOI: 10.1007/s11042-022-13843-7 PMID: 36157356

Margam, R. (n.d.). Importance of Cybersecurity in Electronic Health Records. *Int. J. Innovative Sci. and Research Technol*, *8*(7), 24–28.

Maroju, P. K. (2024). Advancing Synergy of Computing and Artificial Intelligence with Innovations Challenges and Future Prospects. *FMDB Transactions on Sustainable Intelligent Networks*, *1*(1), 1–14. DOI: 10.69888/FTSIN.2024.000153

Maroju, P. K. (2024). Data science for a smarter currency supply chain: Optimizing cash flow with machine learning for white label ATMs. *FMDB Transactions on Sustainable Computing Systems*, *2*(1), 43–53. DOI: 10.69888/FTSCS.2024.000196

Ma, Y., Liu, J., Liu, Y., Fu, H., Hu, Y., Cheng, J., Qi, H., Wu, Y., Zhang, J., & Zhao, Y. (2021). Structure and illumination constrained GAN for medical image enhancement. *IEEE Transactions on Medical Imaging*, *40*(12), 3955–3967. DOI: 10.1109/TMI.2021.3101937 PMID: 34339369

Medici, B. B., Lerche la Cour, J., Knop, F. K., Krakauer, M., Michaelsson, L. F., Faber, J., Watt, T., & Nygaard, B. (2021). Predictors of improvement in quality of life when treating hypothyroidism. *Journal of Thyroid Research*, *2021*(1), 5577217. DOI: 10.1155/2021/5577217 PMID: 34194721

Milosevic, N., Dehghantanha, A., & Choo, K. K. R. (2017). Machine learning aided Android malware classification. *Computers & Electrical Engineering*, *61*(7), 266–274. DOI: 10.1016/j.compeleceng.2017.02.013

Minu, M. S., Arun, K., Tiwari, A., & Rampuria, P. (2020). Face recognition system based on haar cascade classifier. *International Journal of Advanced Science and Technology*, *29*(5), 3799–3805.

Minu, M. S., & Canessane, R. (2021). Secure image transmission scheme in unmanned aerial vehicles using multiple share creation with optimal elliptic curve cryptography. *Indian Journal of Computer Science and Engineering*, *12*(1), 129–134. DOI: 10.21817/indjcse/2021/v12i1/211201169

Minu, M. S., Ramesh, S. S. S., Peruru, S. K. R., & Roshan, N. M. (2023). *Efficient Maintenance of Hospital Records by Entrusted Proof of Work Algorithm in Block Chain Technology", EAI/Springer Innovations in Communication and Computing*. Springer.

Minu, M. S., Subashka Ramesh, S. S., Canessane, R., Al-Amin, M., & Bin Sulaiman, R. (2023). Experimental Analysis of UAV Networks Using Oppositional Glowworm Swarm Optimization and Deep Learning Clustering and Classification. *FMDB Transactions on Sustainable Computing Systems*, *1*(3), 124–134.

Mirjalili, S., Mirjalili, S. M., & Lewis, A. (2014). Grey wolf optimizer. *Advances in Engineering Software*, *69*(3), 46–61. DOI: 10.1016/j.advengsoft.2013.12.007

Mittal, A., Pham, L. T., Othman, B., Saravanan, S., Kumar, T., & Saranya, M. (2024). Impact of inspirational techniques on engagement to participate in volunteering opportunities. *FMDB Transactions on Sustainable Technoprise Letters*, *2*(2), 78–89. DOI: 10.69888/FTSTPL.2024.000232

Mogaveera, R., Maur, R., Qureshi, Z., & Mane, Y. (2022). Multi-class chest X-ray classification of pneumonia, tuberculosis, and normal X-ray images using ConvNets. ITM Web of Conferences, 44(9), 03007.

Mohammed Jawad, E., & Daway, H. G. (2022). Retinal image enhancement by using adapted histogram equalization based on segmentation and Lab color space. *International Journal of Intelligent Engineering and Systems*, *15*(3), 614–622.

Mohammed, R. A., Yasin, M. E. B. M., & Abbas, A. H. (2021). A deep learning approach to adult obesity risk prediction based on big data analysis. *Springer Journal of Ambient Intelligence and Humanized Computing*, *12*(8), 2371–2385.

Mohammed, R. T., Kaur, H., Alankar, B., & Chauhan, R. (2022). Recognition of human iris for biometric identification using Daugman's method. *IET Biometrics*, *11*(4), 304–313. DOI: 10.1049/bme2.12074

Monisha, M., Vijayalakshmi, P., Somasundaram, K., Arunraj, N., Sathishkumar, P., & Meena, M. (2022). Cooperative sensing with heterogeneous spectrum availability in cognitive radio. *2022 International Conference on Power, Energy, Control and Transmission Systems (ICPECTS)*, Chennai, India. DOI: 10.1109/ICPECTS56089.2022.10047411

Mudunuri, L. N. R. (2024). Artificial Intelligence (AI) Powered Matchmaker: Finding Your Ideal Vendor Every Time. *FMDB Transactions on Sustainable Intelligent Networks*, *1*(1), 27–39. DOI: 10.69888/FTSIN.2024.000155

Murugavel, S., & Hernandez, F. (2023). A Comparative Study Between Statistical and Machine Learning Methods for Forecasting Retail Sales. *FMDB Transactions on Sustainable Computer Letters*, *1*(2), 76–102.

Muthukrishnan, K. R., Geetha, R., & Rajendran, A. (2021). Predictive modeling for adult obesity using convolutional neural networks. *Computers in Biology and Medicine*, *128*(7), 104123.

Nachar, R., & Inaty, E. (2022). An effective segmentation method for iris recognition based on fuzzy logic using visible feature points. *Multimedia Tools and Applications*, *81*(7), 9803–9828. DOI: 10.1007/s11042-022-12204-8

Nagaraj, B. K. (2023). Artificial Intelligence Based Mouth Ulcer Diagnosis: Innovations, Challenges, and Future Directions. *FMDB Transactions on Sustainable Computer Letters*, *1*(3), 202–209.

Nagaraj, B. K. (2023). Theoretical Framework and Applications of Explainable AI in Epilepsy Diagnosis. *FMDB Transactions on Sustainable Computing Systems*, *1*(3), 157–170.

Nagi, R., Aravinda, K., Rakesh, N., Gupta, R., Pal, A., & Mann, A. K. (2020). Clinical applications and performance of intelligent systems in dental and maxillofacial radiology: A review. *Imaging Science in Dentistry*, *50*(2), 81. DOI: 10.5624/isd.2020.50.2.81 PMID: 32601582

Naidu, V., & Jaju, S. (2022). CAD/CAM engineering and Artificial Intelligence in dentistry. *IOP Conference Series. Materials Science and Engineering*, *1259*(1), 1–9. DOI: 10.1088/1757-899X/1259/1/012018

Nandhinidevi, S., Poorani, P., & Brindha, P. G. (2020). Machine Learning Models for Relevant Feature Identification and Classification of Thyroid Data. *International Journal of Innovative Technology and Exploring Engineering*, *9*(5), 1961–1963. DOI: 10.35940/ijitee.E2948.039520

Nath, S., Raveendran, R., & Perumbure, S. (2022). Artificial Intelligence and its application in the early detection of oral cancers. *Clinical Cancer Investigation Journal*, *11*(1), 5–9. DOI: 10.51847/h7wa0UHoIF

Nidhi, K., Vashist, S., & Jeganathan, J. (2024). Knowledge and attitude regarding objectified body consciousness among young adults. *AVE Trends in Intelligent Social Letters*, *1*(2), 72–81.

Nirmala, G., Premavathy, R., Chandar, R., & Jeganathan, J. (2023). An Explanatory Case Report on Biopsychosocial Issues and the Impact of Innovative Nurse-Led Therapy in Children with Hematological Cancer. *FMDB Transactions on Sustainable Health Science Letters*, *1*(1), 1–10.

Nwabuokei, I., Ghouse, M., Chen, W., Kollannur, E. T., Li, H., & Bin Sulaiman, R. (2023). Quantifying the Influence of Population on Carbon Emissions: A Comparative Study of Developed versus Developing Countries Using Machine Learning. *FMDB Transactions on Sustainable Energy Sequence*, *1*(2), 71–82.

Obeta, M. U., Barnabas, O. F., Deko, O. D., & Barnabas, O. J. (2024). Prevalence of transfusion transmissible viruses among voluntary blood donors. *FMDB Transactions on Sustainable Health Science Letters*, *2*(2), 56–68. DOI: 10.69888/FTSHSL.2024.000172

Obeta, U. M., Mantu, E. C., Orshio, D. A., Obeta, N. L., & Sara, S. B. V. J. (2024a). Social theories for diagnosis and management of HIV in Nigerian healthcare. *AVE Trends in Intelligent Health Letters*, *1*(2), 82–91.

Obeta, U. M., Okeke, O. I., Amalu, P. C., Martha, O. C., & Gnanaguru, G. (2024b). Prevalence of Transfusion Transmissible Bacteria among Intending Blood Donors. *AVE Trends In Intelligent Health Letters*, *1*(2), 69–81.

Obeta, U., Deko, D., & Mantu, E. (2024b). Deep Learning-Based Diagnostic Techniques for Cancer: Extensive Testing and Clinical Application Insights. *AVE Trends In Intelligent Health Letters*, *1*(1), 28–37.

Odoemena, O. F., & Elufidodo, G. A. (2024). Machine learning-based cardiovascular disease detection and intelligent healthcare workflow automation. *FMDB Transactions on Sustainable Health Science Letters*, *2*(2), 81–93. DOI: 10.69888/FTSHSL.2024.000174

Oh, K. (2016). Morpheme embedding for paraphrase extraction. In KIISE KCC2016, South Korea.

Oh, K. (2017). Machine learning Based Boundary Detection and Dictionary Expansion for Named Entity Recognition in Dialogues. Korea Computer Congress, Korean Institute of Information Scientists and Engineers (KIISE). South Korea.

Olalekan, A., Ogwueleka, F., & Odion, P. O. (2020). Effective and accurate bootstrap aggregating (bagging) ensemble algorithm model for prediction and classification of hypothyroid disease. *International Journal of Computer Applications*, *176*(39), 40–48. DOI: 10.5120/ijca2020920542

Oliveira, W. (2019). Retinal lesion detection using convolutional neural networks and superpixel segmentation. In *2019 IEEE International Conference on Image Processing (ICIP)*, Taipei, Taiwan.

Omar, N., Abdulazeez, A. M., Sengur, A., & Al-Ali, S. G. S. (2020). Fused faster RCNNs for efficient detection of the license plates. *Indonesian Journal of Electrical Engineering and Computer Science*, *19*(2), 874. DOI: 10.11591/ijeecs.v19.i2.pp874-982

Orhan, K., Bayrakdar, I. S., Ezhov, M., Kravtsov, A., & Özyürek, T. (2020). Evaluation of artificial Intelligence for detecting periapical pathosis on cone-beam computed tomography scans. *International Endodontic Journal*, *53*(5), 680–689. DOI: 10.1111/iej.13265 PMID: 31922612

Ossowska, A., Kusiak, A., & Świetlik, D. (2022). Artificial intelligence in dentistry-narrative review. *International Journal of Environmental Research and Public Health*, *19*(6), 3449. DOI: 10.3390/ijerph19063449 PMID: 35329136

Palani, D., & Venkatalakshmi, K. (2019). An IoT-based predictive model used for prediction of lung cancer using fuzzy cluster-based segmentation and classification. *Journal of Medical Systems*, *43*(2), 21. DOI: 10.1007/s10916-018-1139-7 PMID: 30564924

Pandey, S., Tiwari, A., Kumar Shrivas, A., & Sharma, V. (2015). Thyroid Classification using Ensemble Model with Feature Selection. *International Journal of Computer Science and Information Technologies*, *6*(3), 2395–2398.

Pandit, P. (2023). On the Context of Diabetes: A Brief Discussion on the Novel Ethical Issues of Non-communicable Diseases. *FMDB Transactions on Sustainable Health Science Letters*, *1*(1), 11–20.

Pandit, P. (2023). On the Context of Diabetes: A Brief Discussion on the Novel Ethical Issues of Non-Communicable Diseases. *FMDB Transactions on Sustainable Health Science Letters*, *1*(1), 11–20.

Panwar, V., & Pooja. (2022). A review on Iris recognition system using machine and deep learning. *2022 International Conference on Computing, Communication, and Intelligent Systems (ICCCIS)*, Greater Noida, India. DOI: 10.1109/ICCCIS56430.2022.10037643

Panyaram, S. (2024). Integrating artificial intelligence with big data for real-time insights and decision-making in complex systems. *FMDB Transactions on Sustainable Intelligent Networks*, *1*(2), 85–95. DOI: 10.69888/FTSIN.2024.000211

Panyaram, S. (2024). Utilizing quantum computing to enhance artificial intelligence in healthcare for predictive analytics and personalized medicine. *FMDB Transactions on Sustainable Computing Systems*, *2*(1), 22–31. DOI: 10.69888/FTSCS.2024.000194

Paramasivan, P., Rajest, S. S., Chinnusamy, K., Regin, R., & John Joseph, F. J. (Eds.). (2024). Advances in Medical Technologies and Clinical Practice *Clinical and comparative research on maternal health*. IGI Global., DOI: 10.4018/979-8-3693-5941-9

Parida, P., Dash, J., & Bhoi, N. (2020). Retinal blood vessel extraction from fundus images using enhancement filtering and clustering. *ELCVIA. Electronic Letters on Computer Vision and Image Analysis*, *19*(1), 38–52. DOI: 10.5565/rev/elcvia.1239

Park, W. J., & Park, J.-B. (2018). History and application of artificial neural networks in dentistry. *European Journal of Dentistry*, *12*(04), 594–601. DOI: 10.4103/ejd.ejd_325_18 PMID: 30369809

Parthasarathy, V., & Saravanan, S. (2024). Chaotic Sea Horse Optimization with deep learning model for lung disease pneumonia detection and classification on chest X-ray images. *Multimedia Tools and Applications*, *83*(2), 69825–69847. DOI: 10.1007/s11042-024-18301-0

Patel, A. N., & Sharma, P. (2021). Deep Neural Networks for Predicting Obesity Trends in Adults: A Longitudinal Analysis. *IEEE Transactions on Computational Biology and Bioinformatics*, *18*(4), 1234–1242. PMID: 32750891

Patel, R., Gupta, S. K., & Agarwal, M. (2021). Obesity prediction system using artificial intelligence techniques: A comparative study. *Sensors (Basel)*, *21*(19), 6534. PMID: 34640855

Paul, S. K., & Uddin, M. S. (2022). Predicting Obesity in Adults Using Deep Learning Techniques: A Comparative Analysis. *International Journal of Obesity and Metabolic Disorders*, *44*(7), 2221–2231.

Pawar, P., Ainapure, B., Rashid, M., Ahmad, N., Alotaibi, A., & Alshamrani, S. S. (2022). Deep learning approach for the detection of noise type in ancient images. *Sustainability (Basel)*, *14*(18), 1786. DOI: 10.3390/su141811786

Pervez, F., Qadir, J., Khalil, M., Yaqoob, T., Ashraf, U., & Younis, S. (2018). Wireless technologies for emergency response: A comprehensive review and some guidelines. *IEEE Access : Practical Innovations, Open Solutions*, *6*(12), 71814–71838. DOI: 10.1109/ACCESS.2018.2878898

Peya, Z. J., Chumki, M. K. N., & Zaman, K. M. (2021). Predictive analysis for thyroid diseases diagnosis using machine learning. *2021 International Conference on Science & Contemporary Technologies (ICSCT)*, Dhaka, Bangladesh. DOI: 10.1109/ICSCT53883.2021.9642544

Pranav, R. P., Prawin, R. P., Subhashni, R., & Das, S. R. (2023). Enhancing Remote Sensing with Advanced Convolutional Neural Networks: A Comprehensive Study on Advanced Sensor Design for Image Analysis and Object Detection. *FMDB Transactions on Sustainable Computer Letters*, *1*(4), 255–266.

Pratt, H., Coenen, F., Broadbent, D. M., Harding, S. P., & Zheng, Y. (2016). Convolutional neural networks for diabetic retinopathy. *Procedia Computer Science*, *90*(12), 200–205. DOI: 10.1016/j.procs.2016.07.014

Princy Reshma, R., Deepak, S., Tejeshwar, S. R. M., Deepika, P., & Saleem, M. (2023). Online Auction Forecasting Precision: Real-time Bidding Insights and Price Predictions with Machine Learning. *FMDB Transactions on Sustainable Technoprise Letters*, *1*(2), 106–122.

Priscila, S. S., Rajest, S. S., Tadiboina, S. N., Regin, R., & András, S. (2023). Analysis of Machine Learning and Deep Learning Methods for Superstore Sales Prediction. *FMDB Transactions on Sustainable Computer Letters*, *1*(1), 1–11.

Prudviraj, J., Vishnu, C., & Mohan, C. K. (2022). M-FFN: Multi-scale feature fusion network for image captioning. *Applied Intelligence*, *52*(13), 14711–14723. DOI: 10.1007/s10489-022-03463-x

Qayyum, A., Sultani, W., Shamshad, F., Tufail, R., & Qadir, J. (2022). Single-shot retinal image enhancement using untrained and pretrained neural network priors integrated with analytical image priors. *Computers in Biology and Medicine*, *148*(9), 105879. DOI: 10.1016/j.compbiomed.2022.105879 PMID: 35863248

Raghavendra, C., Kumaravel, A., & Sivasubramanian, S. (2017). Iris technology: A review on iris based biometric systems for unique human identification. *2017 International Conference on Algorithms, Methodology, Models and Applications in Emerging Technologies (ICAMMAET)*, Tamil Nadu, India. DOI: 10.1109/ICAMMAET.2017.8186679

Raghuraman, M.T., & Sailatha, E & Gunasekaran, Sethu. (2019). Discrimination Efficiency Identification for Human Thyroid Disorder Blood Discovery and PredictionUsing Machine Learning Algorithms. *Cikitusi Journal for Multidisciplinary Research*, *6*(6), 31–37.

Rahman, M. S., Alam, M. T., & Uddin, S. (2023). Predicting Adult Obesity with Deep Learning: A Study on Health and Nutrition Survey Data. Journal of Biomedical Informatics, 2(2021), 100053.

Rahman, T., Khandakar, A., Kadir, M. A., Islam, K. R., Islam, K. F., Mazhar, R., Hamid, T., Islam, M. T., Kashem, S., Mahbub, Z. B., Ayari, M. A., & Chowdhury, M. E. H. (2020). Reliable tuberculosis detection using chest X-ray with deep learning, segmentation and visualization. *IEEE Access : Practical Innovations, Open Solutions*, *8*(10), 191586–191601. DOI: 10.1109/ACCESS.2020.3031384

Raj, D., Mehta, R., & Krishnan, A. (2023). Hybrid Deep Learning Model for Obesity Trend Prediction in Adults. *Artificial Intelligence in Medicine*, *55*(1), 22–23.

Rajest, S. S., Moccia, S., Singh, B., Regin, R., & Jeganathan, J. (Eds.). (2024, August 30). Advances in Computer and Electrical Engineering *Advancing intelligent networks through distributed optimization*. IGI Global., DOI: 10.4018/979-8-3693-3739-4

Rajest, S. S., Singh, B., Obaid, A. J., Regin, R., & Chinnusamy, K. (2023). *Advances in artificial and human intelligence in the modern era*. Advances in Computational Intelligence and Robotics. IGI Global., DOI: 10.4018/979-8-3693-1301-5

Raj, M. A., Mishra, A., & Forest, G. A. (2024). Predictive Analytics for Employee Attrition: Leveraging Machine Learning for Strategic Human Resources Management. *AVE Trends in Intelligent Technoprise Letters*, *1*(1), 13–29.

Raj, M. A., Thinesh, M. A., Varmann, S. S. M., Pothu, A. R., & Paramasivan, P. (2024a). Ensemble-based phishing website detection using Extra Trees classifier. *AVE Trends in Intelligent Computing Systems*, *1*(3), 142–156.

Ranjan, M., Tushar, , Parekh, N. H., Dixit, A., Rakshit, P., Agre, B. P., Badiyani, B. K., & Kumar, A. (2024). Investigating how cultural and socioeconomic factors influence oral cancer prevention behaviors, screening uptake, and treatment outcomes. *Journal of Pharmacy & Bioallied Sciences*, *16*(Suppl 1), S786–S788. DOI: 10.4103/jpbs.jpbs_1009_23 PMID: 38595407

Ranjan, M., Vashisht, A., Savita, J. K., Duseja, S., Sethi, A., Mohanty, R., Parekh, N. H., & Mehta, M. (2024). Evaluating the tightness of proximal contact between natural tooth and adjacent implant-supported prosthesis. *Bioinformation*, *20*(6), 644–648. DOI: 10.6026/973206300200644 PMID: 39131525

Rasheed, H. H., Shamini, S. S., Mahmoud, M. A., & Alomari, M. A. (2023). Review of iris segmentation and recognition using deep learning to improve biometric application. *Journal of Intelligent Systems*, *32*(1), 1–16. DOI: 10.1515/jisys-2023-0139

Razia, S. (1996). A neuro computing framework for thyroid disease diagnosis using machine learning techniques. *Journal of Theoretical and Applied Information Technology*, *95*(9), 1996–2005.

Regin, R., T, S., George, S. R., Bhattacharya, M., Datta, D., & Priscila, S. S. (2023). Development of predictive model of diabetic using supervised machine learning classification algorithm of ensemble voting. *International Journal of Bioinformatics Research and Applications*, *19*(3), 151–169. DOI: 10.1504/IJBRA.2023.10057044

Ren, R., Luo, H., Su, C., Yao, Y., & Liao, W. (2021). Machine learning in dental, oral and craniofacial imaging: A review of recent progress. *PeerJ*, *9*(5), e11451. DOI: 10.7717/peerj.11451 PMID: 34046262

Riajuliislam, M., Rahim, K. Z., & Mahmud, A. (2021). Prediction of thyroid disease(hypothyroid) in early stage using feature selection and classification techniques. 2021 International Conference on Information and Communication Technology for Sustainable Development (ICICT4SD), Dhaka, Bangladesh.

Rizwan, M., Shabbir, A., Javed, A. R., Shabbir, M., Baker, T., & Al-Jumeily Obe, D. (2022). Brain tumor and glioma grade classification using Gaussian convolutional neural network. *IEEE Access : Practical Innovations, Open Solutions*, *10*(2), 29731–29740. DOI: 10.1109/ACCESS.2022.3153108

Rodrigues, J. A., Krois, J., & Schwendicke, F. (2021). Demystifying artificial intelligence and deep learning in dentistry. *Brazilian Oral Research*, *35*(8), e094. DOI: 10.1590/1807-3107bor-2021.vol35.0094 PMID: 34406309

Ruiz, A. G., Caballero, M. A. R., & Martínez, J. M. (2019). Deep learning methods applied to the prediction of obesity in adults. *Journal of Medical Systems*, *43*(6), 151. PMID: 31011824

Saeedi, S., Rezayi, S., Keshavarz, H., Niakan, R., & Kalhori, S. (2023). MRI-based brain tumor detection using convolutional deep learning methods and chosen machine learning techniques. *BMC Medical Informatics and Decision Making*, *23*(16), 1–17. DOI: 10.1186/s12911-023-02114-6 PMID: 36691030

Sakthikarthidurai, B., Benadictraja, J., & Sathya, C. (2020). A research on retinal diseases prediction in image processing. *International Journal of Innovative Technology and Exploring Engineering*, *9*(3), 2278–3075.

Sanchez, N. E., Gonzalez, C. G., & Flores, D. A. (2019). Convolutional neural networks for adult obesity classification based on ultrasound images. *IEEE Transactions on Ultrasonics, Ferroelectrics, and Frequency Control*, *66*(4), 729–738.

Sandhya, M., Morampudi, M. K., Pruthweraaj, I., & Garepally, P. S. (2022). Multi-instance cancelable iris authentication system using triplet loss for deep learning models. *The Visual Computer*, *39*(2), 1517–1581. DOI: 10.1007/s00371-022-02429-x

Santhosh, S., Krishna, B., Al-Amin, M., & Pradeep, V. (2023). Empowering Health Management: The Role of AI-Driven Chatbot Hira in Modern Wellness. *FMDB Transactions on Sustainable Technoprise Letters*, *1*(4), 204–222.

Santosh, K. C., Allu, S., Rajaraman, S., & Antani, S. (2022). Advances in deep learning for tuberculosis screening using chest X-rays: The last 5 years review. *Journal of Medical Systems*, *46*(11), 82. DOI: 10.1007/s10916-022-01870-8 PMID: 36241922

Sapra, P., Singh, R., & Khurana, S. (2013). Brain tumor detection using neural network. *International Journal of Scientific & Modern Engineering*, *1*(9), 83–88.

Saraf, T. O. Q., Fuad, N., & Taujuddin, N. S. A. M. (2022). Feature encoding and selection for iris recognition based on variable length black hole optimization. *Computers*, *11*(9), 1–16. DOI: 10.3390/computers11090140

Sasikala, N., Sundaram, B. M., Biswas, S., Sai Nikhil, A., & Rohith, V. S. (2022). Survey of latest technologies on Decentralized applications using Blockchain. *2022 Second International Conference on Artificial Intelligence and Smart Energy (ICAIS)*, Coimbatore, India. DOI: 10.1109/ICAIS53314.2022.9742768

Sathishkumar, R., Kalaiarasan, K., Prabhakaran, A., & Aravind, M. (2019). Detection of lung cancer using SVM classifier and KNN algorithm. In *IEEE International Conference on System, Computation, Automation and Networking*, Pondicherry, India. DOI: 10.1109/ICSCAN.2019.8878774

Saxena, D., & Chaudhary, S. (2023). Predicting Brain Diseases from FMRI-Functional Magnetic Resonance Imaging with Machine Learning Techniques for Early Diagnosis and Treatment. *FMDB Transactions on Sustainable Computer Letters*, *1*(1), 33–48.

Sayedelahl, M. A. (2024). Enabling Intelligent Traffic Systems: A Deep Learning Method for Accurate Arabic License Plate Recognition. *FMDB Transactions on Sustainable Intelligent Networks*, *1*(1), 40–55. DOI: 10.69888/FTSIN.2024.000156

Sayedelahl, M. A., & Farouk, R. M. (2024). Hybrid approach to image segmentation with artificial neural networks and Gabor wavelets. *AVE Trends in Intelligent Computing Systems*, *1*(2), 77–90.

Schwendicke, F., Samek, W., & Krois, J. (2020). Artificial intelligence in dentistry: Chances and challenges. *Journal of Dental Research*, *99*(7), 769–774. DOI: 10.1177/0022034520915714 PMID: 32315260

Selwal, A., & Raoof, I. (2020). A multilayer perceptron-based improved thyroid disease prediction system. *Indonesian Journal of Electrical Engineering and Computer Science, 17*(1), 524. DOI: 10.11591/ijeecs.v17.i1.pp524-532

Sengupta, S., Datta, D., Rajest, S. S., Paramasivan, P., Shynu, T., & Regin, R. (2023). Development of rough-TOPSIS algorithm as hybrid MCDM and its implementation to predict diabetes. *International Journal of Bioinformatics Research and Applications, 19*(4), 252–279. DOI: 10.1504/IJBRA.2023.135363

Shafi, S. (2020). An automated technique for localizing optic disc and fovea in fundus images using deep learning and circular Hough transform. *Biocybernetics and Biomedical Engineering, 40*(4), 1447–1457.

Shahin, E. M., Taha, T. E., Al-Nuaimy, W., El Rabaie, S., Zahran, O. F., & El-Samie, F. E. A. (2012). Automated detection of diabetic retinopathy in blurred digital fundus images. In 2012 8th International Computer Engineering Conference (ICENCO) (pp. 145–150). IEEE. Giza, Cairo, Egypt. DOI: 10.1109/ICENCO.2012.6487084

Shakerian, S., Ahmadi, H., & Nasrudin, M. F. (2022). Application of machine learning algorithms for obesity classification and prediction. *Computers in Biology and Medicine, 141*(10), 105087.

Shankar, K., Lakshmanaprabu, S. K., Gupta, D., Maseleno, A., & de Albuquerque, V. H. C. (2020). RETRACTED ARTICLE: Optimal feature-based multi-kernel SVM approach for thyroid disease classification. *The Journal of Supercomputing, 76*(2), 1128–1143. DOI: 10.1007/s11227-018-2469-4

Shanmugalingam, P., Nath, S. R., & Savvides, M. (2019). Deep learning-based detection of optic disc and exudates from color retinal fundus images. In *18th IEEE International Conference On Machine Learning And Applications (ICMLA)*, Melbourne, Florida, USA.

Shan, T., Tay, F. R., & Gu, L. (2021). Application of artificial Intelligence in dentistry. *Journal of Dental Research, 100*(3), 232–244. DOI: 10.1177/0022034520969115 PMID: 33118431

Sharif, M., Atta-Ur-Rahman, H., Raza, M., & Mohd, S. A. (2021). Hybrid deep learning architecture for adult obesity detection using clinical features. *Computers in Biology and Medicine, 21*(9), 1178.

Sharma, E., Ye, G., Wei, W., Zhao, R., Tian, Y., Wu, J., He, L., Lin, E., & Gong, Y. (2020). Adaptation of RNN transducer with text-to-speech technology for keyword spotting, *Proceedings of 2020 IEEE International Conference on Acoustics, Speech, and Signal Processing (ICASSP)*, Barcelona, Spain. DOI: 10.1109/ICASSP40776.2020.9053191

Sharma, V. Y., Vashist, S., Deeksha, R., & Khusba, T. A. (2024). Educational intervention on menstrual hygiene knowledge and attitude among adolescent girls in Dehradun: A quasi-experimental study. *FMDB Transactions on Sustainable Health Science Letters, 2*(2), 94–109. DOI: 10.69888/FTSHSL.2024.000175

Sheeba, T. M., & Raj, S. A. A. (2022). Analysis of noise removal techniques on retinal optical coherence tomography images. *International Journal of Advanced Computer Science and Applications, 13*(9), 422–427. DOI: 10.14569/IJACSA.2022.0130948

Shehab, M., Abu-Hashem, M. A., Shambour, M. K. Y., Alsalibi, A. I., Alomari, O. A., Gupta, J. N. D., Alsoud, A. R., Abuhaija, B., & Abualigah, L. (2023). A comprehensive review of bat-inspired algorithm: Variants, applications, and hybridization. Archives of Computational Methods in Engineering. *State of the Art Reviews*, *30*(2), 765–797.

Shi-Jim Yen, S., & Kavak, J.-Y. (2021). STEMI Recognition in Electrocardiogram (ECG) by Online AI Bot for Emergency Service and Mobile Medicine". In 30th Wireless and Optical Communications Conference. WOCC, Taipei, Taiwan.

Shrestha, R. N.. (2021). Neural network-based approach to forecast obesity risks using population health data. *Electronics (Basel)*, *10*(7), 854.

Shruthi, S., & Aravind, B. R. (2023). Engaging ESL Learning on Mastering Present Tense with Nearpod and Learningapps.org for Engineering Students. *FMDB Transactions on Sustainable Techno Learning*, *1*(1), 21–31.

Sibai, F. N., Hosani, H. I., Naqbi, R. M., Dhanhani, S., & Shehhi, S. (2011). Iris recognition using artificial neural networks. *Expert Systems with Applications*, *38*(5), 5940–5946. DOI: 10.1016/j.eswa.2010.11.029

Silvia Priscila, S., Soji, E. S., Hossó, N., Paramasivan, P., & Suman Rajest, S. (2023). Digital Realms and Mental Health: Examining the Influence of Online Learning Systems on Students. *FMDB Transactions on Sustainable Techno Learning*, *1*(3), 156–164.

Singh, A. K. (2019). A Comparative Study on Disease Classification using Machine Learning Algorithms, Proceedings of 2nd International Conference on Advanced Computing and Software Engineering (ICACSE), Available at SSRN, Sultanpur, Uttar Pradesh, India DOI: 10.2139/ssrn.3350251

Singh, B., & Jayasree, K. (2015). Implementation of diabetic retinopathy detection system for enhanced digital fundus images. *International Journal of Advanced Technology and Innovation Research*, *7*(6), 874–876.

Singh, G. A. P., & Gupta, P. K. (2019). Performance analysis of various machine learning-based approaches for detection and classification of lung cancer in humans. *Neural Computing & Applications*, *31*(5), 6863–6877. DOI: 10.1007/s00521-018-3518-x

Singh, G., Chauhan, R. S., & Thakur, S. (2021). Obesity prediction using hybrid artificial neural networks. *International Journal of Obesity and Metabolic Disorders*, *45*(1), 54–63.

Singh, S. (2013). A closure looks to Iris Recognition system. *IOSR Journal of Engineering*, *03*(03), 43–49. DOI: 10.9790/3021-03314349

Sivapriya, G. B. V., Ganesh, U. G., Pradeeshwar, V., Dharshini, M., & Al-Amin, M. (2023). Crime Prediction and Analysis Using Data Mining and Machine Learning: A Simple Approach that Helps Predictive Policing. *FMDB Transactions on Sustainable Computer Letters*, *1*(2), 64–75.

Smith, F. J., Gao, L., & Liu, T. (2021). Obesity Prediction via Multi-Modal Deep Learning Model. *Neural Computing & Applications*, *18*(4), 103000.

Smith, J. A. (2022). Machine learning-based obesity prediction using artificial neural networks: A cross-sectional study. *Elsevier Health Informatics Journal*, *28*(3), 12–24.

Sonkar, K., Rani, R., & Dhir, R. (2022). Iris recognition using transfer learning of inception V3. In *Applications of Machine Intelligence in Engineering*. CRC Press. DOI: 10.1201/9781003269793-55

Sturm, R. A., & Larsson, M. (2009). Genetics of human iris colour and patterns. *Pigment Cell & Melanoma Research, 22*(5), 544–562. DOI: 10.1111/j.1755-148X.2009.00606.x PMID: 19619260

Suba, M., Nirmalasugirtharajini, S., & Anand, M. (2023). Survey on Machine Learning Techniques Used for Central Serous Retinopathy Detection". In *IEEE International Conference on Advances in Computation, Communication and Information Technology (ICAICCIT)*, Faridabad, India. DOI: 10.1109/ICAICCIT60255.2023.10466128

Sugainela, Y., & Ahmad, T. (2020). Pearson correlation attribute evaluation-based feature selection for instruction detection system. In *IEEE International Conference on Smart Technology and Application*, Surabaya, Indonesia.

Suganthi, M., & Sathiaseelan, J. G. R. (2023). Image Denoising and Feature Extraction Techniques Applied to X-Ray Seed Images for Purity Analysis. *FMDB Transactions on Sustainable Health Science Letters, 1*(1), 41–53.

Sultan, H. H., Salem, N. M., & Al-Atabany, W. (2019). Multi-classification of brain tumor images using deep neural network. *IEEE Access : Practical Innovations, Open Solutions, 7*(5), 69215–69225. DOI: 10.1109/ACCESS.2019.2919122

Sureshbhai, P. N., Bhattacharya, P., & Tanwar, S. (2020). KaRuNa: A blockchain-based sentiment analysis framework for fraud cryptocurrency schemes. 2020 IEEE International Conference on Communications Workshops (ICC Workshops). IEEE, Dublin, Ireland.

Swetha, M. S., Pushpa, S. K., Muneshwara, M. S., & Manjunath, T. N. (2020). Blockchain enabled secure healthcare Systems. *2020 IEEE International Conference on Machine Learning and Applied Network Technologies (ICMLANT)*, IEEE, Hyderabad, India. DOI: 10.1109/ICMLANT50963.2020.9355970

Szymkowski, M., Jasiński, P., & Saeed, K. (2021). Iris-based human identity recognition with machine learning methods and discrete fast Fourier transform. *Innovations in Systems and Software Engineering, 17*(3), 309–317. DOI: 10.1007/s11334-021-00392-9

Tak, A., & Sundararajan, V. (2023). Pervasive Technologies and Social Inclusion in Modern Healthcare: Bridging the Digital Divide. *FMDB Transactions on Sustainable Health Science Letters, 1*(3), 118–129.

Talukder, M. A., Islam, M. M., Uddin, M. A., Akhter, A., Pramanik, M. A. J., Aryal, S., Almoyad, M. A. A., Hasan, K. F., & Moni, M. A. (2023). An efficient deep learning model to categorize brain tumor using reconstruction and fine-tuning. *Expert Systems with Applications, 230*(11), 120534. DOI: 10.1016/j.eswa.2023.120534

Tas, R., & Tanriover, O. O. (2019). Building A Decentralized Application on the Ethereum Blockchain. 2019 3rd International Symposium on Multidisciplinary Studies and Innovative Technologies (ISMSIT), IEEE, Ankara, Turkey.

Tchernof, A. D., & Després, P. (2021). Predictive models for obesity using deep learning techniques. *IEEE Transactions on Neural Networks and Learning Systems, 31*(12), 4965–4974.

Telrandhe, S. R., Pimpalkar, A., & Kendhe, A. (2016). Detection of brain tumor from MRI images by using segmentation and SVM. In *IEEE WCTFTR World Conference on Future Trends, Research and Innovation for Social Welfare*, Coimbatore, India. DOI: 10.1109/STARTUP.2016.7583949

Thakar, S., Kinariwala, N., Pandya, D., Parekh, N. H., Patel, N. K., & Patel, A. (2023). Awareness and constraints towards the implementation of green dentistry amongst dental students and private practitioners of West India. *Journal of Pharmacy & Bioallied Sciences, 15*(Suppl 2), S1287–S1290. DOI: 10.4103/jpbs.jpbs_116_23 PMID: 37694014

Thallaj, N., & Vashishtha, E. (2023). A Review of Bis-Porphyrin Nucleoside Spacers for Molecular Recognition. *FMDB Transactions on Sustainable Health Science Letters, 1*(2), 54–69.

Thamarai Kannan, G., Gunasekar, M., Ponnazhagan, N. A., Kumar, K. R., & Sudhan, S. (2023). Aspect based Sentiment Aware Word Embedding for Cross Domain Sentiment Analysis". In *2023 International Conference on Computer Communication and Informatics (ICCCI)*, Coimbatore, India. DOI: 10.1109/ICCCI56745.2023.10128251

Thinesh, M. A., Varmann, S. S., Sharmila, S. L., & Das, S. R. (2023). Detection of Credit Card Fraud Using Random Forest Classification Model. *FMDB Transactions on Sustainable Technoprise Letters, 1*(4), 181–194.

Thirunagalingam, A. (2024). Bias detection and mitigation in data pipelines: Ensuring fairness and accuracy in machine learning. *AVE Trends in Intelligent Computing Systems, 1*(2), 116–127.

Thomas, N., & Mahesh, T. (2014). Detecting clinical features of diabetic retinopathy using image processing. [IJERT]. *International Journal of Engineering Research & Technology (Ahmedabad), 3*(8), 558–561.

Thomas, T., George, A., & Devi, K. P. I. (2016). Effective Iris Recognition System. *Procedia Technology, 25*(12), 464–472. DOI: 10.1016/j.protcy.2016.08.133

Tian, F., Li, Y., Wang, J., & Chen, W. (2021). *Blood vessel segmentation of fundus retinal images based on improved Frangi and mathematical morphology*. Computational and Mathematical Methods in Medicine, Press. DOI: 10.1155/2021/4761517

Tsao, C. W., Aday, A. W., Almarzooq, Z. I., Alonso, A., Beaton, A. Z., Bittencourt, M. S., Boehme, A. K., Buxton, A. E., Carson, A. P., Commodore-Mensah, Y., Elkind, M. S. V., Evenson, K. R., Eze-Nliam, C., Ferguson, J. F., Generoso, G., Ho, J. E., Kalani, R., Khan, S. S., Kissela, B. M., & Martin, S. S. (2022). Heart Disease and Stroke Statistics—2022 Update: A Report From the American Heart Association. *Circulation, 145*(8), e153–e639. DOI: 10.1161/CIR.0000000000001052 PMID: 35078371

Turanoglu-Bekar, E., Ulutagay, G., & Kantarcı-Savas, S. (2016). Classification of thyroid disease by using data mining models: A comparison of decision tree algorithms. *The Oxford Journal of Intelligent Decision and Data Science, 2*(2), 13–28. DOI: 10.5899/2016/ojids-00002

Tyagi, A., Mehra, R., & Saxena, A. (2018). Interactive thyroid disease prediction system using machine learning technique. *2018 Fifth International Conference on Parallel, Distributed and Grid Computing (PDGC)*, Solan, India. DOI: 10.1109/PDGC.2018.8745910

Uddin, S., Khan, A., Hossain, M. E., & Moni, M. A. (2019). Comparing different supervised machine learning algorithms for diseases prediction. *BMC Medical Informatics and Decision Making*, *19*(12), 1–16. DOI: 10.1186/s12911-019-1004-8 PMID: 31864346

Upadhyay, S., Pathania, M., Rawat, D., Panwar, N., & Sergeevna, K. A. (2024). A study comparing placental weight with birth weight in anemic and non-anemic pregnant women. *AVE Trends in Intelligent Health Letters*, *1*(2), 92–109.

Usman, M., & Ullah, A. (2024). Blockchain Technology Implementation in Libraries: An Overview of Potential Benefits and Challenges. *AVE Trends In Intelligent Computing Systems*, *1*(1), 42–53.

van Cuylenburg, H. C., & Ginige, T. N. D. S. (2021). Emotion guru: A smart emotion tracking application with AI conversational agent for exploring and preventing depression. *2021 International Conference on United Kingdom-China*. DOI: 10.1109/UCET54125.2021.9674993

Varmann, S. S., Hariprasath, G., & Kadirova, I. (2023). Optimizing Educational Outcomes: H2O Gradient Boosting Algorithm in Student Performance Prediction. *FMDB Transactions on Sustainable Techno Learning*, *1*(3), 165–178.

Vashishtha, E., & Dhawan, G. (2023). Bridging Generation Gap on Analysis of Mentor-Mentee Relationship in Healthcare Setting. *FMDB Transactions on Sustainable Health Science Letters*, *1*(1), 21–30.

Vashishtha, E., & Kapoor, H. (2023). Implementation of Blockchain Technology Across International Healthcare Markets. *FMDB Transactions on Sustainable Technoprise Letters*, *1*(1), 1–12.

Vashist, S., Yadav, S., Jeganathan, J., Jyoti, D., Bhatt, N., & Negi, H. (2023). To Investigate the Current State of Professional Ethics and Professional Spirit Among Nurses. *FMDB Transactions on Sustainable Health Science Letters*, *1*(2), 82–91.

Vemula, V. R. (2024). Cognitive artificial intelligence systems for proactive threat hunting in AI-driven cloud applications. *AVE Trends in Intelligent Computing Systems*, *1*(3), 173–183.

Venkatasubramanian, S., Sakthikeerthika, T., & Saltanat Yerbolovna, K. (2023). Examine the Relationship Between Online Learning Students' Screen Time, Digital Fatigue, and Mental Health Issues. *FMDB Transactions on Sustainable Techno Learning*, *1*(4), 179–188.

Vidhushavarshinisathiyabhama, B. (2017). *A Comparison of Classification Techniques on Thyroid Detection Using J48 and Naive Bayes Classification Techniques*.

Vignesh Raja, A. S., Jasper, K. D., Aljaafreh, R., Yogeshwarran, S. K., & Saleem, M. (2023). A Comprehensive Exploration of Blockchain-Based Decentralized Applications and Federated Learning in Reshaping Data Management. *FMDB Transactions on Sustainable Computer Letters*, *1*(4), 228–240.

Vijayan, S. (2020). Fine-tuned VGG19 convolutional neural network architecture for diabetic retinopathy diagnosis. *Indian Journal of Computer Science and Engineering*, *11*(5), 615–622. DOI: 10.21817/indjcse/2020/v11i5/201105266

Vijayan, T., & Karthik, B. (2020). Trainable WEKA segmentation of retinal fundus images for global eye disease diagnosis application. *International Journal of Emerging Trends in Engineering Research*, *8*(9), 5750–5754. DOI: 10.30534/ijeter/2020/136892020

Vijayan, T., Sangeetha, M., & Karthik, B. (2020). Efficient analysis of diabetic retinopathy on retinal fundus images using deep learning techniques with Inception V3 architecture. *Journal of Green Engineering, 10*(10), 9615–9625.

Vijayan, T., Sangeetha, M., Kumaravel, A., & Karthik, B. (2020). Feature selection for simple color histogram filter based on retinal fundus images for diabetic retinopathy recognition. *Journal of the Institution of Electronics and Telecommunication Engineers, 69*(2), 987–994. DOI: 10.1080/03772063.2020.1844082

Wali, G. (2024). Evaluating centralized and decentralized maintenance strategies for improved operational efficiency. *AVE Trends in Intelligent Technoprise Letters, 1*(2), 91–99.

Wan, C.. (2021). Retinal image enhancement using cycle-constraint adversarial network. *Frontiers in Medicine, 8*(1), 793726. PMID: 35096883

Wang, X., Jia, J., Cao, Y., Du, J., Hu, A., Liu, Y., & Wang, Z. (2023). Application of data storage management system in blockchain-based technology. 2023 IEEE 2nd International Conference on Electrical Engineering, Big Data and Algorithms (EEBDA). IEEE, Changchun, China.

Wang, J. (2022). Automated segmentation of choroidal neovascularization in fundus images based on CNN optimized active contour model. *Biomedical Signal Processing and Control, 71*(6), 103253.

Wang, J., Zhao, X., & Li, J. (2019). Deep neural network-based obesity risk prediction from wearable sensor data. *Sensors (Basel), 19*(7), 1595. PMID: 30986985

Wang, P., Yang, Q., He, Z., & Yuan, Y. (2023). Vision transformers in multimodal brain tumor MRI segmentation: A review. *Meta-Radiology, 1*(6), 100004. DOI: 10.1016/j.metrad.2023.100004

Wang, X., Cheng, M., Eaton, J., Hsieh, C.-J., & Wu, S. F. (2022). Fake node attacks on graph convolutional networks. *Journal of Computational and Cognitive Engineering, 1*(4), 165–173. DOI: 10.47852/bonviewJCCE2202321

Wang, X., Yang, Q., & Zhang, J. (2021). Leveraging Convolutional Neural Networks for Predicting Obesity Trends in Large-Scale Population Data. *Sensors (Basel), 344*(3), 123371.

Wei, Y., Zhang, X., Zeng, A., & Huang, H. (2022). Iris recognition method based on parallel Iris localization algorithm and deep learning Iris verification. *Sensors (Basel), 22*(20), 7723. DOI: 10.3390/s22207723 PMID: 36298074

Wenjing, L.. (2022). Retinal vessel segmentation based on B-COSFIRE filters in fundus images. *Frontiers in Public Health, 10*(1), 1–14. PMID: 36159307

Wiggers, K. L., Britto, A. S., Heutte, L., Koerich, A. L., & Oliveira, L. S. (2019). Image re-trieval and pattern spotting using Siamese neural network. In *International Joint Confer-ence on Neural Networks.* IJCNN.

William, M. P., Priscila, S. S., Kiruba, S. B., Dayana, T. R. N., & Velavan, P. (2024). A comprehensive comparison of Adaboost, LightGBM, and CatBoost for Alzheimer's disease classification. *FMDB Transactions on Sustainable Health Science Letters, 2*(3), 175–187. DOI: 10.69888/FTSHSL.2024.000253

Wu, B., Zhu, W., Shi, F., Zhu, S., & Chen, X. (2017). Automatic detection of microaneurysms in retinal fundus images. *Computerized Medical Imaging and Graphics*, *55*(1), 106–112. DOI: 10.1016/j.compmedimag.2016.08.001 PMID: 27595214

Wu, H., Tan, L., & Yang, F. (2021). Predictive Models for Obesity Using Artificial Neural Networks: A Systematic Review. *IEEE Access : Practical Innovations, Open Solutions*, *24*(12), e40589.

Yadav, D. C. (2020). Calculating diagnose odd ratio for thyroid patients using different data mining classifiers and ensemble techniques. *International Journal of Advanced Trends in Computer Science and Engineering*, *9*(4), 5463–5470. DOI: 10.30534/ijatcse/2020/186942020

Yang, X.-S. (2014). Bat algorithms. In *Nature-inspired optimization algorithms*. Elsevier in Amsterdam. DOI: 10.1016/B978-0-12-416743-8.00010-5

Yang, Y., & Song, X. (2022). Research on face intelligent perception technology integrating deep learning under different illumination intensities. *Journal of Computational and Cognitive Engineering*, *1*(1), 32–36. DOI: 10.47852/bonviewJCCE19919

Yaseliani, M., Hamadani, A. Z., Maghsoodi, A. I., & Mosavi, A. (2022). Pneumonia detection proposing a hybrid deep convolutional neural network based on two parallel visual geometry group architectures and machine learning classifiers. *IEEE Access : Practical Innovations, Open Solutions*, *10*(6), 62110–62128. DOI: 10.1109/ACCESS.2022.3182498

Yau, J. W., Rogers, S. L., Kawasaki, R., Lamoureux, E. L., Kowalski, J. W., & Bek, T.Meta-Analysis for Eye Disease (META-EYE) Study Group. (2012). Global prevalence and major risk factors of diabetic retinopathy. *Diabetes Care*, *35*(3), 556–564.

Yenduri, S., Perveen, N., Chalavadi, V., & Mohan, K. (2022). Fine-grained action recognition using dynamic kernels. *Pattern Recognition*, *122*(2), 108282. DOI: 10.1016/j.patcog.2021.108282

Ye, T., Wang, J., & Yi, J. (2021). A deep learning network for parallel self-denoising and segmentation in visible light optical coherence tomography of human retina. *IEEE Transactions on Medical Imaging*, *14*(11), 6088–6099. PMID: 38021135

Yoon, H., Park, M., Lee, H., An, J., Lee, T., & Lee, S.-H. (2024). Deep learning framework for bovine iris segmentation. *Journal of Animal Science and Technology*, *66*(1), 167–177. DOI: 10.5187/jast.2023.e51 PMID: 38618036

Younis, A., Qiang, L., Nyatega, C. O., Adamu, M. J., & Kawuwa, H. B. (2022). Brain tumor analysis using deep learning and VGG-16 ensembling learning approaches. *Applied Sciences (Basel, Switzerland)*, *12*(14), 7282. DOI: 10.3390/app12147282

Yuan, C. T., & Chen, K. S. (2022). Deep Learning for Obesity Detection Based on Daily Habits and Biometric Data. *Journal of Personalized Medicine*, *21*(9), 11178.

Yu, K. H., Zhang, C., Berry, G. J., Altman, R. B., Ré, C., Rubin, D. L., & Snyder, M. (2016). Predicting non-small cell lung cancer prognosis by fully automated microscopic pathology image features. *Nature Communications*, *7*(8), 1–10. DOI: 10.1038/ncomms12474 PMID: 27527408

Zahoor, M. M., Qureshi, S. A., Bibi, S., Khan, S. H., Khan, A., Ghafoor, U., & Bhutta, M. R. (2022). A new deep hybrid boosted and ensemble learning-based brain tumor analysis using MRI. *Sensors (Basel), 22*(7), 2726. DOI: 10.3390/s22072726 PMID: 35408340

Zeebaree, D. Q., Haron, H., Abdulazeez, A. M., & Zebari, D. A. (2019). Trainable model based on new uniform LBP feature to identify the risk of breast cancer. In *2019 International Conference on Advanced Science and Engineering*, Zakho - Duhok, Iraq. DOI: 10.1109/ICOASE.2019.8723827

Zhang, M., Wu, H., & Zhou, X. (2020). Deep Learning-Based Obesity Prediction Using Lifestyle Data. *Computers in Biology and Medicine, 112*(8), 102926.

Zhang, W., Yang, C., Cao, Z., Li, Z., Zhuo, L., Tan, Y., He, Y., Yao, L., Zhou, Q., Gong, Q., Sweeney, J. A., Shi, F., & Lui, S. (2023). Detecting individuals with severe mental illness using artificial intelligence applied to magnetic resonance imaging. *EBioMedicine, 90*(4), 104541. DOI: 10.1016/j.ebiom.2023.104541 PMID: 36996601

Zhao, J., Zhang, L., & Wang, T. (2020). Predicting adult obesity using machine learning algorithms and neural network models. *Journal of Obesity Research & Clinical Practice, 14*(5), 335–342.

Zhao, Q., Zhang, H., & Shang, J. (2022). Interpretable sentiment analysis based on sentient words' syntax information". In *2022 International Conference on Industrial Automation*, Chengdu, China.

Zhao, T., Liu, Y., Huo, G., & Zhu, X. (2019). A deep learning Iris recognition method based on capsule network architecture. *IEEE Access : Practical Innovations, Open Solutions, 7*(1), 49691–49701. DOI: 10.1109/ACCESS.2019.2911056

Zhong, Y., Chen, T., Zhong, D., & Liu, X. (2024). Vessel segmentation in fundus images with multiscale feature extraction and disentangled representation. *Applied Sciences (Basel, Switzerland), 14*(12), 5039. DOI: 10.3390/app14125039

Zhou, M., Jin, K., Wang, S., Ye, J., & Qian, D. (2018). Color retinal image enhancement based on luminosity and contrast adjustment. *IEEE Transactions on Biomedical Engineering, 65*(3), 521–527. DOI: 10.1109/TBME.2017.2700627 PMID: 28475043

Zhou, M., & Li, Y. (2020). Predictive models for adult obesity using neural networks with genetic optimization. *AI in Medicine, 117*(4), 87–98.

Zhou, Z., Liu, Y., Zhu, X., Liu, S., Zhang, S., & Li, Y. (2022). Supervised contrastive learning and intra-dataset adversarial adaptation for iris segmentation. *Entropy (Basel, Switzerland), 24*(9), 1276. DOI: 10.3390/e24091276 PMID: 36141162

Ziller, C. (2020). Superpixel guided convolutional networks for optic disc and cup segmentation. *Medical Image Analysis, 63*(2), 101696.

About The Contributors

Ferdin Joe John Joseph is currently an Assistant Professor with the faculty of information technology, Thai Nichi Institute of technology Bangkok. He graduated his bachelor and masters degrees in computer science and engineering from Anna University Chennai during 2009 and 2011 respectively. He got his PhD in Computer Science and Information Systems from the National Institute of Development Administration Bangkok during 2015. His area of research includes deep learning, IoT and Blockchain technology. He has nearly a decade experience in teaching. He has published in peer reviewed international conferences and journals. He is certified as the "Most Valuable Professional" (MVP) with Alibaba Cloud since 2021. He is teaching as per academic curriculum to students, recognizing, nurturing the creative potential of each student. Teach students using a systematic instructional methodology comprising lecture plans (following the credit allotted to each subject), discussion groups, seminars, case studies, field assignments, and independent and/or group projects. Recently, he has been the technique program committee, the technique reviews, and the track chair for international conferences published by Springer Series. He is serving in the editor in chief, the editorial board of international journals, and he authored/edited different books and filed so many Patents. Finally, he is a member of ISTE, IET, Etc…

Karthikeyan Chinnusamy, Sr Principal with more than 25 years of experience in IT, Product Dev, R&D and Education fields. Fellow IETE, Fellow IE, Sr Member IEEE,Sr Member ACM, Project management Institute (PMI), Reviewer, Editorial Board Member of R&D Journals. Board Member & Program Director SF DAMA. SME in Data Governance, GDPR, HIPAA Compliance, Data Management, Data Architecture, Master Data, Data Quality, AI/ML, Analytics and reporting in Payment processing, Customer, Finance, CRM and License domains. Mentor in SFDC Mig, Data.com, ERP, Architecture, R&D, Embedded systems, VLSI,Adv Information processing. I am also reviewer for IEEE Silicon Valley Sr Member Elevation and Speaker, Volunteer for SFBay ACM. Reviewer of Journals in Springer Nature.

Joseph Jeganathan earned his Ph.D. in Psychiatric Nursing from Rajiv Gandhi University of Health Sciences, National Consortium for Ph.D. Nursing, (Indian Nursing Council), Bangalore, Karnataka, India in 2019. He completed his Postgraduate studies at the National Institute of Mental Health and Neurosciences, Bangalore, Karnataka, India 2011. He is working as an assistant professor in the Mental Health Nursing Department at the University of Bahrain, Kingdom of Bahrain. He has more than 16 years of Undergraduate and Postgraduate teaching experience. He has worked as a Professor at SGT University, Gurugram, Dept. of Nursing, IES University, Bhopal; Associate Professor Akal College of Nursing, Eternal University, Baru Sahib, India; and also worked as a teaching faculty in various nursing colleges in India and Nepal. Dr. Joseph Jeganathan has published many research articles in National and international Nursing Journals. His areas of research interest are Adolescent mental health, Life skills training, and Substance use disorders.

Ahmed J. Obaid is a Faculty Member at Dept. of Computer Science and Mathematics Faculty of Computer Science and Mathematics University of Kufa, Iraq Ahmed J. Obaid, is a Asst. Professor at the Department of Computer Science, Faculty of Computer Science and Mathematics, University of Kufa, Iraq. Dr. Ahmed holds a Bachelor's in Computer Science, a degree in – Information Systems from the College of Computers, University of Anbar, Iraq (2001-2005), and a Master's Degree (M. TECH) in Computer Science Engineering (CSE) from School of Information Technology, Jawaharlal Nehru Technological University, Hyderabad, India (2010-2013), and a Doctor of Philosophy (Ph.D.) in Web Mining from College of Information Technology, University of Babylon, Iraq (2013-2017). He is a Certified Web Mining Consultant with over 14 years of experience working as a Faculty Member at the University of Kufa, Iraq. He has taught courses in Web design, Web Scripting, JavaScript, VB.Net, MATLAB Toolbox, and other courses on PHP, CMC, and DHTML from more than 10 international organizations and institutes in the USA and India. Dr. Ahmed is a member of the Statistical and Information Consultation Center (SICC), at the University of Kufa, Iraq. His main line of research is Web mining Techniques and Applications, Image processing in Web Platforms, Image processing, Genetic Algorithms, information theory, and Medical Health Applications. Ahmed J. is an Associated Editor in the Brazilian Journal of Operations & Production Management (BJO&PM) and an Editorial Board member in the International Journal of Advance Study and Research Work (IJASRW), Journal of Research in Engineering and Applied Sciences(JREAS), GRD Journal for Engineering (GRDJE), International Research Journal of Multidisciplinary Science & Technology (IRJMST), The International Journal of Technology Information and Computer (IJTIC), Career Point International Journal Research (CPIJR). Ahmed J. was an Editor in Many International Conferences such as ISCPS_2020, MAICT_2020, IHICPS_2020, IICESAT_2021, IICPS_2020, ICPAS_2021, etc. (Scopus Indexed Conferences). He has edited Some books, such as Advance Material Science and Engineering (ISBN: 9783035736779, Scientific.net publisher), Computational Intelligence Techniques for Combating COVID-19 (ISBN: 978-3-030-68936-0 EAI/Springer), A Fusion of Artificial Intelligence and Internet of Things for Emerging Cyber Systems (ISBN: 978-3-030-76653-5 Springer). Ahmed J. has supervised several final projects for Bachelor's and Master's in his main line of work and authored and co-authored several scientific publications in journals, Books, and conferences with more than 75+ Journal Research Articles, 5+ book Chapters, 15+ Conference papers, 10+ Conference proceedings, 8+ Books Editing, 2+ Patent. Ahmed J. is also a Reviewer in many Scopus, SCI, and ESCI Journals e.g., CMC, IETE, IJAACS, IJIPM, IJKBD, IJBSR, IET, IJUFKS, and many others. Dr. Ahmed attended and participated as Keynote Speakers (60+ Conferences), Webinars (10+), and Session Chairs (10+),

S. Suman Rajest is the Dean of Research and Development (R&D) and International Student Affairs (ISA) at Dhaanish Ahmed College of Engineering, Chennai, Tamil Nadu, India. He is an Editor in Chief of the International Journal of Human Computing Studies and The International Journal of Social Sciences World, He is the Chief Executive Editor of the International Journal of Advanced Engineering Research and Science, International Journal of Advanced Engineering, Management and Science, The International Journal of Health and Medicines, The International Journal of Management Economy and Accounting Fields and The International Journal of Technology Information and Computer and also he is an Editorial Board Member in International Journal of Management in Education, Scopus, Inderscience, EAI Endorsed Transactions on e-Learning, and Bulletin of the Karaganda university Pedagogy series. He is also a Book Series Editor at IGI Global Publisher, Springer, etc. All of his writing, including his research, involves elements of creative nonfiction in the Human Computing learning system. He is also interested in creative writing and digital media, Learning, AI, student health learning, etc. He has published 400 papers in peer-reviewed international journals. He has authored and co-authored several scientific book publications in journals and conferences and is a frequent reviewer of international journals and conferences. He also reviews Inderscience, EAI Journals, IGI Global, Science Publications, etc....

***

T. Vijayan is working as a associate Professor, Department of Electronics and Communication Engineering, Bharath Institute of Higher Education and Research, Chennai. His current research interests include artificial intelligence, machine learning, soft computing, digital image processing, signal processing and communication systems. He is a member of IEEE, and IAENG.

Index

X

www.ingramcontent.com/pod-product-compliance
Lightning Source LLC
LaVergne TN
LVHW060302011026
849161LV00011B/2757